Innovations in Neonatal-Perinatal Medicine

Innovative Technologies and Therapies that have
Fundamentally Changed the Way We Deliver Care
for the Fetus and the Neonate

Innovations in Neonatal–Perinatal Medicine

Innovative Technologies and Therapies that have
Fundamentally Changed the Way We Deliver Care
for the Fetus and the Neonate

editors

Oommen Mathew
Jatinder Bhatia

Medical College of Georgia, USA

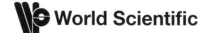

World Scientific

NEW JERSEY · LONDON · SINGAPORE · BEIJING · SHANGHAI · HONG KONG · TAIPEI · CHENNAI

Published by

World Scientific Publishing Co. Pte. Ltd.

5 Toh Tuck Link, Singapore 596224

USA office: 27 Warren Street, Suite 401-402, Hackensack, NJ 07601

UK office: 57 Shelton Street, Covent Garden, London WC2H 9HE

British Library Cataloguing-in-Publication Data
A catalogue record for this book is available from the British Library.

Cover photo by Phil Jones, Medical College of Georgia.

ISBN-13 978-981-4280-04-4
ISBN-10 981-4280-04-6

Typeset by Stallion Press
Email: enquiries@stallionpress.com

Printed in Singapore.

Contents

Preface

The last few decades have brought major innovations in medicine. Life expectancy in the US improved by 25 years during the last century, infant mortality rate decreased by 90%, and maternal mortality decreased by 99%. The focus of this book is to highlight, not to catalog, the impact of innovations in the field of neonatal-perinatal medicine. There are numerous important mile stones in neonatology. However, the principles of life support for the premature infants can be summarized by few seminal observations which set the stage for the evolution of neonatology. These include Silverman's observation on the effect of hypothermia on neonatal mortality, Usher's "radical" use of intravenous fluids in preterm infants, Gregory's report on the effect of continuous positive airway pressure (CPAP) in respiratory distress syndrome (RDS) and successful surfactant replacement therapy for RDS by Fujiwara.

Louise Joy Brown, the poster child of *in vitro* fertilization (IVF), is the world's first successful "test tube" baby and her birth heralded a new era in perinatal medicine. Unlike all other previous experimental pregnancies, the fertilized egg was implanted in the uterine wall and the pregnancy evolved without apparent complications. In 1999, Natalie, her sister, became the first test tube baby to have a baby of her own. Over 100,000 IVF babies have been born by 2004 in the US alone. As Caplan, a renowned bioethicist, once said "You can't buy a baby in the US but you can buy the sperm, buy the egg and you can rent a uterus."

The first chapter discusses the impact of healthcare innovations on neonatal and infant mortality from a global perspective. The impact of IVF, a major innovation in the field of perinatal medicine, and other assisted reproductive technologies is discussed in Chapter 2. Advances in fetal diagnosis including preimplantation genetics, chorionic villous sampling and amniocentesis are summarized in Chapter 3. These innovations help us diagnose chromosomal abnormalities and biochemical disorders at an early gestation *in utero* and cope with the consequences.

Today, fetal and neonatal imaging has become a routine, but vital, part of obstetric and neonatal care. Fetal ultrasound gives us a window into the health and well being of the fetus. Role of imaging in fetal congenital heart disease and neonatal brain development and its complications is addressed in Chapters 4 and 5. Survival of extremely premature infant is commonplace today. Their increased survival can be attributed to several factors. These include noninvasive monitoring techniques (Chapter 6), better regulation of the environment (Chapter 7), better nutrition (Chapter 8), and ventilatory support (Chapter 9). One has to keep in mind that the greatest impact may come from innovations that are perceived as mundane. For example, keeping the preterm infant warm and providing optimal nutrition fall in this category but continue to be a challenge for the critically ill and extremely premature infants.

Drugs designed to treat unique conditions in the neonate also had immense impact on the survival of neonates. Development of surfactant to treat respiratory syndrome in preterm infants (Chapter 10) and inhaled nitric oxide to treat hypoxic respiratory failure in term and near-term infants (Chapter 11) are excellent examples of drugs in this category. Several hundred thousands of infants have been saved by these miracle drugs. Treatment of women during labor with common and inexpensive antibiotics such as penicillin has substantially reduced infections in the immediate neonatal period in developed countries. Still, over a million neonates die from infection worldwide, mostly in developing countries. As in other areas of medicine, surgical innovations have benefited neonates as well. These innovations extend from laser surgery for retinopathy of prematurity which saves thousands of preterm infants from blindness to staged repair of hypoplastic left heart syndrome, an otherwise fatal disease (Chapter 12). The ethical and moral issues raised by IVF and other advanced life sustaining measures of extremely premature and critically ill newborns is discussed throughout the book.

We hope that the readers will find this unique collection of reviews by authors who are experts in their respective fields interesting and worthwhile.

Oommen Mathew
Jatinder Bhatia

List of Editors and Contributors

Editors

Oommen P. Mathew, MD
Division of Neonatology
Professor of Pediatrics
Medical College of Georgia
Augusta, GA

Jatinder S. Bhatia, MD
Chief, Division of Neonatology
Professor of Pediatrics
Medical College of Georgia
Augusta, GA

Contributors

David H. Adamkin, MD
Chief, Division of Neonatology
Professor of Pediatrics
University of Louisville
Louisville, KY

Stephen Baumgart, MD
Professor of Pediatrics
GWU School of Medicine and Health Sciences
Children's National Medical Center
Division of Neonatology
Washington, DC

Joshua A. Copel, MD
Professor
Obstetrics, Gynecology, and Reproductive Science, and of Pediatrics
Vice Chair, Obstetrics
Yale University School of Medicine
New Haven, CT

Adelina M. Emmi, MD
Professor, Obstetrics and Gynecology
Section of Reproductive Endocrinology, Infertility and Genetics
Medical Director, Reproductive Laboratories of Augusta
Medical College of Georgia
Augusta, GA

Katherine B. Geiersbach, MD
Assistant Medical Director
Cytogenetics and Molecular Cytogenetics
ARUP Laboratories Inc.
Visiting Instructor
University of Utah, School of Medicine
Department of Pathology
Salt Lake City, UT

Olivera Kontic-Vucinic, MD PhD
Associate Professor
Obstetrics and Gynecology
University of Belgrade School of Medicine
Belgrade, Serbia

Ana A. Murphy, MD
Greenblatt Professor and Chair
Department of Obstetrics and Gynecology
Medical College of Georgia
Augusta, GA

T. Michael O'Shea, MD MPH
Chief, Section of Neonatology
Professor
Department of Pediatrics
Wake Forest University School of Medicine
Winston-Salem, NC

Anjali Parish, MD
Assistant Professor
Department of Pediatrics
Medical College of Georgia
Augusta, GA

Rangasamy Ramanathan, MD
Professor of Pediatrics
Associate Division Chief and Section Head
USC Division of Neonatal Medicine
Keck School of Medicine
University of Southern California
Los Angeles, CA

Sarah South, PhD
Assistant Professor, Department of Pediatrics
Adjunct Professor, Department of Pathology
University of Utah, School of Medicine
Medical Director, Cytogenetics, Genetics Processing and
Molecular Cytogenetics
ARUP Laboratories, Inc.
Salt Lake City, UT

Suzanne Touch, MD
Associate Professor of Pediatrics
Drexel University School of Medicine
St. Christopher's Hospital for Children
Division of Neonatology
Philadelphia, PA

Dharmapuri Vidyasagar, MD MSc FAAP FCCM
Professor Emeritus
Department of Pediatrics
University of Illinois at Chicago
Bloomberg School of Public Health
Johns Hopkins University
Baltimore, MD

Christopher T. Whitlow, MD PhD
Fellow in Neuroradiology
Department of Radiology
Wake Forest University School of Medicine
Winston-Salem, NC

Chapter 1

Medical Innovations in the 20th Century and Their Impact on Neonatal-Perinatal Medicine: A Global Perspective

Dharmapuri Vidyasagar*

1.1 Introduction

The twentieth century has seen the greatest progress in healthcare than any other time in history. Several reviewers in the field have recounted the progress made in different fields of medicine at the end of the 20th century. For example, the Center for Disease Control (CDC) declared that the 20th century made major progress in the ten most important areas of health during 1900 and 1999.[1] Of these gains, improved maternal and child health was noted to be the most impressive gain. During this period, the life expectancy improved by 25 years, infant mortality rate (IMR) decreased by 90%, and maternal mortality decreased by 99% in USA. It further stated that these gains "resulted from better hygiene and nutrition, availability of antibiotics, greater access to healthcare and technologic advances in maternal and neonatal medicine."

Whereas the statement reflected the progress made in USA, the same can be said of the gains made in Western industrialized countries during

*Professor Emeritus, Department of Pediatrics, University of Illinois at Chicago; Bloomberg School of Public Health, Johns Hopkins University.

1

this same period. Although the progress has been slow in the developing countries, it is unquestionable that the benefits of these technological advances have been percolating slowly but surely during the later half of the 20th century. In spite of these observations, the history of neonatal medical technologies and their impact on *global* neonatal and infant mortality has not received much of scholarly attention. Subsequent chapters of this book detail the history of medical innovations that changed the way we deliver care to the fetus and the newborn during the last century. In this chapter I will attempt to summarize the evolution of numerous healthcare technologies and their overall impact on *global* neonatal mortality rate (NMR) and IMR. The subject is daunting however, because of the difficulty in collecting information on the vast number of innovations that have developed during the last century.

1.2 Innovations that Influenced Population Health

Technological innovations of the 20th century that influenced the health outcome of people include those that improved agricultural products, as well as water purification and sanitation. These innovations are known to have had the greatest impact on population health, especially child health. They were the most responsible for the decrease in overall mortality and child mortality and an increase in life expectancy. Development of newer medical technologies on the other hand has made a direct impact on neonatal and perinatal outcome. These include biomedical technologies such as vaccines, pharmacologic technologies such as antibiotics, and instrumentation such as ventilators. Of the ten most important advances declared by CDC, vaccination, or control of infectious diseases, has made the most impact on IMR/NMR. Innovation of medical technologies in isolation would have no benefit unless they are made accessible to the public and are utilized in countries around the world. To understand the mechanisms of the impact of technology on global health, we need to understand the methods of transferring technology from "bench to bedside" in a country of innovation and then "diffusion" of medical technology from a country of innovation to countries with limited resources.

The model in Fig. 1.1A shows the pathways of development of medical technology in a developed country and its diffusion. There is usually

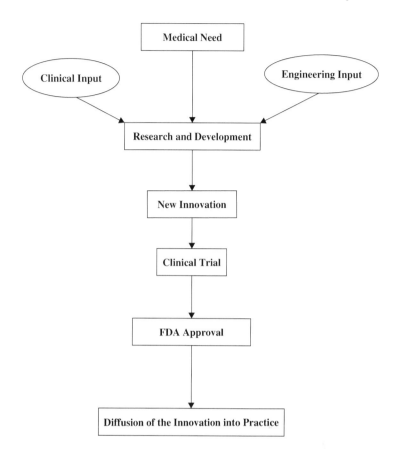

Fig. 1.1A. The pathways of drug/device innovations. The need for new drugs/devices is usually identified by the medical community and the scientists who work in the industry. After the innovation is perfected, it goes through several testing and clinical trials before an approval by the FDA. See text for details.

a lag period for the experimental drug/innovation to diffuse from "bench to bedside" even in the developed countries. It is estimated that it takes 10 to 15 years and about 400 to 800 million US dollars for the discovery of a drug to reach the market for public use.[2] Similarly medical devices take a long time, from innovation, to diffuse into the market and to the practitioners.[3] There is a further lag period of years to decades for the innovation to diffuse from country of innovation to resource poor countries. While industrialized nations are the immediate beneficiaries, the rest of the less developed countries (LDC) and developing countries have to wait for decades to benefit from the life-saving medical technologies.

Global diffusion of medical technology from countries of innovation to resource poor countries depends on multiple limiting factors/barriers (Fig. 1.1B). The limitations include: restriction on cross-country trade,

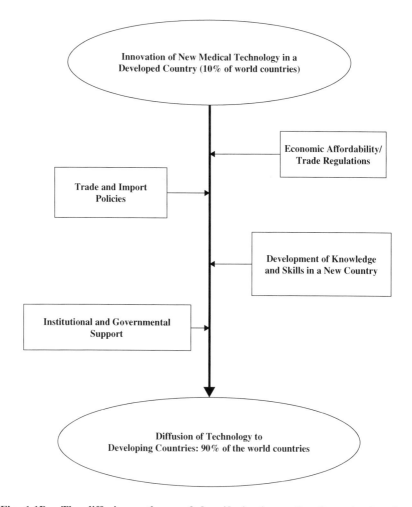

Fig. 1.1B.   The diffusion pathway of drug/device innovation from developed to developing countries.   The side boxes show different barriers to smooth and even diffusion of innovations. Note that only 10% of the world countries are capable of investing funds in research and development.

regional economics, and availability of skilled and experienced professionals who can use the new innovation in the care of their patients. The latter depends on the rate of diffusion of new knowledge and skill development of professionals (capacity building) in the recipient country. These unavoidable steps slow down the rate of diffusion of medical technology. Fortunately, the 20th century also has benefited from political, economic, and technological dividends, which have, in fact, accelerated the diffusion of technology to resource poor countries. Political dividends in the form of democratization of countries and economic dividends in the form of free trade have been the hallmark of globalization in the later half of the 20th century. Economists believe that when domestic and global markets are completely accessible, health services also become easily accessible. The process of globalization was further accelerated through the "technologic dividend" in the later part of the 20th century. The "technological dividend" in the form of the rapid growth of internet technology (IT) has accelerated the diffusion of knowledge resulting in "knowledge dividend". Cumulative effects of these dividends have made a major impact on global health.

1.3 Growth and Influence of Internet Technology

At this juncture, a discussion of the growth of internet technology and its effect on diffusion of knowledge is pertinent. Internet technology itself has grown by geometric progression within the last 25 years (Figs. 1.2A and 1.2B). Figure 1.2 shows the growth of websites in the world since the 1990s. The data is staggering. Over 238 million websites are known to have existed in the world in 2007.[4] They have been growing ever so rapidly that it is indeed difficult to get accurate real time data on the number of existing websites. Currently, the estimated number of web pages is thought to be a staggering one trillion! Most websites are database in the developed countries; nevertheless, developing countries are catching up fast in the usage of internet technology.

Although it is logical to think that internet technology has made a great impact on dissemination of health and medical information, there is no accurate data on the number of health related websites, nor there is evidentiary data to the role of health related websites and impact on

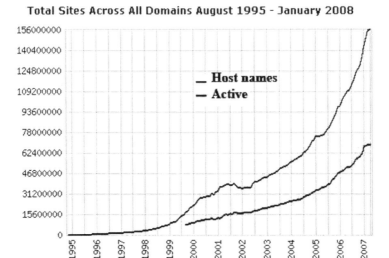

Fig. 1.2A.   This growth of global internet websites from 1995–2008. (Modified from Ref. 4.) After a slow increase up to 2000, there a geometric progression in the number of IT websites reaching an ultimate number of 238 million in 2008. The lower line indicates the active websites during this same period. See text for details.

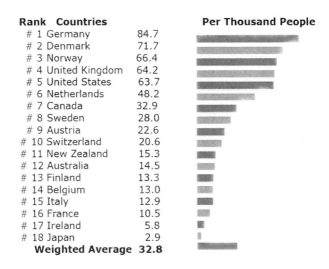

Rank	Countries	Per Thousand People	
# 1	Germany	84.7	
# 2	Denmark	71.7	
# 3	Norway	66.4	
# 4	United Kingdom	64.2	
# 5	United States	63.7	
# 6	Netherlands	48.2	
# 7	Canada	32.9	
# 8	Sweden	28.0	
# 9	Austria	22.6	
# 10	Switzerland	20.6	
# 11	New Zealand	15.3	
# 12	Australia	14.5	
# 13	Finland	13.3	
# 14	Belgium	13.0	
# 15	Italy	12.9	
# 16	France	10.5	
# 17	Ireland	5.8	
# 18	Japan	2.9	
	Weighted Average	**32.8**	

Fig. 1.2B.   The number of websites in 18 industrialized nations. Germany had the most number of websites per 1,000 people while Japan had the lowest. See text for details. *Source*: OECD, Communications Outlook 2003, Nationmaster.com.

individual or population health. There is a need for research in this area. There is a critical limitation for such a study. Accounting for the number of health related websites has been difficult due to the lack of a definition for "health related websites", thus it has become difficult to quantitate the impact of internet technology on the dissemination of medical knowledge. Even so, internet technology has been found to be highly useful to medical professionals around the world. It is the main paperless source of information to health professionals in the remotest parts of the world. Many electronic medical journals have sprouted with free access to readers worldwide (for example, the *International Journal of Pediatrics*). Also, many well-established medical journals are accessible through IT, enabling a fast diffusion of new medical, nursing, and public health information around the world. In summary, internet technology is playing a great role in disseminating the ever evolving medical information to developing countries.

1.4 Health Related Technologies

Health and medical technologies can be classified into two categories: preventive technologies and curative technologies. Preventive technologies include public health measures such as improvements in water purification systems, sanitation, and vaccine technologies. Examples of curative technologies include antibiotics and life-saving medical technologies. The preventive technologies of water purification and sanitation were critical to improving overall mortality and child survival in late 19th century and early 20th century. A discussion of these public health interventions and their impact on IMR in Western developed countries are presented below.

1.4.1 *Preventive public health technologies*

Cutler *et al.* analyzed the changes in mortality during the 20th century.[5] They noted that overall mortality dropped by 40% at an average rate of 1% per year. Life expectancy also rose from 47 to 63 years. Nearly all the reduction in mortality estimated is due to a decline in infectious diseases. In their analysis, they demonstrated that large scale public health measures of water purification and sanitation reduced overall mortality in 13 major cities of USA during 1900–1940. Fifty percent of overall mortality, 75% of IMR, and 66.7% of child mortality reduction was attributed to clean water technology. The dividends of these technologies continue to benefit the population in developed countries. Unfortunately, after a century of proven benefits of clean water and sanitation in improving child survival, many developing countries still do not have access to these technologies. They continue to suffer from unacceptably high NMR and IMR.

1.4.2 *Role of medical technologies*

The 20th century has seen major scientific progress in the field of medicine. This is evident in every region of the world. During this century, we have seen a major reduction in overall mortality and an increase in life expectancy. In particular, the reduction in infant mortality and maternal mortality rates (IMR and MMR) has been dramatic. The reduction is more evident in Western countries than in developing countries, in fact much less so in developing countries. In the beginning of the 20th century, even the Western industrialized countries suffered from high IMR, which decreased with improved sanitation and clean water technologies.[6] Improvements were observed in European cities following improvements in water and sanitation. Neonatal mortality continued to remain a major component of IMR. Further improvements in IMR did not occur until after the introduction of antibiotics, oxygen therapy, and nutritional support in 1940s and 1950s. Even in the mid-20th century, IMR was high in all regions of the world including the developed countries. However, developing regions had far higher IMR than developed regions. This wide difference showed "divergence" of IMR among different regions of the world.[7] A steady overall reduction of IMR was observed among all regions during the last part of the century, leading to a change in IMR from a "divergence" to "convergence" (Fig. 1.3). The improved outcomes during this period were not only because of economic growth but also because of the scientific dividends that transcended the geopolitical borders. Many technologies were responsible for the reduction in IMR and NMR to lowest levels in the Western developed world by the end of 20th century. Figure 1.4 and Table 1.1 show the timeline of various innovations during the past century that contributed to a decrease in NMR/IMR in USA. Among these innovations, incubators to

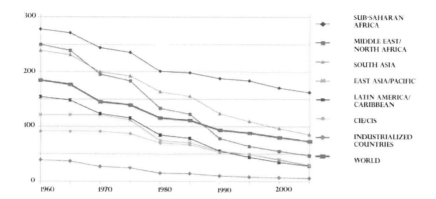

Fig. 1.3.   Global trends in infant mortality rate in the different regions of the globe, 1952–2000. (Modified from Ref. 7.) The IMR in all regions was higher in 1950 with a wide variation (divergence). Starting from the 1980s, the IMR decrease significantly. In the year 2000, there was a decrease in IMR in all the regions analyzed and there was minimal variation (convergence) of infant mortality. For details, read the text.

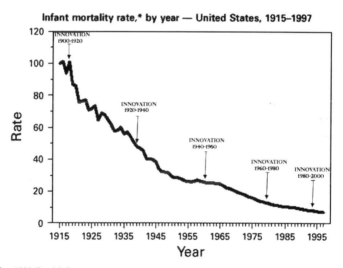

*Per 1000 live births.

Fig. 1.4.   The graph shows the IMR trend in USA 1900–1999. (Modified from Ref. 1.) The boxes with arrows indicate the time duration during which major technologic interventions were introduced. The subsequent decrease in IMR indicates the impact of technology introduced in the preceding decade. See also Table 1.1. It must be noted that many other innovations and policies were introduced that also contributed to reduction of IMR but could not be listed due to space constraints. For details, see the text.

Table 1.1.   Timeline of major technologic interventions introduced during 1900–1999 that were responsible for reduction of IMR in subsequent decades. Please see the accompanying Fig. 1.4

Major innovations are listed according to timeline:

1900–1920

- Forty of the 47 states of USA had established health departments (1900)
- First continuous municipal use of chlorinate water in all over USA (1915)
- Increased awareness of newborn care, aseptic techniques of feeding
- Use of incubators

1920–1940

- Establishment of premature care center (Michael Reese Hospital Chicago)
- Improved protocols to decrease infections of newborns
- Isolation nurseries to decrease newborn infections in the hospital

1940–1960

- First use of penicillin in an adult in USA (1942)
- Increased use of antibiotics in newborns
- Exchange transfusions for erythroblastosis

1960–1980

- Apgar score
- Systematic neonatal resuscitation
- Establishment of neonatal intensive care units (NICU)
- Neonatal electronic monitoring HR, RR, BP
- Ventilator care
- Introduction of CPAP
- Introduction of noninvasive $TcPO_2$ and oxygen saturation monitors
- Introduction of total parenteral nutrition
- Antenatal steroids to prevent RDS

1980–2000

- Regionalization of perinatal care
- Maternal and infant transport system
- High frequency ventilation
- Inhaled nitric oxide
- Prenatal AZT treatment to decrease mother to baby transmission of HIV

maintain thermoregulation of the premature infants stand out as the earliest technology innovation that improved NMR. Further this was followed by an introduction of oxygen therapy, use of antibiotics, intravenous fluids, parenteral nutrition, respiratory support, CPAP, and surfactant therapy. With the introduction of each new technology, there was a significant reduction in neonatal mortality. Development and impact of these technologies are further discussed in subsequent chapters. In this chapter, the impact of technologic innovations on global IMR/NMR is described.

1.4.3 *Diffusion of medical technologies in developed countries*

For students of medical history, it is important to know that the diffusion of medical technology even in the industrialized countries was very slow. The story of incubators was narrated by several authors. It took long a time for the technology and the concept to cross international borders in Europe and then across the Atlantic to North America.[8] Similarly, it took a long time for other innovations to become a useful clinical tools used for diagnosis and/or treatment after their approval. In a study of medical technology development during 1850–1940, Howell found that there was a gap of several decades between the invention of new technology and its diffusion into general medical practice.[9] Mike and his colleagues in a study of the use of "Transcutaneous Oxygen Monitoring in Neonatal Intensive Care Unit" during 1980s concluded that physicians were very quick to adopt new technology such as the $tcPO_2$ monitor for clinical use.[10] Similarly, the use of pulmonary surfactant for treatment of neonatal respiratory disease (RDS/HMD) took less than a decade from the first use to obtaining FDA approval for general use. In 1980, the first report of clinical use of surfactant was published.[11] After further extensive clinical trials in USA, several surfactant preparations were approved by FDA: a synthetic surfactant Exosurf was the first surfactant to be approved in 1990; Survanta, a bovine derived natural surfactant was approved in 1991, Infasurf in 1998 and Curosurf in 1999.[12] These are the examples of rapid adaptations of new drugs innovations for clinical use. They show that the diffusion of technology from "bench to bedside" was much more rapid in the later half of 20th century. Surfactant for use in premature infants for the treatment of RDS was one of the most well studied innovations prior to common usage. This new innovation also has had the greatest impact on neonatal survival in industrialized countries.

Finally, regionalization of perinatal care in 1970s facilitated the diffusion of neonatal medical technologies from "innovations" to "practical interventional" tools for use in patients in the community. The concept of the development of neonatal intensive care and regionalization of perinatal care was advocated first in Canada in the 1960s and in USA in 1970s.[13–15] This model was created to use the newly developed technologies effectively for a larger population of sick newborns in the community. The hallmark of this model was to develop an efficient maternal transport, "*in utero* transport" of the unborn high risk fetus, and neonatal transport from Level I community hospitals to designated Level III tertiary NICUs in the region. There is convincing evidence that regionalization of perinatal care has made a significant contribution to improved neonatal survival.[16] This model is an example of the cost effective collective utilization of expensive neonatal medical technologies for a larger population. With time, the concept of regionalization of perinatal care has been adopted as a health policy across the globe in many other developing countries with good results.[17,18]

1.4.4 *Diffusion of medical technologies to resource poor countries*

Once the innovations are proven to be of significant clinical value, there is a demand on the local as well as global market. The process of acquiring new technology in resource poor countries is usually a long one. As stated earlier in the chapter, rapid globalization has accelerated the diffusion of medical technology to developing countries as well. However, the rate of diffusion has been slow and evidence for the positive impact is scarce. There are few studies providing such information.[19] Papageorgiou *et al.* studied the evidence of the impact of the diffusion of medical technology on general mortality and infant mortality rate (IMR) in resource poor countries. They analyzed the impact of medical technology diffusion from developed countries to developing countries extensively. They showed that globally there are only 13 developed countries which are capable of investing in research, development, and production of medical technology. The rest of the countries in the world are solely dependant on imports of medical technology. The way to diffusion of medical technology into developing countries is via imports. But imports are modulated through economic constraints of the country. The authors studied the pattern of medical technology imports during a period of 10 years in 73 countries that are dependant on imported medical technologies.

The technologies selected for analysis were broadly grouped into: (1) medicinal and pharmaceutical products; (2) medical instruments: dental, surgical, orthopedic, and optical goods; (3) laboratory hygiene and pharmacology articles; (4) insecticides. They also studied overall mortality, the male mortality, and IMR in each of the 73 countries during the study period. The data showed that there was a direct negative correlation with increasing medical technology imports among these 73 countries (Fig. 1.5). It was

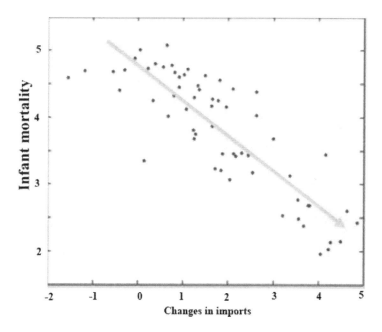

Fig. 1.5.   The figure shows a scattered graph of IMR of 73 countries analyzed during the study period. (Modified from Ref. 19.) The x-axis shows the changes in imports of medical technology to the countries and the y-axis shows infant mortality rate. Note: the arrowed line shows the general trend of a drop in infant mortality with increasing imports. Coefficient of correlation is 0.79. See the text for details.

found that the technologies developed in the advanced countries had benefited not only the countries of origin of innovation, but also other developing countries in improving their health outcome. The degree of benefits was dependant on imports of technologies. What is more interesting is that the benefits of imports of medical technologies had independent effects on IMR and other health indices outside the increase in per capita income in the countries studied. Although the authors did not analyze the data specific to neonatal medical technologies, they found that medical technology diffusion had a direct impact on IMR in all the 73 countries studied, thus establishing a direct relationship of medical technology on IMR. This study is unique in that for the first time it establishes the impact of medical technology on IMR in developing countries. There is a need for studies to focus on impact of medical technology specific to neonatal care.

1.4.5 *Considerations in making decision to acquire new equipment*

Increased imports of medical technology alone do not influence health outcomes in the resource poor country. Countries importing new technology must take into consideration the economic and operational factors into their plans for better utilization of their funds in the purchase of the equipment. Before acquiring new expensive equipment, one must answer the questions "Will the new drug or equipment improve survival or quality of care given to infants? If so what is the cost effectiveness?" One must look for simplicity of operation and ease of maintenance of the equipment. The equipment should have an overall low cost of ownership and life cycle cost. Other pertinent guidelines for acquiring new equipment are given in Table 1.2.

The recommended economic considerations are essential to making appropriate business plans and proper decisions in purchasing the drug/equipment. The operational guidelines assure appropriate training of healthcare professionals in the use of new technology and "capacity building", which is a prerequisite for successful technology diffusion. It also serves the best interests of the patient care. At the same time the manufacturers must assure technical support, required operation, and

Table 1.2.   Guidelines for acquiring new technologies and successful utilization

---

A. Economic Considerations

Make provision of adequate budget for the required purchase of the required
    technology

Make provision for recurring cost of maintenance

Include service and parts supply in contract

Make a business plan to offset the cost

Assess the cost effectiveness

B. Operational Considerations

Availability of appropriately trained personnel to use the equipment

Assigning an individual (MD/Nurse) to maintain equipment

Uninterrupted availability of power for operation of equipment

Availability of sufficient trained nursing staff

Availability of maintenance staff trained in equipment repair (engineers)

Providing continuing education year round

Maintenance of data on the equipment operation and function

Periodic review of performance of personnel and for quality improvement

---

maintenance of the equipment. These commitments are critical to the sustainability of the usage of imported technologies in resource limited countries. An example is the support needed after the import of neonatal ventilators in the developing countries. Ventilator purchase by hospitals in the developing countries requires that the purchase is backed by a service contract for repair and maintenance. Further, other support systems such as monitoring technologies and supplies including oxygen supply and other paraphernalia are available all year round. Personnel (doctors and nurses) who are trained in the use of the ventilator are essential for sustainability. Our experience in different countries, including China, India and Poland, over the last three decades shows that capacity building is critical to successful technology transfer to resource poor countries. Various methods of "knowledge and skill transfer" have been used in the medical and health fields. Among these models, capacity building is best achieved through an "institution to institution" collaboration between interested institutions.[18] Table 1.3 lists various programs implemented in different countries by our group at the University of Illinois during the last 30 years. These programs were aimed at capacity building, developing

Table 1.3.   Development of programs to facilitate knowledge and skill diffusion to different countries, China, Poland, and India: Experience at Division of Neonatology at UIC Chicago

---

A. Programs for Capacity Building

Leadership Training Program for Senior Neonatologists and nurses from different countries and different institutions
Onsite conduct of didactic lectures and workshops
Multiple CME Programs in the host country
Multiple bilateral faculty exchanges

B. Developing Specific Programs

Introduction of Neonatal Resuscitation Program
Establishment of Regional Perinatal Center
Neonatal/Perinatal transport system
Hospital pharmacy services
Nursing education
Hospital administration
Neurosurgery
Orthopedic surgery
Women's health program

C. Research and Education

Joint publication of *Textbook of Neonatology* in Poland
Publication of research in peer reviewed journals
Development of collaborative research
Obtaining NIH Global Network Grant
Obtaining grants from MOD

---

specific clinical programs to improve perinatal patient care and enhancing scholarly activity of the faculty in research and education in the collaborating institutes in each country: China, Poland, India and Uzbekistan.

1.4.6 *Review of NICU technology diffusion in developing countries*

Neonatal intensive care units (NICU) in the developing countries have been slowly but steadily expanding. Since the development of NICU is based on acquiring high cost of medical technologies and capital investments, their growth has been uneven among the countries. Rapidly emerging economies such as China and India are moving faster than other countries in Africa and Latin America. India and China started to initiate their NICU programs in the early 1980s, followed by countries with slower economic growth such as Malaysia, Indonesia and more recently in Ghana. In China, the first children's intensive care program was established by the Ministry of Health of People's Republic of China and United Nations Children's Fund in 1983. The author was one of the first neonatologists to establish relationship between China Medical College Shenyang and University of Illinois in this endeavor.[20] The establishment of NICUs in China in the early 1980s has shown steady improvement in premature infants requiring ventilation and overall neonatal survival. A survey of 23 tertiary care NICUs showed significant improvement in LBW infants requiring ventilation. The utilization of all modern ventilators including HFV has increased. The downside is that the cost of NICU care has also increased.[21]

Assisted ventilation for neonates started in India in mid-1980s at major teaching institutions.[22] The first surfactant administration in India was given in 1987 at AIIMS. However, since the 1990s, several private and corporate hospitals have developed well-equipped units that meet the Western standards of Level III NICUs. In 1997, it was noted that half of the units surveyed reported 50–70% survival of the ventilated babies. In 2002, a survey of 27 Level III units showed results comparable to Western units, and at almost all birth weight groups these units are managed by highly qualified medical and nursing personnel.

Similarly, reports from Pakistan show the benefits of diffusion of neonatal technologies in improving neonatal outcomes there.[23,24] In Malaysia, the first NICU was established in 1987 with six ventilators which later expanded in 1993.[25] An analysis of their outcome data from their NICU in 2003 showed a significant increase in survival after establishing ventilator care. In South Africa in a recent survey of eight hospitals in one province, two were providing Level II care and three others were providing Level III care.[26] These units were well equipped and were well staffed with skilled nursing and medical staff. A report from Ghana showed that establishment of a ventilator support in the NICU at a teaching hospital led to dramatic decrease in mortality of infants admitted to the unit.[27] The significance of this report was that the major single intervention in already existing NICU was very effective in reducing neonatal mortality. One time capital investment for the addition of ventilators and improved physical facilities was the only intervention. No new nurses were added, however, the existing staff was given on-site additional training in ventilator care. All these observations suggest that it is possible to develop NICUs with ventilatory support even in developing countries with minimum investments. However, the success of utilization of the technology was dependant on the availability of skilled nursing and medical staff. Therefore, technology diffusion without skill and knowledge diffusion will be ineffective in achieving the intended objective of reduction of NMR/IMR. These data also demonstrate that in spite of economic barriers, neonatal medical technology is spreading steadily into the developing countries.

Augmenting the availability of oxygen with the use of oxygen concentrators, using infant warmers to avoid hypothermia, and devices such as CPAP and pulse oximeters are examples of relatively low-cost, high-yield technologies. In addition, training of healthcare workers in the effective use of these technologies will yield very good results, as shown in several programs described above.

Availability of oxygen in rural hospitals is a major problem in developing countries.[28] Oxygen is normally supplied in pressurized tanks. This is an expensive method and has no reliability of constant supply in remote health facilities with poor transport systems. Oxygen concentrators are alternate options. Oxygen concentrators absorb nitrogen from air and supply oxygen concentrators up to 85–95% at different flow rate. The devices are highly economical over oxygen cylinders. The cost of oxygen-stored cylinders for one year exceeds the initial cost of oxygen concentrator. A typical oxygen concentrator has a life span of seven years and is maintenance-free for first 26,400 hours of use. A great advantage in developing countries!

The concerns regarding the high cost of medical technology transfer to low economy countries must be acknowledged. The question remains "whether it is justifiable to invest country's meager resources to benefit a few sick infants". As a public policy matter, one would first implement low-cost, high-yield innovations.

1.5 Technology Assessment and Public Policy

Although development of medical technologies has improved the health outcomes in industrialized countries, methodical assessment of medical technology is lacking. Such information forms the basis for "development of a sound public policy" regarding the general use of the technology for an intended purpose. In the absence of technology assessment, widespread use of technology will add to the unnecessary healthcare cost. Battista *et al.* summarized their findings of technology assessment of the six most commonly used technologies in eight developed countries (Australia, USA, UK, Canada, Germany, France, Netherlands and Sweden), all of which had similar economic status and had similarities in utilization of newer healthcare technologies.[17] Their analysis included the following medical technologies which have made a major impact on health outcome: cardiac bypass surgery, imaging technologies, laparoscopic surgery, breast cancer treatment, end-stage renal disease, and neonatal intensive care services. They concluded that new medical technologies have had a major impact on the care of patients as well as improved survival. Table 1.4 shows a summary of the findings. Neonatal intensive care services were found to be provided in all eight countries through an organized system. It should be noted that assessing the impact of NICU implies assessment of the "cumulative impact" of neonatal medical technologies used in the NICU. The definition of NICU however, may vary from center to center depending on the component of services provided. It is difficult to study the precise effect of diffusion of individual medical technology on NMR or IMR. Assessment of neonatal medical technology was least assessed compared to other widely used technologies. Except in Canada, the impact of NICU has not been well studied in the eight countries. As for USA, they commented that "the United States of America is striking for its high level of such services combined with a high infant mortality rate compared with other industrialized countries."

Despite the fact that newer medical technologies have made a major contribution to improved health of populations at large, they are not universally accessible because of economic constraints. These observations underscore the difficulties of making public policies regarding adaptation of new technologies on a global scale.

Table 1.4.   Relative impact of technology adoption and diffusion

Impact of TA	CABG/ PTCA	CT/MRI	LC	ESRD	NICU	Breast Cancer
			Case Study Technologies			
Highest	Sweden	Sweden	Sweden	Sweden	Canada	UK
				Canada		Sweden
	Canada	UK	Australia		Netherlands	Canada
		Canada	Netherlands			Netherlands
			France			
	UK		UK		UK	
	France	Netherlands	Canada	France	France	
	Netherlands	France	US	Netherlands	Sweden	US
	Australia	Australia	Germany	Australia	Australia	Australia
				UK		France
Lowest	US	US		US	US	
	Germany	Germany		Germany	Germany	Germany

Key: Breast cancer: screening programs for breast cancer, CABG: coronary artery bypass grafting, CT/MRI: computerized tomography and magnetic resonance imaging, ESRD: treatments for end-stage renal disease, LC: laparoscopic cholecystectomy techniques, NICU: neonatal intensive care units and EMCO, PTCA: percutaneous transluminal coronary angioplasty, TA: technology adoption.
Note: Joined cells suggest that there is little to distinguish the countries in the list.
Source: Ref. 17.

1.5.1 *Low cost technologies and child survival in developing countries*

The discussions so far in this chapter has focused on the evolution and utilization of high cost medical technology in the care of sick newborns. It was also mentioned that the modern NICU care is very expensive, therefore not always affordable particularly in the developing countries. Thus it is critical that those countries adopt low cost but high yield medical technologies which are cost effective and this aspect will have appeal for universal usage. The evidence for such low cost interventions was provided recently by Jones *et al.*[29]

In an article devoted to understanding the causes of neonatal mortality and how they can be prevented, the authors reviewed the evidence for the effectiveness of interventions used to reduce child mortality in low income countries.[29] Interventions were grouped into "preventive" and "treatment" categories. They were also classified according to the "effectiveness" of the intervention according to the available evidence: The designation of Level 1 evidence was given if there was sufficient evidence for the intervention to be effective in preventing or treating the intended illness/disease, Level 2 evidence suggested that there was limited evidence, and Level 3 evidence indicated that there was inadequate evidence for the intervention to be effective in preventing or treating the intended purpose. Table 1.5 provides a list of the interventions and their level of evidence of their effectiveness in preventing/decreasing the illness thus

Table 1.5. Evidence for the effectiveness of selected interventions in reducing child survival. (Modified from Ref. 29)

Level 1 Evidence
  Preventive Interventions
    Water/sanitation
    Vaccines
    Nutritional supplements
    Antenatal treatments: HIV, malaria, tetanus toxoid
    Clean delivery
  Treatment Interventions
    Oral dehydration
    Antibiotics for pneumonia, dysentery and sepsis
    Antimalarials
    Nutritional support zinc, vitamin A
Level 2 Evidence
  Preventive interventions
    Antibiotics for PROM
    Temporary management of NB
    Treatment interventions
    Neonatal resuscitation

Key: Level 1 Evidence: Sufficient evidence, Level 2 Evidence: Limited evidence.
It should be noted that designated Level 2 evidence for the impact of neonatal temperature management and neonatal resuscitation on child survival as presented in this paper does not negate the true impact of these interventions. It simply indicates that there was no sufficient evidence particularly from the low income countries, at the time of analysis. However, since then, more evidence is gathering in support of effectiveness of these interventions in reducing NMR. (See Fig. 1 for more details.)

decreasing the IMR. Their observations indicate that there are several proven low cost interventions available now that could be employed in resource poor countries and make a vast improvement in child survival across the globe.

1.5.2 *Ethical dilemmas*

It is the developing countries that have the highest NMR/IMR and therefore stand to benefit the most from newer technologies. Yet, they can least afford the cost of the new technology. In our opinion, ideally countries with very high IMR (>45) would benefit the most from basic neonatal care and improved public health measures: clean water technology and sanitation, since these measures are indeed very cost effective. Countries with mid-level IMR (30–46) would benefit faster with the addition of low cost technologies, for example, infant warmers resuscitation equipment, oxygen therapy, and CPAP. High cost technology oriented NICU will be appropriate in countries which have achieved IMR of <30.[30]

It was interesting that Papageorgiou noted that imports of medical technologies in the resource poor countries had an impact in improving IMR independent of per capita income.[19] This finding in theory justifies adopting a public policy of acquiring appropriate medical technologies even in resource poor countries.

The high cost of new technologies, even though life saving, may put an unjustified strain on national economies with low yield in health benefits. Further, efficacy studies of new innovations in resource poor countries, unless planned with serious consideration of all ethical issues, may be considered as exploitation of the developing country. One note of caution must be heeded here in regard to conducting studies or introducing newer innovations into developing countries. Several ethical questions were raised in the HIV treatment studies in Africa and surfactant trials in South America.[31] The experience of these studies emphasizes the need for following the guidelines established for studies in resource poor countries.

It should be noted as a public policy matter, low cost medical technologies such as oxygen saturation monitor, CPAP devices, and antenatal steroids will have far higher impact than expensive technologies such as surfactant treatment or ventilator care and ECMO. Therefore, implementation of low-cost, high-yield technologies will be of greater importance for developing countries.

The following statement by Jones *et al.* sums up what we need to do in utilizing the innovations we already know are effective in reducing IMR and child mortality across the globe.[29] *"There is no need to wait for new vaccines or drugs or new technology, although all these must remain on our agenda. The main challenge today is to transfer what we already know into action: deliver the interventions we have in hand to the children, mothers and the families who need them, and thus achieve the millennium development goal of reducing under-5 mortality by two-thirds by 2015."*

We must work towards overcoming these challenges.

References

1. CDC. (1999) Achievements in public health, 1900–1999: healthier mothers and babies. *MMWR* 48: 849–858.

2. DiMasi JA, Hansen RW, Grabowski HG. (2003) The price of innovation: new estimates of drug development costs. *J Health Econ* 22: 151–185.

3. Kaplan AV, Baim DS, Smith JJ, Feigal DA, Simons M, Jeffreys D, *et al.* (2004) Medical device development: from prototype to regulatory approval. *Circulation* 109: 3068–3072.

4. WWW FAQS: How many websites are there in the world? Boutell.Com, Inc. 2007 Feb. http://www.boutell.com/newfaq/misc/sizeofweb.html

5. Cutler D, Miller G. (2005) The role of public health improvements in health advances: the twentieth-century United States. *Demography* 42: 1–22.

6. Burstrom B, Macassa G, Oberg L, Bernhardt E, Smedman L. (2005) Equitable child health intervention: the impact of improved water and sanitation on inequalities in child mortality in Stockholm, 1878 to 1925. *Am J Public Health* 95: 208–214.

7. Moser K, Shkolnikov V, Leon DA. (2005) World mortality 1950–2000: divergence replaces convergence from the late 1980s. *Bull World Health Organ* 83: 202–209.

8. Baker JP. (1996) The machine in the nursery: incubator technology and the origins of newborn intensive care. Baltimore: Johns Hopkins University Press.

9. Howell JD. (1987) Cardiac physiology and clinical medicine? Two case studies. In: Geison, GL, ed. *Physiology in American Context*, 1850–1940. Bethesda, MD: Lippincott Williams and Wilkins; 279–292.

10. Mike V, Krauss AN, Ross GS. (1993) Reflections on a medical innovation: transcutaneous oxygen monitoring in neonatal intensive care. *Technology and Culture* 34: 894–922.

11. Fujiwara T, Maeta H, Chida S, Morita T, Watabe Y, Abe T. (1980) Artificial surfactant therapy in hyaline-membrane disease. *Lancet* 1(8159): 55–59.

12. FDA/Center for Drug Evaluation and Research. Drugs@FDA. 2009. Access at: www.accessdata.fda.gov/Scripts/cder/DrugsatFDA. Accessed June 30, 2009.

13. Usher R. (1977) Changing mortality rates with perinatal intensive care and regionalization. *Semin Perinatal* 1(3): 309–319.

14. Committee on Perinatal Health. (1993) Toward improving the outcome of pregnancy: the 90s and beyond. White Plains, N.Y.: National Foundation-March of Dimes.

15. Butterfield LJ. (1976) Newborn country USA. *Clin Perinatol* 3(2): 281–295.

16. Clement MS. (2005) Perinatal care in Arizona 1950–2002: a study of the positive impact of technology, regionalization and the Arizona Perinatal Trust. *J Perinatol* 25: 503–508.

17. Battista RN, Banta HD, Jonsson E, Hedge M, Gelband H. (2004) Lessons from the eight countries. In: Banta HD, Battista RN, Gelband H, Jonsson E, eds. *Health Care Technology and Its Assessment in Eight Countries*. Office of Technological Assessment United States Congress; pp. 335–354.

18. Vidyasagar D. (2009) International perspectives: models of technology transfer to developing countries: experience of three decades. *NeoReviews* 10: e1–e9.

19. Papageorgiou C, Savvides A, Zachariadis M. (2007) International Medical Technology Diffusion. *J Int Econ* 72(2): 409–427.

20. Wei KL. (China Medical College, Shenyang PRC). Personal Communication.

21. Li J, Wei K. (2005) Management of infants with chronic lung disease of prematurity in China. *Early Hum Dev* 81(2): 151–154.

22. Vidyasagar D, Singh M, Bhakoo ON, Paul VK, Narang A, Bhutani V, Beligere N, Deorari A. (1997) Evolution of neonatal and pediatric critical care in India. *Crit Care Clin* 13(2): 331–346.

23. Bhutta ZA, Yusuf K, Khan IA. (1999) Is management of neonatal respiratory distress syndrome feasible in developing countries? Experience from Karachi (Pakistan). *Pediatr Pulmonol* 27(5): 305–311.

24. Moazam F, Lakhani M. (1990) Ethical dilemmas of health care in the developing nations. *J Pediatr Surg* 25(4): 438–441.

25. Ho JJ, Chang ASM. (2007) Changes in the process of care and outcome over a 10 year period in a neonatal nursery in a developing country. *J Trop Pediatr* 53: 232–237.

26. Adhikari SA. (Department of Pediatrics and Child Health. Nelson R. Mandela School of Medicine University of Kwazulu Natal, South Africa). Personal Communication.

27. Enweronu-Laryea CC, Nkyekyer K, Rodrigues OP. (2008) The impact of improved neonatal intensive care facilities on referral pattern and outcome at a teaching hospital in Ghana. *J Perinatol* 28(8): 561–565.

28. Mokuolo OA, Ajayi OA. (2002) Use of an oxygen concentrator in a Nigerian neonatal unit: economic implications and reliability. *Ann Trop Pediatr* 22: 209–212.

29. Jones G, Steketee RW, Black RE, Bhutta ZA, Morris SS, Bellagio Child Survival Study Group. (2003) How many child deaths can we prevent this year? *Lancet* 362: 65–71.

30. Knippenberg R, Lawn JE, Darmstadt GL, Begkoyian G, Fogstad H, Walelign N, Paul VK; Lancet Neonatal Survival Steering Team. (2005) Systematic scaling up of neonatal care in countries. *Lancet* 365(9464): 1087–1098.

31. National Bioethics Advisory Commission. (2001) Ethical Considerations in the Design and Conduct of International Clinical Trials. In: *Ethical and Policy Issues in International Research: Clinical Trials in Developing Countries*. Bethesda, MD; 19–34.

Chapter 2

Assisted Reproductive Technologies

Adelina M. Emmi* and Ana A. Murphy*

On July 25, 1978, the field of reproductive medicine and infertility changed forever with the birth of Louise Brown in England by *in vitro* fertilization (IVF). Her birth gave hope to many couples not able to conceive conventionally. The initial indication for IVF was tubal factor or pelvic adhesive disease as IVF bypasses the fallopian tubes by using controlled ovarian hyperstimulation (COH), egg retrieval, and insemination with ultimate embryo transfer. COH produces large numbers of mature eggs for insemination extracorporally. Intracytoplasmic sperm injection (ICSI) injects a single sperm into the cytoplasm of an egg. It has revolutionized the treatment of men with oligospermia or azoospermia in whom intratesticular sperm are present. The success rate of IVF with ICSI approaches the pregnancy rate with conventional IVF for non-male factor etiologies. Women with premature ovarian failure, decreased ovarian reserve, or age factor infertility, can chose to undergo an IVF cycle with donor oocytes and enjoy excellent pregnancy rates.

2.1 Initial Evaluation for IVF

The initial evaluation includes a review of the couples' medical, surgical, and infertility history and informed consent process is obtained.

---

*Department of Obstetrics & Gynecology, Medical College of Georgia.

Topics of discussion should include:

- Genetic screening, testing, and counseling.
- Controlled ovarian stimulation, retrieval techniques, and risk factors.
- Fresh and frozen embryo transfer procedures.
- A discussion of nonselective reduction.
- ICSI and its indications.
- An estimate of the number of embryo(s) to be transferred.
- An estimate of the individual couple's pregnancy rate with IVF.
- Potential adverse events such as cancellation of cycles, gamete/fertilization problems, and pregnancy risk (multiple gestation, spontaneous abortion, and ectopic pregnancy).
- The couple has access to referrals for psychological testing. In cases of donor egg and surrogacy, psychological referral is mandatory.

IVF is the assisted reproductive modality of choice. Gamete intrafallopian transfer (GIFT) and zygote intrafallopian transfer (ZIFT) are alternatives to conventional IVF. GIFT places retrieved oocytes and sperm into the fallopian tube via laparoscopy or laparotomy where fertilization takes place, while ZIFT places fertilized oocytes created by IVF, at the stage prior to cleavage, into the fallopian tube. ZIFT and GIFT require at least one normal fallopian tube. For religious reasons, some couples prefer GIFT rather than IVF because fertilization occurs in the fallopian tube and not in the laboratory.

With the advent of ICSI, assisted hatching, and advanced laboratory techniques (i.e., culture media and embryo day 3 or 5 transfers), IVF success rates exceed ZIFT/GIFT rates and very few of these procedures are performed.

2.2 Patient Selection for IVF

Although tubal factor infertility was the original indication for IVF, the indications for IVF have now been expanded to make this the final step in virtually all infertile couples.[1] Tubal factor infertility can arise from various etiologies, including pelvic inflammatory disease, endometriosis, prior abdominopelvic surgery (including tubal ligations), ectopic pregnancy, or a ruptured appendix. This diagnosis is made by hysterosalpingogram (HSG) or laparoscopy. Although surgical therapy may be a reasonable option in young patients, IVF may be the best option for women with significant tubal damage, older women, or those with multiple factor infertility. The poor prognosis for repeat tuboplasty makes IVF the treatment of choice.

Treatment of male factor infertility has been drastically advanced by IVF and ICSI. Men who have a motile sperm count below 10×10^6 with poor morphology have a significant reduction in pregnancy rates. ICSI has been used to treat severe male factor infertility, with pregnancy and fertilization rates similar to couples with normal semen parameters who are undergoing conventional IVF. Oligospermic and selected azoospermic males, who have intratesticular sperm, have high fertilization and pregnancy rates with ICSI, regardless of motility, morphology, or sperm concentrations.

Reduced fertility with advancing maternal age seems to be more common as women delay childbearing. In non-contracepting populations, fertility starts to decrease at age 30, the decline escalating in the late 30s, with a severe decrease in fertility after age 40. This decline is manifested as an age-related decrease in ovarian follicles and decline in oocyte quality.[2] Women over 35 have a significantly decreased chance of pregnancy, compared to younger patients. Data from women of all ages, who have received oocytes from young donors, have excellent pregnancy rates independent of the recipient's age. This implies that the uterus does not age.

Women with diminished ovarian reserve (DOR), regardless of their age, have significantly lower pregnancy rates with any modality. They also have an increased risk of aneuploid pregnancy and spontaneous miscarriage compared to patients with normal ovarian reserve.

Day 3 or basal follicles-stimulating hormone (FSH) and the clomiphene challenge test (CCT), correlate best with conception using assisted reproductive technologies (ARTs), and are also applicable to an infertility population.[3] Typically, an abnormal day 3 FSH is about > 12.6 IU/L. These values are dependent on the particular assay used and are patient population-dependent. Infertile patients who are older than 43 years or have an elevated FSH, have decreased pregnancy rates per cycle, and may be encouraged to pursue donor egg or adoption.

Endometriosis affects 30% to 40% of infertile women. Endometriosis involving the ovaries, fallopian tubes, and pelvis may cause anatomic distortion and adhesion of the tubes and ovaries, hampering ovum pickup. Patients with moderate to severe endometriosis (stage III and IV) are encouraged to attempt IVF early, especially those with severe adhesive disease. Many of these patients have had one or more conservative surgeries and have not achieved pregnancy despite optimal debulking of their disease. Surgery prior to IVF to improve pregnancy rates is not recommended. Surgical excision of endometrioma prior to stimulation may improve stimulation and optimize oocyte retrieval. However, this is controversial.

Many couples who fail clomiphene citrate (CC) and gonadotropin therapy eventually require IVF. Patients under 36 years of age, World Health Organization (WHO) Infertility group I and II, frequently try three to four cycles of CC or gonadotropins with intrauterine insemination (IUI). Of patients who become pregnant with CC and IUI, over 85% become pregnant within the first four cycles of treatment.

Patients with unexplained infertility are by definition ovulatory, with normal fallopian tubes and uterine cavity, and a normal semen analyses by WHO criteria. The majority of these patients have already attempted other therapeutic strategies such as timed intercourse, CC, or gonadotropins with IUI. Women with unexplained infertility have a combined per cycle IVF pregnancy rate of approximately 20% compared to 8% and 17% for CC with IUI and gonadotropin with IUI, respectively. In 2000, IVF pregnancy rates for unexplained infertility were appreciably higher indicating this technique should be more rapidly offered. The FASTT Trial (2009), a prospective randomized trial funded by the NIH, demonstrated that progression directly from Clomid with insemination to IVF is the most cost effective treatment strategy in patients with unexplained fertility.[4]

Premature ovarian failure (POF) is defined as hypergonadism prior to the age of 40. Causes of premature loss of oocytes include gonadal dysgenesis, failure of germ cell migration in fetal life, and postnatal germ cell loss (castration, autoimmune disease, infections). Iatrogenic oocyte loss occurs with chemotherapy, radiotherapy, and ovarian surgery for benign disease. Patients with POF have excellent success when receiving donor oocytes. There is no decrease in pregnancy or delivery rates with increasing age or the diagnosis of the recipient (i.e., POF, surgical castration, previous IVF failure, menopause, DOR). Thus, endometrial receptivity does not appear to be altered by recipient age or diagnosis. Using young donor oocytes optimizes success rates and improves chances of transferring healthy embryos.

2.3 Testing Prior to Assisted Reproduction

Previous IVF cycles should be reviewed in detail focusing on the method of stimulation, number and quality of embryos, the method of insemination (conventional versus ICSI), follicular and endometrial development, estradiol levels throughout the stimulation, length of the stimulation, and the pregnancy outcome. In addition, we review the method and number of embryos transferred. Frozen embryo transfer cycles are also assessed, noting the endometrial stimulation, day of transfer, and embryo quality after thawing.

Evaluation should also consider thyroid disease (thyroid-stimulating hormone), hyperprolactinemia (prolactin), a glucose and insulin test to screen for diabetes and hyperinsulinemia (if indicated), blood type and Rh. An infectious disease panel consists of hepatitis B and C, syphilis, human immunodeficiency virus (HIV 1, 2), and rubella titer.

Initial selected genetic tests for carrier status are offered and may include Tay-Sachs disease (Ashkenazi Jews), sickle cell anemia (African descent), β-thalassemia (Mediterranean/Chinese), α-thalassemia (Southeast Asians), and cystic fibrosis (Caucasians) as well as other necessary screening.

2.3.1 *Ovarian reserve testing*

Testing for ovarian reserve is useful for all IVF patients.[1,3] These tests are inexpensive, noninvasive, help in determining medication dosing, and predictive of ultimate outcome with ART. Most IVF programs routinely check all patients as per American Society for Reproductive Medicine guidelines and to help determine protocols in patients with risk factors such as those with multiple surgeries, severe endometriosis, severe adhesive disease, and cigarette smokers.

A day 3 basal FSH is obtained during a natural cycle. Based on our laboratory assay, a day 3 FSH >12.6 mIU/mL predicts a decreased chance of achieving a pregnancy with IVF. In order to counsel patients effectively, each institution and laboratory must establish their own critical cutoff point, above which, a pregnancy becomes highly unlikely.

Both FSH and estradiol have been shown to be excellent predictors of IVF performance. As a "single predictor", basal FSH is better than age at predicting a successful pregnancy, until age 43, after which IVF success rates appear to have an extremely poor prognosis.[5] Regardless of age or fertility history, women with diminished ovarian reserve, as manifested by an elevated day 3 FSH, ultimately conceive with a high rate of first trimester pregnancy loss. Significant intercycle variability can be found among basal FSH values. This variability reflects the physiologic inability of the follicle cohort to suppress FSH as a result of declining follicular health. FSH levels rise as granulosa cell production of inhibin-B decreases. Inhibin exerts negative control on the pituitary. Once a patient has an isolated elevated day 3 FSH, even among normal cycles, her chance for IVF pregnancy is poor.

The clomiphene challenge test (CCT) uses day 3 FSH value, and a provoked day 10 response to 100 mg of clomiphene citrate, administered cycle days 5 through 9. The CCT can be interpreted in various ways looking at day 3 and 10 values, but carries the same prognosis as an abnormal day 3. An elevated day 3 basal FSH value, or an abnormal CCT, predicts a less than 5% chance of pregnancy with ART. Unexplained infertility comprises 52% of the patients with an abnormal CCT.

Recent evidence suggests that anti-Mullerian hormone (AMH) is produced by small preantral and small antral follicles. These follicles cease to produce AMH when they reach dominance. With the decrease in antral follicles with age, serum levels are also diminished. AMH becomes undetectable by menopause. In contrast to other markers of ovarian reserve, AMH can be used independent of phase of the menstrual cycle. AMH follicle count may be a better test of ovarian reserve.[6,7]

2.3.2 *Evaluation of the uterus and fallopian tubes*

A sonohysterogram (HSG) or office hysteroscopy should be done before starting IVF. An HSG aids in the diagnosis of hydrosalpinges or an intrauterine filling defect, both of which decrease IVF pregnancy rates. Since patients can develop uterine or tubal pathology in intervening years, a repeat study should be considered if the previous uterine evaluation is more than one year old. A complete pelvic ultrasound, a trial embryo transfer, vaginal cultures, and a Pap smear are done on all patients. During the ultrasound, the adnexae are evaluated for ovarian cysts, endometrioma, and hydrosalpinges. Leiomyoma and polyps may be noted in the uterus. Sonohysterography is almost as accurate as hysteroscopy, and more sensitive and specific than transvaginal ultrasound or HSG in diagnosing intracavitary pathology. Additionally, sonohysterograpy is less invasive, relatively inexpensive, and does not require the use of contrast dyes.

2.3.2.1 Hydrosalpinges and IVF

Tubal disease is one of the main indications for IVF with hydrosalpinges accounting for 10% to 30% of tubal factor infertility. Compared to other types of tubal pathology, women with hydrosalpinges (including surrogate carriers) have reduced IVF success. Hydrosalpinges decrease IVF implantation, pregnancy, and delivery rates while increasing early pregnancy loss. This has been confirmed by large meta-analyses as well as numerous retrospective studies.

Only two randomized, prospective studies have evaluated whether prophylactic salpingectomy of hydrosalpinges prior to IVF improves pregnancy rates.[8,9] Pregnancy rates after a single IVF cycle are approximately 37% in women after salpingectomy and 24% when the hydrosalpinx were not removed. Subgroup evaluation of these patients revealed that women with bilateral hydrosalpinges, visible on ultrasound, had a significant increase in implantation and delivery rates after salpingectomy compared to the non-intervention group. Ultimate delivery rates more than doubled in patients with ultrasound visible hydrosalpinges after salpingectomy.

Many mechanisms have been proposed to explain the adverse effects of hydrosalpinges on IVF success rates. Fluid that accumulates in the hydrosalpinx can enter the uterine cavity. Markers of endometrial receptivity have been shown to be decreased in patients with hydrosalpinges as inflammatory cytokines within the fluid may act as inhibitors. Salpingectomy is recommended when the Fallopian tubes have visible fluid within the tube(s) on sonogram. Polyps, Müllerian anomalies, intrauterine synechiae, and leiomyoma are all associated with reproductive loss or failure. In women undergoing IVF, a midfollicular office sonohysterogram (intrauterine saline infusion) can further delineate the nature of the lesion(s). After the lesion is identified, a diagnostic or operative hysteroscopy should be performed to correct the abnormality.

Uterine leiomyoma may contribute to infertility and miscarriage but the data are limited by the uncontrolled retrospective nature of the reports. Most IVF studies distinguish between submucosal (leiomyoma that distort the uterine cavity), intramural (confined to the myometrium with no cavity distortion), and subserosal (leiomyoma protruding from the serosal surface). Subserosal leiomyoma, which are not adjacent to the endometrium, do not decrease pregnancy rates or increase miscarriages rates. Submucosal leiomyoma, which protrude into the uterine cavity, have been shown to decrease IVF implantation and pregnancy rates when compared to non-protruding intramural and subserosal leiomyoma. Prior to starting an IVF cycle, removal of submucosal distorting leiomyoma is strongly recommended. Depending on the location, leiomyoma are removed abdominally or hysteroscopically.

There is significant controversy in the literature regarding the removal of intramural leiomyoma prior to an IVF cycle, especially if they do not distort the endometrial cavity. In retrospective studies of patients under 40 years of age with intramural leiomyoma, there is a significant decrease in implantation rate. There is also a trend toward decreased live-birth rates in women with intramural leiomyoma, independent of the size of the leiomyoma volume.

Debate remains as to whether endometrioma should be removed prior to IVF. The few retrospective studies performed have not shown an increase in pregnancy rates with removal of endometrioma. However, other studies have shown a decrease in peak estradiol levels, fertilization, and implantation rates with advanced stages of endometriosis, including endometrioma. In older patients, most experienced clinicians do not remove endometrioma prior to IVF. However, in young women with endometriosis there appears to be a significant improvement in the recruitment of follicles. Debulking endometriosis is not warranted before IVF except in cases of large endometrioma or pelvic pain.

2.3.3 *Evaluation of male factor infertility*

Male factor infertility will affect 50% of infertile couples in some fashion. In the vast majority of cases, this diagnosis is known prior to IVF. During the initial IVF consultation, the male partner is encouraged to be present so we can review his medical history and any prior semen analyses. Men suspected of male factor infertility are typically evaluated with regard to the following:

- infertility history
- sexual history
- childhood and developmental history
- medical history
- surgical history
- prior infections
- gonadotoxins
- family history
- review of systems.

Multiple semen analyses should be evaluated in addition to any appropriate hormonal and genetic screening.

2.3.3.1 *Semen analysis and sperm preparation*

Semen samples should be collected after an abstinence interval of two to three days. WHO criteria are a rough guideline for evaluation of semen samples. These criteria include assessment of volume, sperm concentration, motility, morphology, pH, and total sperm count. Sperm morphology has become an useful indicator of successful fertilization with IVF. Kruger coined the term "strict criteria", in order to strictly grade normally shaped sperm. In studies using strict morphologic criteria, men with greater than 14% normal forms had normal fertilization rates *in vitro*. For patients with 4% to 14% normal forms, intermediate fertilization rates are seen, while men with less than 4% normal forms had fertilization rates of 7% to 8%. ICSI should be recommended for any factor or combination of factors that are abnormal, including count, motility and score, as well as sperm morphology. In men with poor sperm parameters, ICSI produces fertilization and pregnancy rates similar to conventional IVF.

If the semen analysis is normal, a fresh sample for insemination will be produced on the day of oocyte retrieval. Semen samples need to be washed and processed prior to their use in IVF. Washing techniques isolate motile capacitated sperm for insemination. Sperm isolation may be performed on ejaculated semen, sperm retrieved from the epididymis or testes, as well as cryopreserved samples. Several isolation techniques are currently used. The "swim-up" method is used for samples with normal concentration and motility. For low motility and decreased sperm counts, the semen sample is layered over discontinuous Percoll gradients (45% and 90%) and centrifuged. The resulting pellet separates normal spermatozoa from lymphocytes, epithelial cells, abnormal sperm, cell debris, and bacteria.

Many tests have been proposed to evaluate sperm function, however, these tests have poor inter- and intra-laboratory reproducibility. Moreover, the information gained from these studies rarely changes management.

2.3.3.2 *Genetic and hormonal evaluation of infertile male*

Developments in genomic medicine will likely explain much of what is now considered idiopathic male infertility. Indeed, our understanding of the genetic defects that cause infertility is no longer confined to chromosomal aneuploidies (e.g., Klinefelter syndrome) and single-gene defects (cystic fibrosis and congenital absence of the vas deferens). The past decade has seen that isolated Y-chromosomal loci can influence spermatogenesis (AZF regions) and that the human X chromosome is likely to be an important source of spermatogenesis genes. More recently, the finding that faulty recombination occurs in male infertility has large implications not only for the cause of the infertility but also for the use of affected gametes. Indeed, as our understanding of genetic infertility matures, so too will the importance and complexity of genetic counseling and testing for patients who use assisted reproduction.[10,11]

Men who have obstructive azoospermia, with congenital bilateral absence of the vas deferens (CBAVD), require testing for mutations in the cystic fibrosis gene. Ninety percent of patients with CBAVD will have gene aberrations. Since these genes are transmitted in an autosomal recessive fashion, genetic counseling is advised for these men and their families.

Evaluation of oligospermic and azoospermic men requires serum measurements of LH, FSH, prolactin, testosterone, and usually a karyotype. Serum Inhibin B values may also be helpful.[12] These tests often aid in the diagnoses of testicular resistance or failure, and hypogonadotropic hypogonadism.

2.4 Preparation for IVF

A trial or "mock" embryo transfer should be performed with the same catheter used during the actual embryo transfer. This enables the physician to measure the uterine length and note the curvature of the cervix and uterus. The goal of this pre-cycle trial transfer is to facilitate a non-traumatic embryo transfer which has been shown to increase pregnancy and implantation rates. If there is cervical stenosis precluding easy access to the uterine cavity, it will be detected before undergoing an IVF cycle. Severe cases of cervical stenosis may require dilation of the cervix with hysteroscopic guidance prior to starting the IVF cycle.

2.5 Fetal Safety of Drugs in Pregnancy

Clomiphene citrate was the first drug to be used commonly as first line drug therapy for patients with ovulatory problems. It is a racemic mixture of enclomiphene that clears relatively quickly and zuclomiphene that clears slowly. This drug has agonist/antagonist properties that may result in accumulation of CC with increased use. With continued use of CC, endometrial atrophy may be seen as well as a significant decrease in cervical mucus. Both of these effects significantly decrease pregnancy rates.

Uncontrolled case reports raised the possibility that CC may be associated with the possible risk of neural tube defect. Medveczky *et al.*[13] found an odds ratio (OR) of 2.1 (95% CI 1.0–4.5) with CC and neural tube defect (NTD). A more recent study by Wu *et al.*[14] found an OR of 11.7 (95% CI 2.0–44.8). The number of CC cycles in the 12 months prior to conception was higher in mothers of infants with NTDs than in controls (mean 5.7 versus 2.6 cycles, $P = 0.01$). There appears to be weak association between CC and NTD.

Since CC is similar to DES, concern was raised that there may be an increased risk for hypospadias. Sorenson *et al.*[15] compared cases of hypospadias and matched control male births. Clomiphene does not appear to be associated with an increase in hypospadias [OR of 0.48 (95% CI 0.15–1.54)]. However, within a cohort of patients with preconceptual exposure to CC, Meijer *et al.*[16] noted a severe form of hypospadias, a penoscrotal hypospadias that is significantly higher (6.08, CI 95% 1.4–26.33).

Aromatase inhibitors are well known in the cancer area. However, Mittwally and Casper[17] were the first to suggest aromatase inhibitors for ovulation induction of women with polycystic ovarian syndrome. Elizur and Tulandi[18] reported outcome of newborns who were conceived with letrozole ($n = 514$) and CC ($n = 397$). Miscarriage rates were not different. Another study by Forman *et al.*[19] compared 112 newborns following letrozole treatment to 271 newborns following CC treatment and 94 newborns achieved spontaneously. The rates of malformations were 0, 2.6%, and 3.2%. These data would suggest that its use for ovulation induction is very unlikely to be associated with teratogenesis.

Progesterone was first studied as a contraceptive and later used to support the luteal phase. In 1988, the Food and Drug Administration approved its use in the US. It is widely used for luteal support in IVF cycles.

In 1958, gonadotropins were extracted from human pituitaries to induce follicular growth in amenorrheic women. Human urinary menopausal gonadotropins replaced human pituitary gonadotropins-hCG. A review of 1160 babies born following ovulation induction with hMG-hCG, 63 infants with malformations were identified for an overall incidence of 54.3 per 1000 (major malformation 21.6 of 1000 and minor malformations 32.7 of 1000). These data do not suggest evidence of teratogenicity.

2.6 IVF Protocols

Many protocols have been described for COH designed to increase the number of mature follicles for retrieval. All protocols aim to maximize the number of mature oocytes retrieved per stimulation cycle. The information needed to make a protocol decision is based on:

- medical and surgical history,
- results from laboratory tests (i.e., ovarian reserve testing, semen analysis),
- review of previous assisted reproductive cycles (stimulation response, embryo quantity and quality, fertilization rate, embryo transfer).

In general, patients fit into one of three groups — normal, high, and poor responders. Patients with a high response to gonadotropin stimulation are typically young and often have PCOS. They are at risk for producing elevated estradiol levels with multiple follicles. This results in cycle cancellation (withholding hCG), to avoid the development of ovarian hyperstimulation syndrome (OHSS). Poor responders recruit fewer oocytes than normal responders. Patient characteristics that predict a poor response include women over 40 years of age, a prior cancelled IVF cycle and diminished ovarian reserve. Normal responders are often patients with tubal disease, or male factor infertility.

2.6.1 *COH medication and strategies*

Gonadotropin releasing hormone-agonists (GnRH-a) revolutionized the use of gonadotropin-based stimulation protocols.[1] Monitoring for the luteinizing hormone (LH) surge was necessary before the use of GnRH-a because as many as 15% of IVF cycles were cancelled because of a premature LH surge. GnRH-agonists, like leuprolide acetate, substitute amino acids at position 6 and 10 on the GnRH molecule. This decreases the degradation rate and increases the binding affinity of the agonist to the GnRH receptor. GnRH-a initially produce a surge or flare response that increase circulating LH and FSH levels. The flare is then followed by down-regulation and desensitization, which results in suppression and a hypogonadal state with eventual withdrawal bleeding. This suppression of endogenous gonadotropins prevents the spontaneous LH surge prior to oocyte retrieval. IVF agonist protocols can capitalize on both of these effects. The long lupron protocol uses the GnRH-a down-regulation effect. The microdose protocols begin GnRH-a one to two days prior to the start of gonadotropin administration and utilizes the flare effect first and then the down-regulation effect to suppress ovulation to try to enhance follicular formation in patients who may be poor responders to stimulation.

The majority of IVF cycles use GnRH-a protocols. GnRh antagonists are increasing in use for COH in IVF. Third-generation antagonists (ganirelix and cetrorelix) are more complex than agonists in their action, having substitutions on the GnRH molecule at positions 1, 2, 3, 6 and 10. They bind competitively to the GnRH receptor, decreasing gonadotropin secretion within 4 to 8 hours in a dose-dependent manner. GnRH antagonists also prevent the risk of a premature LH surge and are used in either single-dose or multiple-dose protocols.

In a meta-analysis comparing long agonist protocols to antagonist protocols, antagonists significantly reduced the incidence of OHSS and the amount of gonadotropins needed for stimulation, but appeared to have lower pregnancy rates associated with their stimulation cycles.[20] There are many benefits to their use in IVF. These protocols are simpler for patients to follow and appear to be less expensive. Their use, therefore, warrants further investigation. While the ideal stimulation protocol has yet to be developed, GnRH agonist and antagonist protocols will continue to be universally used.

Gonadotropin stimulation in IVF will also continue to be used because meta-analyses have shown that IVF pregnancy rates are significantly improved with gonadotropin use because of the increased numbers of oocytes retrieved. There are two major classes of gonadotropins, urinary-derived human menopausal gonadotropins (hMG) which contain both LH and FSH, and recombinant gonadotropin, pure FSH. The goal of any gonadotropin therapy is to maximize follicular recruitment for oocyte retrieval. The urinary hMG typically has 75 IU of FSH and 75 IU of LH per ampule. The newer recombinant gonadotropins are genetically engineered by inserting the human gene for FSH in cultured immortal mammalian cells. Mammalian cells are needed as bacteria are unable to glycosylate FSH and glycosylation is required for FSH to be biologically active. Recombinant gonadotropin products (r-FSH) are devoid of LH and are tolerated well upon injection. Pregnancy rates appear to be comparable between the two products. However, more large randomized controlled trials are needed to assess the difference between hMG and r-FSH.

Metformin, an insulin-sensitizing agent, has been successfully used to induce ovulation in women with polycystic ovary syndrome (PCOS), although it is not considered a first line agent for ovulation induction in these patients. Metformin appears to decrease OHSS rates in PCOS patients who undergo IVF,[21,22] but more randomized controlled trials are necessary to determine if metformin improves live-birth and pregnancy rates.[23]

Young, normal and high responder patients can use leuprolide (1.0 mg subcutaneous daily) in the "long protocol". This is started either in the mid-luteal phase (seven days after a positive LH surge) of the menstrual cycle preceding their stimulation, or patients are placed on oral contraceptive pills for cycle control and/or gonadotropin suppression, which can be important prior to an IVF start, and then their pills are simply overlapped with their leuprolide for one to two days. The leuprolide dose is decreased to 0.5 mg per day on the day gonadotropin stimulation is initiated. Gonadotropin stimulation is initiated when patients are adequately suppressed.

The starting dosage of gonadotropin is based on multiple factors including prior stimulation cycles and the patient's diagnosis. The daily dose of gonadotropins is fixed initially and then adjusted according to individual patient response. When at least three follicles reach maturity, ovulation is triggered with hCG and the leuprolide is discontinued. Oocytes are retrieved within 35–38 hours after hCG injection.

Microdose luprolide protocols are frequently utilized in women in older age groups, or patients who may respond less vigorously to stimulation. These patients are usually placed on oral contraceptives the cycle prior to stimulation and then stop their pills with 3–4 days break off medication before institution of their stimulation protocol.

After appropriate suppression is diagnosed, stimulation begun with 1–2 days of microdose luprolide usually at 40 μg twice daily and continued until the day of or after hCG injection. Gonadotropin stimulation is usually begun on the third day of luprolide injection. This takes advantage of the initial flare effect of the agonist prior to its suppressive effect.

Agonist protocols are still the most frequently used in IVF centers. However, antagonist protocols have become more frequently used and may become the more frequently used protocols because of their simplicity and decreased cost. There are two commonly used antagonist protocols, a "single-dose" and a "multiple-dose" regimen. In the "multiple-dose" protocols, the antagonist is administered daily from day 6 or 7 of stimulation, or starting when the lead follicles reach approximately 13–14 mm and estradiol levels reach 200–250 pg/ml, until ovulation is triggered. The single dose regime involves the single dose administration of cetrorelix, 3 mg on day 7–8 of stimulation.[24]

Several protocols have been proposed for poor responders. These protocols usually attempt to decrease hormone levels in the cycle prior to stimulation and frequently use high doses of gonadotropins. These may increase the number of follicles and oocytes, but pregnancy rates remain low.

2.6.2 *Oocyte retrieval*

Oocyte retrieval is performed 35–38 hours after hCG injection. Retrieval is performed in either an operating room or more frequently in a procedure room. The perineum and vagina are prepped with warm sterile saline prior to retrieval. Oocytes are retrieved by needle guided vacuum aspiration of follicles under transvaginal ultrasound guidance. Aspirates are collected into 15-mL heated collection tubes. Intravenous sedation is usually administered prior to the procedure with rapid recovery and patient discharge.

In the laboratory, oocytes are placed in culture media. The optimum stage of oocyte maturity is metaphase II, with one polar body extruded. At this stage, conventional insemination or intracytoplasmic sperm injection (ICSI) can be performed. Oocytes are placed into culture media after having any blood removed and cultured for 4–6 hours prior to insemination or ICSI. Each dish can contain more than one egg because eggs do better in group culture. After this, the prepared sperm are placed with the eggs in the culture dish at a concentration of approximately 50–150,000 sperm/dish. A check for fertilization is performed between 17–19 hours after insemination. When ICSI is performed, oocytes are examined under a dissecting microscope and cumulus granulosa cells are stripped to judge maturity. ICSI can only be performed on metaphase II oocytes. ICSI is performed by injection of a sperm individually into an egg by a micromanipulation needle ensuring the egg's polar body is at a 12 o'clock position and the injection is done at a 3 o'clock position in order to avoid the spindle. Again, 17–19 hours later, observation for fertilization is performed. Improvements in culture media now allow for the culture of embryos to the blastocyst stage. Embryo transfers are usually performed on either day 3 or 5 post retrieval. Day 5 blastocyst transfer, in appropriately selected patients, allows for the selection of better quality embryos and for a reduced number of embryos to be transferred.[1]

2.6.3 *Luteal progesterone support after oocyte retrieval*

The reasoning behind the use of exogenous hormonal support in the luteal phase of the IVF cycle is based on the fact that during oocycte retrieval, the follicle is aspirated and the oocyte along with the cumulus and some granulosa cells are removed. This may lead to the loss of cells that are necessary for adequate corpus luteum formation. The use of exogenous progesterone, during the luteal phase of an IVF cycle, to increase pregnancy rates is supported by large meta-analyses. Progesterone prepares the endometrial lining for implantation and pregnancy maintenance.[25] The timing of progesterone supplementation has been debated. It is usually started either the day of retrieval or the day after retrieval.[26] Intramuscular progesterone has remained the standard, although some newer forms of vaginal progesterone support have increased in use, such as vaginal tablets. Studies will be necessary to compare their efficacy to IM progesterone.

Progesterone is usually continued until 8–10 weeks of gestation when pregnancy occurs, or during the entire time that the corpus luteum would support the pregnancy. Many programs also support the luteal phase with estrogen supplementation after retrieval during the first few weeks of pregnancy. This is done with either estradiol patches, vaginal or oral estradiol and is usually continued until at least a fetal heart is noted on ultrasound.

2.6.4 *ICSI and sperm retrieval techniques for severe male factor*

ICSI is a microinsemination technique which has allowed men with severe male factor infertility, which was previously untreatable, the ability to reproduce. ICSI delivers a single sperm into the cytoplasm of an egg through the zona pellucida and egg membrane. Pregnancy rates with ICSI using viable, motile spermatozoa are almost those of conventional IVF with standard insemination.

Sperm retrieval techniques have given hope to men with obstructive and non-obstructive azoospermia.[1] It is important to diagnose the etiology of azoospermia prior to IVF and evaluate and counsel patients appropriately concerning possible genetically related conditions and the need for possible chromosome analysis. The kind of azoospermia may influence the method of sperm extraction. Sperm can be extracted from either the epididymis or testis by needle aspiration or surgical methods. The least invasive and simplest method should be attempted first until there are more randomized clinical trials to show a clear benefit from any of the presently available techniques. Adequate numbers of sperm can sometimes be retrieved allowing for cryopreservation of some sperm for future ICSI cycles. Patients need to be counseled that sperm retrieval techniques may fail to recover sperm and they may then need to opt for use of donor sperm.

ICSI uses a single washed sperm placed into a viscous solution which impedes sperm movement. The spermatozoa flagellum is crushed, which causes immobilization. The morphologically normal sperm is aspirated tail-first into an injecting pipette. The sperm is injected through the zona pellucida and into the ooplasm with the polar body at 12 o'clock.

There have been conflicting reports concerning the possible increased risk of birth defects associated with ICSI.[27,28] Studies have not determined if the risk is due to the ICSI procedure or inherent to sperm defects necessitating the ICSI procedure. If there is an increased risk, it is relatively low, noted to be about 4.2% compared to 3% in the general population found in one large study.

2.6.5 *Assisted hatching prior to embryo transfer*

The majority of morphologically "normal" embryos do not implant. The embryo "hatches" from the zona pellucida before implantation. Assisted hatching is the process by which the zona pellucida is artificially breached or opened (e.g., drilling). This disruption of the zona pellucida theoretically facilitates the hatching of embryos by opening a hole and allowing blastomeres to be more easily extracted. Studies suggest that a thick and hardened zona may prevent or reduce the efficiency of hatching of otherwise normally developing embryos and, hence, hatching may improve the rate of implantation.[29,30] A thickened or hardened zona has been postulated to result from gonadotropin stimulation, the laboratory environment, culture techniques or age. This "drilling" creates a defect in the zona pellucida. The opening can be made by mechanical or chemical means. Indications for assisted hatching include age greater than 37, an elevated day 3, FSH, a prior failed IVF cycle, increased zona thickness, and excess oocyte fragmentation. Assisted hatching may improve pregnancy rates in women who have had failed IVF cycles, and in older patient, but it may also increase the multiple pregnancy rates.

2.6.6 *Embryo transfer*

Embryo transfer involves the joint effort of both the clinician and laboratory. The success of implantation hinges in part on the success of the embryo transfer. Embryos can be transferred up to six days after fertilization. Many programs successfully transfer embryos at the blastocyst stage. This has the advantage of decreasing the number of embryos transferred to one or two embryos, which reduce the number of high order multiple pregnancies. A review of recent trials found that pregnancy rates appear higher in women undergoing blastocyst transfer than at earlier stages of transfer.[31] However, there is also a higher risk that patients may not have embryos to transfer or freeze if their embryos do not survive until day 5.

There are different grading systems for embryo quality and embryos can be graded on different days from day 3 to day 6. Embryos are graded on the number and evenness of their cells and cleavage rates. The American Society for Reproductive Medicine's, Society for Assisted Reproductive Technologies has guidelines for practice, concerning the number and quality of embryos for transfer,[32] which can be followed. These guidelines vary depending upon the patient's age, the quality of the embryos and the day of transfer. Other factors that may influence the decision as to the number of embryos to transfer are the patient's history, including the number of previous failed IVF cycles, the patient's personal desires and their feelings about fetal reduction.

Embryos can be transferred with a variety of soft catheters which reduce tissue trauma. A full bladder prior to transfer helps straighten out the angle between the uterus and cervix. The cervix and vagina are prepped to decrease blood, mucus, or bacteria from entering the uterus or catheter tip as these contaminants may impede implantation. Using abdominal ultrasound guidance, embryos are deposited between 1 and 1.5 cm from the fundus without actually contacting it. Touching the fundus during transfer may cause uterine contractions thereby increasing the intrauterine pressure and expelling the embryos through the cervix which reduce pregnancy rates. Ultrasound guidance facilitates embryo transfer and confirms that the embryos are placed correctly in the uterus. There appears to be a significant increase in implantation and pregnancy rates using ultrasound-guided embryo transfer. After transfer, the catheter is checked for any retained embryos.

2.6.7 *Oocyte donation*

Oocyte donation consists of oocyte retrieval from a donor female and oocyte fertilization with the sperm of the male partner of the recipient with subsequent embryo transfer to the female partner of the recipient couple. Oocyte donation can be offered to women with:

- premature ovarian failure,
- a history of surgical castration with a uterus,
- diminished ovarian reserve,
- a risk of transmitting a heritable disease to an offspring,
- menopause but are in good physical health and are of reasonable age.

Donor-recipient IVF cycles typically have the highest pregnancy rates among all ARTs and the number of donor-recipient cycles are increasing. In 2006, the CDC (Center for Disease Control) registry reported that 12.2% (16,978) of all ART cycle used donor oocytes.[33]

The success of donor recipient cycles is based on the tenet that the capacity to conceive is not based on uterine aging but on the quality of the oocyte.[34] Younger donors have higher implantation and pregnancy rates when compared to older donors, with a decreased incidence of pregnancy loss. There does not appear to be a decrease in cumulative pregnancy rates as endometrial receptivity does not appear to be altered by advancing maternal age or the etiology of the infertility of the recipient.

Oocyte donors can be known or remain anonymous. Donors must be screened prior to donation as outlined by the Food and Drug Administration regulations for tissue donors. They should also be screened according to the American Society for Reproductive Medicine's guidelines for gamete and embryo donation.[35] These guidelines and regulations are specific in their requirements for screening, testing and the timing of testing, depending on the type of donation and sex of the donor. Psychological assessment by a qualified mental health professional is required. There are potential psychological risks that donors undertake. With appropriate pretreatment screening, these can hopefully be minimized and few donors will have feelings of ambivalence or regret after donation. This is important with both known and anonymous donation. In anonymous donation, once prospective donors complete initial evaluation, they are matched with potential recipients based on both physical and personal characteristics. Donors should be between the ages of 21 and 34 years.

Oocyte donation is not without risks to the donor. Donors are often concerned about the risk of ovulation-inducing drugs and ovarian cancer, although the aggregate of studies does not support any association. With COH, the risk of OHSS is always present because these women receive hCG. Most programs strive to use low dose protocols to stimulate donors understanding that these women are not infertile, attempting to avoid hyperstimulation and retrieval associated complications, such as anesthesia complications, pelvic infection, and intraperitoneal hemorrhage, which are possible, though very rare.

Prior to starting a donor-recipient cycle, recipients have a precycle evaluation that includes an evaluation of the uterine cavity by sonohysterography or office hysteroscopy. If an intracavitary lesion or a hydrosalpinx is noted, surgical removal is conducted prior to embryo transfer.

Recipients over 45 years of age are at an increased risk for obstetrical complication, including gestational diabetes mellitus, hypertensive disorders, Cesarean delivery, intrauterine growth restriction, abruptio placentae, and preterm labor. These patients are referred to maternal-fetal medicine specialist for consultation prior to and after conception with IVF. Since there is an increasing risk of adverse pregnancy outcomes with advanced maternal age, many centers do not perform donation for women over 50 years of age.

Patients with Turner syndrome are not considered good candidates for donor oocytes because fatal aortic dissection has been reported in pregnancies established by oocyte donation in these women. They are infertile due to gonadal dysgenesis, with natural pregnancies occurring in approximately 2% of these women, usually in patients with mosaicism (46XX, 45X).

2.6.8 *Donor oocyte recipient endometrial preparation*

Embryos are transferred into the recipient's uterus after exogenous endometrial preparation using sequential estrogen and progesterone. Some protocols use gonadotropin down-regulation if the recipient is still cycling. This hormonal manipulation primes the endometrium for embryo transfer by mimicking the natural menstrual cycle. Estrogen therapy is initiated, based on the date of anticipated embryo transfer. Transdermal estradiol patches (0.1 mg) or oral estrogen is usually used in increasing doses that mimic the progressively increasing estradiol levels in the follicular phase. The recipient will receive between two to three weeks of estrogen for endometrial preparation. Once the endometrial lining is ≥ 8 mm, the recipient is ready for the pharmacologic conversion to the luteal phase in coordination with the status of the oocyte donor. Both intramuscular and vaginal progesterone are usually administered with the majority of fresh embryos transferred on day 5. If pregnancy occurs, both estrogen and progesterone support are continued until the placental production of hormones becomes evident at about week 10–11 of gestation.

2.6.9 *Cryopreservation*

After COH and fresh embryo transfer, many stimulated IVF cycles will produce excess viable embryos which are available for cryopreservation. Cryopreserved or frozen embryos can be thawed and transferred back into the uterus, during a subsequent frozen embryo transfer cycle. This allows for higher overall pregnancy rates per attempted IVF cycle. Cryopreservation techniques attempt to minimize cell damage to embryos during the freezing and thawing process with the aid of cryoprotectants. Embryos can be cryopreserved either by a slow cooling method or a vitrification method. After they are frozen, they are stored in liquid nitrogen. Typically, cryopreservation results in an 80% survival rate after thawing frozen embryos. Patients should be extensively counseled prior to oocyte retrieval with regard to cryopreserving excess embryos.

Semen is cryopreserved in men who may not be able to produce a sample on the day of oocyte retrieval. Freezing and thawing sperm samples can decrease motility by 50%. This is usually not a problem when the original ejaculate sample contains a large number of sperm. In men with azoospermia, epididymal or testicular samples can be cryopreserved until the day of oocyte retrieval. On the day of oocyte retrieval, the semen sample(s) are thawed, the cryoprotectant removed, and ICSI is performed.

Oocyte freezing is being performed on an experimental basis throughout the world.[36,37] Although there have been over 900 live births reported with established programs reporting good outcomes, a successful and standard method for the cryopreservation of a cell containing such a large amount of cytoplasm has not yet been developed. The ability to harvest autographs of ovarian tissue and stimulate oocyte development from these autographs is present and ongoing research will hopefully one day benefit many different groups of patients.

2.6.10 *Frozen embryo transfer*

Patient preparation of the recipient endometrium prior to frozen embryo transfer is similar to that in the recipient for oocyte donation. The recipient will receive between two and three weeks of estrogen for endometrial preparation. Once the endometrial lining is ≥ 8 mm, intramuscular and vaginal progesterone is started for endometrial support.

The morning of "frozen embryo transfer", embryos are thawed and surviving embryos are again graded. Pregnancy rates for frozen embryo transfer have improved over the past 10 years. This is due to selection of better quality embryos for freezing. Many embryos are now cryopreserved on day 5 or 6 after retrieval. Since fewer embryos survive to day 5 and become blastocysts, these higher quality embryos reduce the number of poor quality embryos stored that might yield a poorer outcome. In 1996, the frozen embryo transfer pregnancy rate reported by the CDC was 16.7%. In 2006, the CDC reported a take home baby rate of 28.9%, showing a trend toward improvement over time.[33]

2.6.11 *Preimplantation genetic diagnosis*

Preimplantation genetic diagnosis (PGD) enables couples who are carriers of genetic diseases to test embryos *in vitro* for genetic abnormalities prior to embryo transfer and select the embryos free of the genetic error for transfer.[38] Traditionally, carrier couples have used chorionic villus sampling and amniocentesis, during the first and second trimesters respectively, to determine if they have a genetically abnormal fetus. The major disadvantage of these types of prenatal diagnosis is the need for second trimester pregnancy termination when genetically abnormal fetuses are detected. PGD provides couples the option to select genetically normal embryos for embryo transfer prior to implantation. It must be emphasized that the specific mutations must be known in the parents before PGD can be performed.

PGD involves performing a blastomere biopsy and then genetic testing to determine the genetic complement of the embryo. Genetic information can be removed either from oocytes or embryos, allowing for biopsy at three different stages — polar body analysis, 6- to 10-cell cleavage stage biopsy, and blastocyst stage biopsy. Cleavage stage biopsy is the most widely used technique (day 3). In order to biopsy a blastomere or polar body, a hole is made in the zona pellucida using micromanipulation instruments. Since these embryos are transferred back into the uterus on day 4 or 5, a genetic diagnosis can be determined within 48 hours. Polar body biopsy evaluates only maternal chromosomes and is not the method of choice performed by most centers offering PGD. Crossover recombination events between homologous chromosomes can create improper diagnoses of heterozygous genetic defects.

Cleavage stage biopsies are performed on one or two blastomeres of 6- to 10-cell stage embryos three days after insemination. When embryos are at the blastocyst stage, they contain up to 300 cells. This allows for more cells to be removed without a detrimental effect on the embryo and improve the chance of an accurate diagnosis. Cryopresevation of embryos biopsied at this stage is more difficult and may be necessary while awaiting a diagnosis. These cells are used for diagnosis with polymerase chain reaction (PCR) or fluorescent *in situ* hybridization (FISH). PCR amplifies fragments of DNA for specific single gene defects. DNA amplification requires careful monitoring to avoid the problems of accidental contamination and allele dropout (ADO) leading to an erroneous genetic diagnosis. ADO or preferential amplification occurs when one of two alleles amplifies preferentially over the other. This could lead to misdiagnosis in a heterozygous cell, the normal allele may be amplified over the abnormal allele and the embryo could be diagnosed as "normal", and then transferred. Fluorescent PCR has been shown to be 1000-fold more sensitive than conventional PCR.[39] It has improved single locus diagnosis by making it more accurate and decreasing the time to diagnosis, which is key in procedures requiring transfer of embryos within 24–48 hours. Multiplex PCR allows for the simultaneous amplification of more than one DNA fragment from the embryonic cell, which provides knowledge of the target gene, as well as parental polymorphisms, allowing for more accurate identification of the amplified DNA fragment, which makes diagnosis more accurate.

PGD has been applied to many single gene disorders including autosomal recessive, dominant, and X-linked diseases. Examples include cystic fibrosis, Tay-Sachs, spinal muscular dystrophy, Huntington disease, Marfan's syndrome, and Fragile X syndrome.

FISH can also be used for preimplantation diagnosis to examine chromosomes in embryos. FISH uses fluorochrome-labeled probes that hybridize to complementary DNA sequences. The fluorescence produced by the probes allows a color and number notation of these probes which aids in diagnosis. FISH is used in the diagnosis of aneuploidy in patients with male factor infertility and in women with advanced maternal age. Common aneuploidies occurring and screened for with FISH include defects in chromosomes 13, 16, 18, 21, 22, X, and Y. FISH is also the method used to diagnose chromosomal translocations.

Although PGD success rates are good, amniocentesis and chorionic villus sampling should still be recommended to patients who have undergone this procedure.

2.7 Risks of IVF

Couples who present for ART are usually healthy with no significant medical history. In the treatment of their infertility, they are asked to take significant risks. The two major complications of ART are OHSS and multiple gestations.[40] There has been a proposed association between ovulation-induction drugs and gynecologic cancers, although this is not supported by well-controlled retrospective trials. Prior to initiating an IVF cycle, the risks and benefits of ART should be discussed, and formal written consent is obtained after complete review of the risks and benefits including counseling patients concerning fetal reduction of high-order multiple pregnancies to decrease perinatal morbidity of infants and mother.

2.7.1 *OHSS*

OHSS (ovarian hyperstimulation syndrome) is a potentially life-threatening complication of gonadotropin-induced COH. Although the signs and symptoms of impending OHSS usually become evident during stimulation, this syndrome does not become fully manifested until after hCG administration and oocyte retrieval. Patients typically resolve the OHSS within 10 to 14 days after onset of their initial symptoms. The syndrome is prolonged if a triggering of hCG is followed by a supplemental dose of hCG or if the patient becomes pregnant and produces her own hCG.

Patients who develop OHSS complain of abdominal bloating and pain due to ovarian enlargement. The pathophysiology of OHSS includes increased capillary permeability with "third spacing" of protein-rich fluid. This can result in hemoconcentration and ascites with dramatic fluid accumulations in the abdomen, pleura, or pericardial spaces. Patients can develop nausea, vomiting, diarrhea, and a decrease in appetite if OHSS progresses. As significant amounts of "third spacing" ensure, we often see shortness of breath and decreased urine output. The precise pathophysiology of OHSS is still not completely understood, though vascular endothelial growth factor (VEGF), also known as "vascular permeability factor", has been implicated. It has been shown that follicular fluid from patients with OHSS produce VEGF in increased quantities which, in a dose-dependant manner, increase vascular permeability.

OHSS can be staged based on clinical signs and symptoms, ultrasound features, and laboratory findings and is used to help predict which women require hospitalization. Patients with mild OHSS present with abdominal discomfort, distention and pain, with ovaries enlarged up to 12 cm. Patients may have nausea, vomiting, or diarrhea. Moderate OHSS includes all the features of mild OHSS, but ultrasonographic evidence of ascites as well. Severe OHSS complicates less than 2% of stimulations. It includes features of mild and moderate OHSS, as well as clinical evidence of ascites or hydrothorax and difficulty breathing. In addition, severe OHSS patients are at risk for hemoconcentration, coagulation and electrolyte abnormalities, diminished renal perfusion and function, and even adult respiratory distress syndrome.

Risk factors for developing OHSS include young age, low body mass index, and elevated estradiol levels with an increased number of stimulated follicles during COH. In addition, women with a previous pregnancy complicated by a history of OHSS are at great risk of recurrence. If early manifestations of OHSS appear (i.e., abdominal pain, rapidly increasing estradiol levels [> 3000 pg/mL], and extensive follicular recruitment) preventive treatment strategies are employed. On rare occasions, when follicular development and estradiol levels are excessively high early in the stimulation protocol, all stimulation medications are stopped and the cycle cancelled. More often, gonadotropin dosages are adjusted so that estradiol levels increase more slowly, or "freeze all" the embryos rather than transfer them as fresh embryos. Alternatively, using a "coast" by withdrawing gonadotropins and withholding hCG until the estradiol level decreases often allows retrieval and transfer of fresh embryos.[41,42]

Once OHSS develops, a complete physical exam and ultrasound are performed including blood tests for sodium, potassium, creatinine, and hematocrit. On physical examination, patients often have abdominal distension and tenderness. Decreased breath sounds may be heard at the bases with pleural effusions. Ultrasound is performed to note the presence of ascites and ovarian size. Patients with OHSS can develop hyponatremia, hemoconcentration, hyperkalemia and even decreased renal perfusion. These patients are monitored as outpatients daily until the condition improves significantly. Patients are instructed to weigh and measure their abdominal girth daily, drink eight glasses of a high sodium drink, and maintain a high protein diet. In addition, they monitor their urine output, and are instructed to report any changes. An increase in abdominal pain or girth, nausea, vomiting, or decreased appetite necessitates a prompt phone call to the healthcare provider and an office visit.

2.7.2 *Multiple pregnancy*

Multiple pregnancies occur with a higher frequency in pregnancies resulting from ART versus spontaneous conception. Since there is a low implantation rate per embryo (10–25%) with IVF, more than one embryo is often placed into the uterus. The goal is to minimize the number of multiple pregnancies while maintaining good pregnancy rates.

Multifetal gestations confer significant morbidity and mortality to both the mother and fetuses because of a high rate of prematurity and *in utero* mortality.[43,44] Maternal risks include preterm labor, placental abruption, placenta previa, Cesarean section, postpartum hemorrhage, gestational diabetes, and preeclampsia.

According to the US Department of Health/Centers for Disease Control and Prevention's 2006 National Summary and Fertility Clinic Reports, a total of 138,198 ART procedures resulted in 41,343 live-birth deliveries and 54,656 infants.[33] Treatment resulted in 44% transfer procedures. Thirty-seven percent of all ART births using fresh non-donor oocytes were multiple births (84% twins and 16% triplets and higher). Fresh embryos from donor eggs result in 54% live births. Risk of multiple-fetus pregnancy and multiple-infant live birth from ART cycles using fresh embryos from donor eggs in 2006 is shown in Fig. 2.1. Less than 3% of births in the general population are multiples.

Patients under 34 years of age with a history of a full-term pregnancy and no history of female infertility have the highest implantation rates

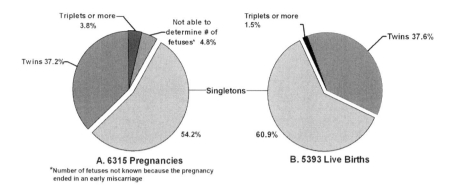

Fig. 2.1. The risk of a multiple-fetus pregnancy (A) and multiple-infant live birth (B) from ART cycles using fresh embryos from donor eggs in 2006. (Modified from Ref. 33.)

with IVF. This includes women with previous tubal ligation, normal ovarian reserve, donor oocyte recipients, and couples with male factor infertility. In contrast, women older than 34 years of age with no pregnancies and extended history of infertility have lower implantation rates. Quite often these patients have a history of poor ovarian reserve and previous failed IVF cycles.

During the initial IVF consultation, IVF success rates and patient's infertility history is reviewed. Based on this information, the number of embryos to be transferred and the number of embryos a couple is willing to accept is defined. The goal is that each patient will preferably have one excellent blastocyst or two good quality embryos replaced, adjusting (up or down) the number of embryos according to embryo quality and each patient's infertility history.

Multifetal pregnancy reduction should be discussed as an option for couples with high-order multiple pregnancy. The aim is to reduce preterm deliveries by decreasing the number of fetuses a woman carries. Besides being an invasive procedure, pregnancy reduction, either transabdominal or transvaginal, risks the loss of the entire pregnancy. In experienced centers, pregnancy loss after transabdominal fetal reduction occurs in 6% to 8% of these pregnancies. However, data suggest that pregnancies reduced to twins proceed as if the fetuses were naturally conceived as twins.

There is a psychological toll on couples who are making decisions regarding multifetal reduction, especially in women who have experienced difficulty becoming pregnant. If fetal reduction is not acceptable to a patient under 40, the decision is based on embryo quality, favorable versus unfavorable, age of embryos 2–3 day versus 5–6 day and patient age. There is evidence of a difference in pregnancy rates between early cleavage embryo transfer (day 2–3; 29.4%) versus blastocyst (day 5–6; 36%) in good prognosis patients.

A significant difference in pregnancy and live-birth rates in favor of blastocyst transfer in good prognosis patients, with high numbers of eight-cell embryos on day 3, is the most favorable group. In selected patients, blastocyst culture may be applicable for single embryo transfer. However, failure to transfer any embryos per couple is significantly higher in day 5–6 embryos versus day 2–3.[45]

High-order multiple pregnancies (triplets and higher) can no longer be viewed as an acceptable risk of IVF and transferring two embryos at most will decrease the risk. Proponents of two-embryo transfers argue that pregnancy rates in large series are equivalent when compared to three-embryo transfers. Multiple pregnancy rates in patients 30 to 35 years of age are significantly increased from approximately 29% when two embryos are transferred to 40% with the transfer of three embryos. However, the twin birth rate with transfers of two and three embryos is 26% and 29%, respectively. Thus, a decrease in embryos transferred from three to two decreases the incidence of high-order pregnancies, but does not reduce the twining rate.

2.7.3 *ART and major birth defects*

More than 1% of US births occur following use of ART. Reefhuis *et al.*[46] analyzed data from the National Birth Defects Prevention Study of infants delivered during the period from 1997–2003. Among singleton births, ART was associated with higher incidence of septal heart defects, cleft lip with or without cleft palate, esophageal atresia and anorectal atresia. However, no such association was seen among multiple births. Other studies have also documented small but increased incidence of birth defects among children born after assisted fertilization.[47–49]

Couples considering ART should be informed of all potential risks and benefits.

2.8 Success Rates

The Fertility Clinic Success and Certification Act of 1992 required all clinics performing ARTs in the US to annually report their success rates to the CDC. The CDC compiles these data and publishes a yearly report which is available on the CDC website. The first year this clinical data became available for review was 1995. There is a three-year lag between the time clinics report to the CDC and the time that these reports are available to the public, which reflects the time for the last delivery in a calendar year and the subsequent time needed to compile and publish the data.

Each clinic reports on their "pregnancy success rates" based on the type of cycle performed (fresh embryos from non-donor eggs, frozen embryos from non-donor eggs, and donor eggs) as well as the age of the women (< 35, 35–37, 38–40, and > 40.) The number of ART cycles in the US has increased as well as success rates. In 1995, 45,906 fresh non-donor IVF cycles were performed as compared to 99,199 in 2006 (Fig. 2.2). Rate of pregnancy and live birth for various procedures in 2006 is shown in Fig. 2.3. In 1996, the overall success rate for live births for each cycle

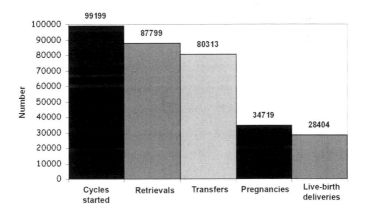

Fig. 2.2. Outcome of ART cycles in 2006 for fresh non-donor eggs or embryos. (Modified from Ref. 33.)

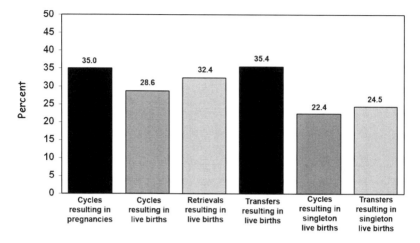

Fig. 2.3.   Live birth rates for ART using fresh non-donor eggs or embryos in 2006 using different measures. (Modified from Ref. 33.)

started was reported to be 28.1% using fresh non-donor embryos and 27.8% in patients who used fresh non-donor embryos which required the ICSI procedure. In 2006, the reported success rates for the same procedures respectively were 37.2% and 34.2% for ICSI embryos. Success rates vary with patient age in patients using their own oocytes, decreasing with increasing age. It is difficult to directly compare the success rates between individual ART programs as they may treat different populations of infertile patients and may focus on specific infertility factors.

References

1. Gardner DK, Weissman A, Howles CM, Shoham Z. (2004) *Textbook of Assisted Reproductive Techniques, Laboratory and Clinical Perspectives.* Informa HealthCare, London.
2. Broekmans FJ, Soules MR, Fauser BC. (2009) Ovarian Aging: mechanisms and clinical consequences. *Endocrine Rev* 30(5): 465–493.
3. Maheshwari A, Gibreel A, Bhattacharya S, Johnson NP. (2008) Dynamic tests of ovarian reserve: a systematic review of diagnostic accuracy. *Fertil Steril* 90(3): 737–743.
4. Reindollar RH, Regan MM, Neurmann PJ, Levine BS, Thornton KL, Alper MM, Goldman MB. (2010) A randomized clinical trial to evaluate optimal

treatment for unexplained infertility: the fast track and standard treatment (FASTT) trial. *Fertil Steril* 94(3): 888–899.

5. Klipstein S, Regan M, Ryley DA, Goldman MB, Alper MM, Reindollar RH. (2005) One last chance for pregnancy: a review of 2,705 *in vitro* fertilization cycles initiated in women age 40 years and above. *Fertil Steril* 84(2): 435–445.

6. Kwee J, Schats R, McDonnell J, Themmen A, de Jong F, Lambalk C. (2008) Evaluation of anti-Müllerian hormone as a test for the prediction of ovarian reserve. *Fertil Steril* 90(3): 737–743.

7. Broer SL, Mol BWJ, Hendriks D, Brockmans Frank JM. (2009) The role of antimullerian hormone in prediction of outcome after IVF: comparison with the antral follicle count. *Fertil Steril* 91(3): 705–714.

8. Strandell A, Lindhard A, Waldenström U, Thorburn J. (2001) Hydrosalpinx and IVF outcome: cumulative results after salpingectomy in a randomized controlled trial. *Hum Repro* 16(11): 2403–2410.

9. Daftary GS, Kayisli U, Seli E, Bukulmez O, Arici A, Taylor HS. (2007) Salpingectomy increases peri-implantation endometrial HOXA10 expression in women with hydrosalpinx. *Fertil Steril* 87(2): 367–372.

10. Disteche C. (2002) Y chromosome infertility: Y chromosome-related azoospermia. *Gene Rev.* Mar 2007.

11. Sadeghi-Nejad H, Oates R. (2008) The Y chromosome and male infertility *Curr Opin Urol* 18: 628–632.

12. Bhasin S. (2007) Approach to the infertile man. *JCEM* 92(6): 1995–2004.

13. Medveczky E, Puhó E, Czeizel EA. (2004) The use of drugs in mothers of offspring with neural-tube defects. *Pharmacoepidemiol Drug Saf* 13(7): 443–455.

14. Wu YW, Croen LA, Henning L, Najjar DV, Schembri M, Croughan MS. (2006) Potential association between infertility and spinal neural tube defects in offspring. *Birth Defects Res A Clin Mol Teratol* 76(10): 718–722.

15. Sørensen HT, Pedersen L, Skriver MV, Nørgaard M, Nørgård B, Hatch EE. (2005) Use of clomifene during early pregnancy and risk of hypospadias: population based case-control study. *BMJ* 330(7483): 126–127.

16. Meijer WM, de Jong-Van den Berg LT, van den Berg MD, Verheij JB, de Walle HE. (2006) Clomiphene and hypospadias on a detailed level: signal or chance? *Birth Defects Res A Clin Mol Teratol* 76(4): 249–252.

17. Mitwally MF, Casper RF. (2003) Aromatase inhibitors for the treatment of infertility. *Expert Opin Investig Drugs* 12(3): 353–371.
18. Elizur SE, Tulandi T. (2008) Drugs in infertility and fetal safety. *Fertil Steril* 89(6): 1595–1602.
19. Forman R, Gill S, Moretti M, Tulandi T, Koren G, Casper R. (2007) Fetal safety of letrozole and clomiphene citrate for ovulation induction. *J Obstet Gynaecol Can* 29(8): 668–671.
20. Al-Inany HG, Abou-Setta AM, Aboulghar M. (2006) Gonadotrophin-releasing hormone antagonists for assisted conception. *Cochrane Database Syst Rev* 3: CD001750.
21. Legro R, Branhart H, Schlaff W, Carr B, Diamond M, Carson S, Steinkampf M, Coutifaris C, McGovern P, Cataldo N, Gosman G, Nestler J, Giudice L, Leppert P, Myers E. (2007) Clomiphene, metformin, or both for infertility in the polycystic ovary syndrome. *N Engl J Med* 356: 551–566.
22. Tso LO, Costello MF, Albuquerque LE, Andriolo, RB, Freitas V. (2009) Metformin treatment before and during IVF or ICSI in women with polycystic ovary syndrome. *Cochrane Database Syst Rev* 2: CD006105.
23. Stadtmauer LA, Toma SK, Riehl RM, *et al.* (2001) Metformin treatment of patients with polycystic ovary syndrome undergoing *in vitro* fertilization improves outcomes and is associated with modulation of the insulin-like growth factors. *Fertil Steril* 75: 505–509.
24. Olivennes F, Belaisch-Allart J, Emperaire JC, *et al.* (2000) Prospective, randomized, controlled study of *in vitro* fertilization-embryo transfer with a single dose of leuteinizing hormone-releasing hormone (LH-RH) antagonist (cetrorelix) or a depot formula of an LH-RH agonist (triptorelin). *Fertil Steril* 73: 314–320.
25. Soliman S, Daya S, Collins J, *et al.* (1994) The role of luteal phase support in infertility treatment: meta-analysis of randomized trials. *Fertil Steril* 61: 1068–1076.
26. Sohn SH, Penzias AS, Emmi AM, Dubey AK, Layman LC, Reindollar RH, DeCherney AH. (1999) Administration of progesterone before oocyte retrieval negatively affects the implantation rate. *Fertil Steril* 71(1): 11–14.
27. American Society for Reproductive Medicine: A Practice Committee Report. (2000) A Committee Opinion. Does intracytoplasmic sperm injection ICSI carry inherent genetic risks? Nov. 2000.

28. Buckett WM, Tan SL. (2005) Congenital abnormalities in children born after assisted reproductive techniques: how much is associated with the presence of infertility and how much with its treatment? *Fertil Steril* 84(5): 1318–1319.

29. Das S, Blake D, Farquhar C, Seif MM. (2009) Assisted hatching on assisted conception (IVF and ICSI). *Cochrane Database Syst Rev* 15(2): CD001894.

30. American Society for Reproductive Medicine: A Practice Committee Report. A Committee Opinion. (2000) The role of assisted hatching in IVF: A review of the literature. Aug. 2000.

31. Blake DA, Farquhar CM, Johnson N, Proctor M. (2007) Cleavage state versus blastocyst stage embryo transfer in assisted conception. *Chochrane Database Syst Rev* (4): CD002118.

32. American Society for Reproductive Medicine: A Practice Committee Report. A Committee Opinion. (1999) Guidelines on number of embryos transferred. Nov. 1999.

33. Centers for Disease Control and Prevention, American Society for Reproductive Medicine, Society for Assisted Reproductive Technology. (2008) 2006 Assisted Reproductive Technology Success Rates: National Summary and Fertility Clinic Reports, Atlanta: US Department of Health and Human Services, Centers for Disease Control and Prevention.

34. Navot D, Drew MR, Bergh PA, *et al.* (1994) Age-related decline in female fertility is not due to diminished capacity of the uterus to sustain embryo implantation. *Fertil Steril* 61: 97–101.

35. American Society for Reproductive Medicine. (2002) Guidelines for gamete and embryo donation. *Fertil Steril* 5(77): 1S–18S.

36. Cao Y, Xing Q, Zhang ZG, Wei ZL, Zhou P, Cong L. (2009) Cryo-preservation of immature and *in vitro* matured human oocytes by vitrification. *Reprod Biomed Online* 19(3): 369–373.

37. Fadini R, Brambillasca F, Renzini MM, Merola M, Comi R, De Ponti E, Dal Canto MB. (2009) Human oocyte cryopreservation: comparison between slow and ultrarapid methods. *Reprod Biomed Online* 19(2): 171–180.

38. Findlay I, Quirke P, Hall J, Rutherford A. (1996) Fluorescent PCR a new technique for PCG of sex and single-gene defects. *J Assist Genet* 13: 96–103.

39. Braude P, Pickering S, Flinter F, Ogilvie C. (2002) Preimplantation genetic diagnosis. *Nat Rev Genet* 3: 941–953.

40. Basatemur E, Sutcliffe A. Follow-up of children born after ART. (2008) *Placenta* 29: S125–S140.

41. Benadiva CA, Davis O, Kligman I, *et al*. (1997) Withholding gonadotropin administration is an effective alternative for the prevention of ovarian hyperstimulation syndrome. *Fertil Steril* 67: 724–727.

42. D'Angelo A, Amso NN. (2007) Embryo freezing for preventing ovarian hyperstimulation syndrome. *Cochrane Database Syst Rev* 3: CD002806.

43. Makhseed M, Al-Sharhan M, Egbase P, Al-Essa M, Grudzinskas JG. (1998) Maternal and perinatal outcomes of multiple pregnancy following IVF-ET. *Int J Gynecol Obstet* 61: 155–163.

44. Halliday J. (2007) Outcomes of IVF conceptions: are they different? *Obstet Gynaecol* 21(1): 67–81.

45. Sunderam S, Chang J, Flowers L, Kulkarni A, Sentelle G, Jeng G, Macaluso M. (2009) Assisted reproductive technology surveillance — United States, 2006. *MMWR Surveill Summ* 58(5): 1–25; PMID: 9521336.

46. Reefhuis J, Honein MA, Schieve LA, Correa A, Hobbs CA, Rasmussen SA. (2009) Assisted reproductive technology and major structural birth defects in the United States. *Hum Repro* 24(2): 360–366.

47. Klemetti R, Gissler M, Sevón T, Koivurova S, Ritvanen A, Hemminki E. (2005) Children born after assisted fertilization have an increased rate of major congenital anomalies. *Fertil Steril* 84(5): 1300–1307.

48. Hansen M, Bower C, Milne E, de Klerk N, Kurinczuk JJ. (2005) Assisted reproductive technologies and the risk of birth defects — a systematic review. *Hum Reprod* 20(2): 328–338.

49. Olson CK, Keppler-Noreuil KM, Romitti PA, Budelier WT, Ryan G, Sparks AET, Van Voorhis BJ. (2005) *In vitro* fertilization is associated with an increase in major birth defects. *Fertil Steril* 84(5): 1388–1076.

Chapter 3

Advances in Fetal Diagnostics for Genomic Alterations

Katherine B. Geiersbach*,‡ and Sarah T. South*,†,‡

3.1 Origin of Genomic Imbalances

Genomic imbalances are a significant source of prenatal and perinatal morbidity and mortality. Between 20% and 60% of first-trimester spontaneous aborted fetuses have chromosomal abnormalities, but only 0.65–0.84% of liveborn infants have major chromosomal abnormalities, due to the high morbidity of most genomic imbalances.[1] The majority of genomic imbalances in the fetus are due to malsegregation of chromosomes during maternal gametogenesis, resulting in aneuploidy (gain or loss of a chromosome). Primary oocytes are generated in the female fetus and are suspended in meiosis I until ovulation, a period which ranges up to 50 years. During this period, there is a cumulative risk for disturbances in meiotic cell division that increases with maternal age. It is thought that the prolonged duration of the first meiotic division also predisposes the female gamete to nondisjunction events in meiosis II. In contrast to autosomal trisomies (gains of chromosomes 1–22) and trisomy X, other sex chromosome imbalances and structural abnormalities are just as likely or more likely to originate in paternal meiosis.

*Department of Pathology, University of Utah.
†Department of Pediatrics, University of Utah.
‡ARUP Laboratories Inc., University of Utah.

The most frequently observed chromosomal abnormalities in the first trimester pregnancy loss are autosomal trisomies, triploidy, and monosomy X (associated with Turner syndrome). Only a small subset of chromosomal disorders are viable. The most frequently observed genomic disorders in newborns are sex chromosome aneuploidy, trisomies for chromosomes 21, 18 and 13, and balanced chromosomal rearrangements.

3.2 Prenatal Screening

3.2.1 *Serum biomarkers and ultrasound screening*

Noninvasive screening by ultrasound and measurement of maternal serum analytes has been a standard of prenatal care since the 1990s. In addition to detecting abnormalities due to the common trisomies, fetal ultrasound can detect fetal abnormalities due to other causes. Screening is aimed at identifying high risk pregnancies in order to reduce the number of women requiring invasive testing. In prenatal screening for Down syndrome, a risk level of about one in 300 or higher is usually accepted as an indication for invasive diagnostic testing. This number is roughly equivalent to the risk of fetal loss due to amniocentesis. The false positive rate of prenatal screening is necessarily high to ensure detection of most affected pregnancies. Therefore, the majority of invasive diagnostic tests performed for an indication of increased risk for Down syndrome will have normal results.

The sensitivity and specificity of maternal serum screening is critically dependent upon the precise determination of gestational age. Ultrasound measurements of biparietal diameter and crown-rump length provide the most reliable estimate for gestational age. Laboratories establish their own median values for each analyte to control for geographic differences and variations in laboratory methods and reagents. Laboratory results are expressed as multiples of the median (MoM) for each analyte, and combined into a final risk estimate for Down syndrome based on the age-adjusted risk for aneuploidy. For integrated and contingent screening methods, risk assessment requires the use of specialized software.

Four maternal serum analytes are commonly used as Down syndrome markers in the second trimester. Alpha fetoprotein (AFP) is produced by the fetal yolk sac and later in gestation by the fetal liver and gastrointestinal tract. Maternal serum AFP has been used for the detection of open neural tube defects (ONTD) since the 1970s, and has since become a valuable marker for Down syndrome as well. Another marker for fetal Down syndrome is hCG, a hormone produced by trophoblastic cells that form the placenta. This hormone is detectable in maternal serum within days of conception. Its levels increase rapidly and then fall by the end of the first trimester, reaching a plateau later in pregnancy. Unconjugated estriol, uE3, is produced by the fetal liver from the steroid precursor, DHEA-S, and is also produced by the mother. Dimeric inhibin A (DIA) is secreted by the placenta during pregnancy and acts to inhibit the production of follicle stimulating hormone (FSH) by the maternal pituitary gland. Down syndrome is characterized by low AFP, low uE3, high hCG, and high DIA in the maternal serum. While levels of these analytes can be abnormal for many other reasons, the four together (known as quadruple screening) provide sensitive detection of Down syndrome in the second trimester.

Early screening for Down syndrome became possible after the addition of a fifth analyte, pregnancy associated plasma protein A (PAPP-A). PAPP-A is a metalloproteinase enzyme produced by the fetus and maternal endometrium during pregnancy, and reduced levels at 10–13 weeks gestation are associated with Down syndrome. In addition, nuchal translucency (NT) measurement by ultrasound between 11 and 14 weeks gestation allowed for substantial improvement in the first trimester screening, such that detection rates were improved over second trimester screening.[2] Three markers, PAPP-A, total hCG, and NT, have since become components of combined screening. First trimester screening allows for early diagnosis and intervention, and is desirable for many.

More recent studies have focused on maximizing sensitivity and limiting the percentage of false positive screening results by combining first and second trimester screening tests. Integrated screening was the first method for providing a risk estimate for Down syndrome based on the results of both first and trimester screening tests.[3] Serum integrated screening is based upon maternal serum screening alone. Full integrated screening combines maternal serum screening with ultrasound measurement of NT. While integrated screening has a high detection rate and low false positive rate, it delays the reporting of a risk estimate until the second trimester. In sequential screening, a provisional risk estimate is reported in the first trimester, followed by a fully integrated risk estimate in the second trimester. Stepwise sequential screening, in which a provisional risk estimate in the first trimester is integrated with a second trimester risk estimate, is superior to independent first and second trimester screening.

The FASTER trial, published in 2005, compared the performance of first and second trimester screening on 38,167 pregnant women at multiple centers in the US.[4] This study demonstrated the equivalent performance of first trimester combined screening and second trimester quadruple screening. The SURUSS trial, conducted in the UK several years earlier, also supported these findings.[5] The FASTER trial data were subsequently used to demonstrate that second trimester screening was unnecessary when risk for Down syndrome is sufficiently low on first trimester screening.[6] This approach, known as contingent screening, decreases the overall number of screening tests performed, but may be logistically difficult for some centers to adopt.

While early screening is desirable for many, measurement of AFP in the second trimester is still necessary to detect open neural tube defects (open spina bifida and anencephaly). Elevation of maternal serum AFP occurs when the neural tube fails to close and fetal proteins leak into the amniotic fluid and maternal circulation. Neural tube defects are multi-factorial. Risk factors include maternal exposure to anticonvulsant medications, inadequate folate intake, and genetic factors. Confirmatory testing requires fetal ultrasound and measurement of AFP and acetylcholinesterase (AChE) levels in amniotic fluid.

The markers used for Down syndrome screening are also abnormal in pregnancies with trisomy 18. Using integrated screening, 90% of pregnancies with trisomy 18 can be detected at a false positive rate of only 0.1%.[7]

In the past, diagnostic testing by amniocentesis or chorionic villus sampling was offered primarily to women aged 35 or older. While advanced maternal age is a key risk factor for Down syndrome, about half of Down syndrome babies are born to mothers under the age of 35, based on recent data.[8] Due to the wide availability of prenatal testing, American College of Obstetrics and Gynecology (ACOG) recommended in 2007 that all women should be offered screening and invasive diagnostic testing for aneuploidy.[9] While universal access to prenatal testing holds great promise for detecting genomic abnormalities in the prenatal period, socioeconomic barriers to basic prenatal care are prevalent in some areas. These factors are associated with late initiation of prenatal care or in some cases lack of prenatal care.

Current Screening Panels for the Detection of Fetal Down Syndrome[4,6]

Panel	Analytes	Trimester	Detection rate at 5% screen positive rate	Screen positive rate at 85% detection rate
Quad	AFP, hCG, uE3, DIA	2nd	81%	7%
First Trimester Combined	PAPP-A, hCG, NT	1st	82–87%	6%
Serum Integrated	PAPP-A + Quad	1st and 2nd	85–88%	3%
Full Integrated	PAPP-A, NT + Quad	1st and 2nd	94–96%	1%
Stepwise Sequential	Combined + Quad	1st and 2nd	95%	2%
Contingent	Combined ± Quad	1st	88–94%	1%

Screen positive is defined as a risk of one in 300 or greater.

3.2.2 *Carrier screening*

Screening couples for population-specific genetic diseases is a relatively recent development in prenatal care. In 2001, the American College of Medical Genetics (ACMG) and ACOG recommended offering cystic fibrosis carrier screening for 25 common mutations to Caucasian and

Ashkenazi Jewish couples.[10] Carrier screening of Ashkenazi Jewish couples for eight additional genetic disorders has also been jointly recommended by the ACMG and ACOG.[11] These tests are ideally performed before conception to allow time for genetic counseling and consideration of reproductive options. However, carrier screening can also be performed during pregnancy.

3.2.3 *Maternal serum screening of circulating fetal nucleic acids*

First trimester fetal gender determination by maternal serum testing for the presence of Y chromosome DNA is one method for managing pregnancies in carriers of X-linked genetic disorders; however, this method is highly sensitive and therefore subject to false positive results. A new development is the discovery of small cell-free fragments of fetally derived nucleic acids in the maternal circulation. Whereas cells from the fetus can remain in the maternal circulation for years, cell free fetal (cff) nucleic acids clear quite rapidly from the maternal circulation after delivery. Cff nucleic acids are remarkably stable, making it feasible to isolate this fraction in the laboratory for testing. Direct detection of fetal trisomy by quantitation of cff nucleic acids is now possible. For DNA testing, it is necessary to enrich for the small proportion of circulating DNA derived from the fetus. Since fetal DNA is highly fragmented (100–300 base pairs), the sample can be enriched for fetal DNA by size fractionation. Aneuploidy detection involves a comparison of DNA levels between chromosomes (relative chromosome dosage) or determination of heterozygous allele ratios at polymorphic loci. Single nucleotide polymorphisms (SNPs) or DNA microsatellites are used for the latter method. RNA based testing does not require enrichment as RNA transcripts specific to the fetus can be selected for analysis; however, RNA is more subject to degradation. Larger studies will be necessary to determine the sensitivity of noninvasive screening methods in comparison to CVS and amniocentesis. For the immediate future, fetal nucleic acid testing will be viewed as an alternate screening method, rather than a diagnostic method. Clinical trials are ongoing to determine the sensitivity and specificity of fetal nucleic acid testing, and if this method performs comparably to maternal serum screening it may become clinically available within a few years.

3.3 Prenatal Diagnostic Testing

3.3.1 *Amniotic fluid*

Amniocentesis involves withdrawal of fluid from the amniotic sac under ultrasound guidance. This method has been used to obtain fetal cells for chromosome analysis since the 1960s. With the development of chromosome banding in the early 1970s, genomic imbalances and rearrangements involving five to 10 million base pairs (5–10 megabases, Mb) of DNA or more could be routinely detected. The optimal period for the retrieval of a sufficient volume of viable cells from amniotic fluid is between 16 and 20 weeks gestation. However, cytogenetic analysis is usually successful when amniocentesis is performed between 15 and 24 weeks gestation. Early amniocentesis (before 15 weeks) is an option if early diagnosis is desirable and chorionic villus sampling cannot be performed. Amniocentesis has been in use since the late 1960s and has low risk for fetal loss (about 0.5% over baseline). The sensitivity and specificity of cytogenetic analysis for detection of abnormalities larger than 5–10 Mb in amniotic fluid is over 99%.[12]

Amniotic fluid contains a mixture of fetal urothelial, gastrointestinal, respiratory, and amnionic epithelial cells, termed "amniocytes". The first aliquot of amniotic fluid may be contaminated with maternal cells and is therefore not used for cytogenetic analysis. Successful cytogenetic analysis of amniotic fluid also requires that the sample is pure, sterile and viable. Amniotic fluid is collected into sterile tubes and remains viable at ambient temperature (20°C to 25°C) for at least 48 hours. Amniotic fluid transported under refrigeration may retain viability. However, once frozen and thawed, the cells will no longer grow in culture. In the laboratory, cells from amniotic fluid are isolated into a pellet by ultracentrifugation, and the supernatant fluid is retained for biochemical testing, including reagent strip testing to identify specimens in which urine was inadvertently collected. Cultured amniocytes will grow as a monolayer in growth medium on the surface of a coverslip or flask. An adequate number of dividing cells can be obtained for chromosome analysis after one to two weeks in culture. During "harvest", the coverslips are treated to suspend dividing cells in metaphase and to spread the chromosomes for better visualization. The coverslips are fixed and stained, and metaphase cells are analyzed *in situ*. If the flask method is used, cells are first detached from the surface of the flask using trypsin and then re-suspended and fixed onto a slide for analysis.

Chromosome analysis is performed on at least 15 colonies if the *in situ* (coverslip) method is used, and on at least 20 metaphase cells if the flask method is used. Each colony on a coverslip represents one amniocyte that attached to the coverslip and divided repeatedly during the incubation period. Therefore, analysis of the best available metaphases from 15 separate colonies ensures that 15 cells from the primary specimen have been analyzed. At the 95% confidence interval, analysis of 15 cell colonies permits exclusion of mosaicism for an abnormal cell line of 20% or greater.[13] With examination of 24 additional colonies from multiple *in situ* cultures, mosaicism of 12% or higher can be excluded at a 95% confidence interval.[13]

Although the karyotype of a metaphase cell from amniotic fluid is assumed to represent the true fetal karyotype, there are a variety of possibilities when two or more karyotypes are observed. If there is a 46,XY population admixed with a 46,XX population, maternal cell contamination is a possibility, but twin gestation and fetal chimerism are also important diagnostic considerations, as the incidence of maternal cell contamination of amniotic fluid is quite low (about 1 in 200 cases).[12] In all other cases, the abnormal population could signify a mitotic error that occurred during fetal development (*in vivo*) or during culture in the laboratory (*in vitro*). True fetal mosaicism due to an *in vivo* mitotic error is thought to occur in 0.1% or fewer pregnancies. However, abnormal metaphase cells are encountered in about 1% of amniotic fluid specimens.[12] The abnormal cells may populate an entire colony or only a portion of one colony. The majority of these abnormalities, termed pseudomosaicism, are due to *in vitro* artifact. It is thought that the artificial growth conditions in culture permit random chromosomal abnormalities to occur in single cells.

Due to the possibility of true fetal mosaicism, additional metaphase cells are usually examined when an abnormal population is observed. The level of work up is dependent upon the chromosome involved. Gains of chromosomes 13, 18, or 21, and gains or losses of sex chromosomes are clearly associated with the possibility of a phenotypically abnormal off-spring in the mosaic or non-mosaic state. Trisomies 8 and 9 are also viable in the mosaic state. Mosaic trisomy for chromosomes 12 or 20 generally cannot be confirmed in blood, and the risk for abnormality in the fetus is relatively low. Additional investigation is also indicated when there is a single cell with an unbalanced structural rearrangement or marker chromosome.[14]

3.3.2 *Chorionic villus sampling*

Chorionic villus sampling (CVS), introduced in the 1980s, allows diagnosis of chromosomal disorders at 9–13 weeks gestation. In the first trimester, the volume of amniotic fluid is insufficient for amniocentesis, but a biopsy of chorionic villi can be obtained under ultrasound guidance. Chorionic villi are transported to the laboratory in sterile medium at ambient temperature. Once received, chorionic villi are cleaned under a dissecting microscope to eliminate contaminating maternal tissue. For long term culture, villi are treated with trypsin to enrich the specimen for mesenchymal cells from the villous core. After dissociation into single cells with collagenase treatment, the specimen is re-suspended in growth medium. The remainder of the procedure is the same as that for amniotic fluid specimens.

Pseudomosaicism and maternal cell contamination can be confounding factors in the cytogenetic analysis of CVS specimens. Another consideration is confined placental mosaicism (CPM), a situation in which the fetal karyotype and the placental karyotype differ. The abnormal cell population may be limited to trophoblasts, mesenchymal cells, or both lineages. While CPM is observed in 1–2% of pregnancies studied by "direct" (short term) culture methods, it is observed in only 0.6% of long term cultures.[12] Since mesenchymal cells of the villous core are most closely related to the embryonic cell line that forms the fetus, long term culture is preferred for accurate representation of the fetal karyotype. When mosaicism is detected, a follow-up study on amniotic fluid is performed to distinguish CPM from true fetal mosaicism.

One of the advantages of CVS over amniocentesis is that genomic imbalances can be detected earlier in pregnancy, when termination of pregnancy is associated with fewer complications. The sensitivity and success rate of CVS is close to that of amniocentesis, but the risk to the fetus is slightly higher. Overall, the fetal loss rate is about 0.8% over the baseline risk without the procedure.

3.3.3 *Fetal blood sampling*

Fetal blood sampling, also known as cordocentesis or percutaneous blood sampling (PUBS), entails needle puncture of a fetal vessel (usually an umbilical vein) under ultrasound guidance and aspiration of blood for genetic, biochemical, and/or hematologic analysis. This procedure is usually performed during the second trimester and is associated with a higher risk for fetal loss than either CVS or amniocentesis (2–5%). The processing time for a fetal blood sample is reduced (2–4 days), but because of the high complication rate, it is not a preferred method for prenatal diagnosis. Fetal blood sampling has been useful in the past when amniotic fluid culture was unsuccessful or to address possible fetal mosaicism. FISH technology allows evaluation of interphase cells in any prenatal specimen and has thus decreased the need for fetal blood sampling.

3.3.4 *Preimplantation genetic diagnosis*

Before implantation, a single cell can be removed from the 6–10-cell embryo for genetic analysis without adverse consequences to the remainder of the conceptus. The first and second polar bodies of the ovum can also be removed for analysis. Genetic analysis of a blastomere or polar body is known as preimplantation genetic diagnosis (PGD) and is used to select healthy embryos when there is a familial risk for a specific genetic condition. In addition to targeted mutation analysis by molecular techniques, fluorescence *in situ* hybridization (FISH) can be performed to detect common aneuploidies and to determine gender. After testing, normal embryos are transferred to the uterus.

3.3.5 *Targeted molecular diagnostic testing*

Molecular testing of amniotic fluid and chorionic villi is now available for a growing list of single gene disorders. Techniques used for postnatal testing of peripheral blood can be equally applied to prenatal specimens, along with testing for possible maternal contamination of the sample. Most genetic disorders are quite rare, and fetal testing is usually targeted to a known familial mutation. The list of single gene disorders continues to grow. Publicly funded websites such as GeneTests (www.genetests.org) are helpful references for available testing.

FISH analysis for specific microdeletion or microduplication syndromes can be performed as clinically indicated on metaphase spreads from amniotic fluid or chorionic villi. One such example is FISH for the 22q11.2 deletion as indicated for certain heart defects. FISH is also very useful to detect imbalanced chromosomal rearrangements resulting from a familial balanced rearrangement.

3.3.6 *Rapid aneuploidy detection technologies*

Trisomy 13, trisomy 18, trisomy 21, and sex chromosome aneuploidy account for 70–80% of clinically significant chromosome abnormalities identified in the newborn population.[15,16] The sensitivity and specificity for the detection of these common aneuploidies by a chromosome analysis of amniotic fluid or CVS material are greater than 99%. However, due to the requirement for culturing the sample in order to obtain metaphase chromosomes, one to two weeks pass between the time of sample acquisition and result. As detection of these common aneuploidies may alter pregnancy management, a more rapid detection for these common aneuploidies is desirable. Furthermore, a targeted detection for just these common aneuploidies is less costly than full chromosome analysis.

The first clinically available rapid aneuploidy detection method for trisomy 13, 18, 21, and sex chromosome aneuploidy utilized fluorescence *in situ* hybridization (FISH) technology with probes for chromosome 13, 18, 21, X and Y. This analysis is performed on uncultured amniocytes or chorionic villi and the result is available within one to two days of sample acquisition. The sensitivity and specificity of FISH for these common aneuploidies is at least 99%,[17] matching that of full chromosome analysis. However, it is standard practice in many countries including the US to perform a full chromosome analysis subsequent to the FISH analysis to both confirm the finding and to identify other large scale aberrations that would not be detected by these FISH probes. Furthermore, the American College of Medical Genetics recommends against therapeutic decisions based upon the result of aneuploidy FISH analysis alone.[18]

Quantitative fluorescence polymerase chain reaction (QF-PCR) is a newer method for detection of trisomy 13, 18, 21 and X/Y aneuploidy. This technique involves amplification of highly polymorphic short tandem repeats on the chromosomes of interest using fluorescently-labeled primers. The size and fluorescent intensity of the PCR products are analyzed to determine whether the sample is monoallelic, diallelic, or triallelic at these short tandem repeats. Results correlate with chromosome copy number. To increase confidence in the result, three to six short tandem repeats on each chromosome with a high level of heterozygosity are analyzed. QF-PCR kits are commercially available and in clinical use in many countries. Large studies indicate that the clinical sensitivity is at least as high as rapid FISH analysis on uncultured amniocytes for these chromosomes.[17,19,20] QF-PCR is less expensive than FISH analysis because the assay is more easily automated. Furthermore, QF-PCR can detect maternal cell contamination in both male and female fetuses, whereas maternal cell contamination by FISH can only be detected in the male fetuses.

Rapid analysis for the common aneuploidies can also be performed by multiplex ligation dependent probe amplification (MLPA). MLPA is another PCR based method with commercial kits available. Additional loci beyond the common chromosome aneuploidies can be assessed within a single reaction and large studies indicate MLPA is also highly effective at detecting the common aneuploidies.[21,22] Maternal cells and male triploidy (69,XXY) may also be detected. However, this assay will not detect female triploidy (69,XXX) which is easily detected by FISH and can also be detected by QF-PCR.

3.4 Prenatal Genomic Microarray

3.4.1 *Utility of a whole genome analysis at high resolution*

For over three decades, chromosome imbalances have been detected in the prenatal population through a standard G-banded chromosome analysis. This technology has been very useful for the detection of the most common viable chromosome rearrangements including trisomy 21, trisomy 13, trisomy 18 and the sex chromosome aneuploidies. Its ability to detect other chromosome rearrangements, however, is largely dependent upon both the size of the chromosome imbalance, the region of the genome that is affected, and the quality of the chromosome preparation as the banding pattern of the chromosomes must be altered. This requirement for a banding pattern alteration has led to a frequently reported resolution of a 5–10 megabase alteration for detection by chromosome analysis. However, this limit of resolution is not always reproducible, again due to location within the genome and quality of banding preparations.

Furthermore, this level of resolution will certainly not detect more subtle abnormalities such as microdeletion/microduplication syndromes which can be more often detected in the postnatal population due to a clinical phenotype suggestive of these syndromes. Therefore, there is interest in a higher resolution whole genome analysis in the prenatal population to allow for detection of these subtle chromosome imbalances that cannot be reliably detected by a standard chromosome study. Based on the incidence of the currently recognized microdeletion/microduplication syndromes and clinically consequential imbalances, it is predicted every one out of 300 to one out of 600 newborns would be affected with one of these conditions.[23] In contrast, the incidence of a poor prognosis chromosome abnormality that would be undetected by rapid aneuploidy detection for chromosomes 13, 18 and 21 is approximately one out of 1600 pregnancies.[23] Therefore, after ruling out a 13, 18 or 21 trisomy, there is significant interest in offering a whole genome screen that could identify both the poor prognosis chromosome abnormalities, plus the recurrent microdeletion/microduplication syndromes.

Genomic microarray technology has shown the promise of providing such a whole genome analysis, with the resolution afforded by fluorescence *in situ* hybridization (FISH) for the recurrent microdeletion/microduplication syndromes. Postnatal studies of individuals with mental retardation or developmental delay indicate at least a two- to three-fold increase in detection of clinically significant imbalances over a standard G-banded chromosome analysis.[24–27] Furthermore, although its resolution is similar to FISH, the design of the platform can allow for literally thousands of loci to be analyzed simultaneously, which precludes the necessity of a previous suspicion for a particular genomic region as is necessary with FISH.

3.4.2 *Technical components of a genomic microarray*

Genomic microarray involves the labeling of patient DNA, isolated from millions of cells from a tissue of interest, which is then hybridized to a slide on which has been spotted either oligonucleotides or cloned segments (both subsequently referred to as targets) of DNA representative of the human genome. The resolution of the array will depend upon the density of the targets within a genomic interval. These targets can be concentrated in gene-rich regions of the genome, or can be spaced at regular intervals throughout the genome to provide a more whole genome analysis, and many commercial platforms in use are a combination of increased density within genes as well as regular spacing of targets between genes.

The intensity of the hybridization of the labeled patient DNA is compared to either an *in silico* control or to a competitively hybridized differentially labeled control. If the patient has a deletion of the target DNA, then relatively less of that patient's DNA will hybridize as compared to the control, whereas duplication in the patient will result in increased hybridization compared to the control. Therefore, by comparing the amount of hybridization, genomic imbalances can be identified in the patient DNA. Balanced rearrangements will not be detected as there is no loss or gain of DNA. Imbalances within the patient's DNA that do not have targets on the array platform will also not be detected, and low level mosaicism may be undetected as it would result in a relatively reduced difference in hybridization between the patient and the control. However, as the vast majority of clinically significant chromosome rearrangements are imbalances that are either non-mosaic or high-level mosaic, genomic microarray affords a greatly enhanced detection rate for clinically significant imbalances.

3.4.3 *Challenges for interpretation*

Although genomic microarray has the ability to detect genomic copy number changes (small genomic imbalances) at a higher resolution than a standard chromosome analysis, copy number changes within or even involving many genes may not have a clinical consequence due to either redundancy within the genome, redundancy within metabolic pathways, or other compensatory mechanisms. Therefore, patients undergoing a prenatal analysis using genomic microarray technology need appropriate genetic counseling as copy number changes of unclear clinical significance will require additional follow-up. A standard algorithm for determining the clinical significance of a copy number change involves accessing the size of the imbalance, genetic content of the imbalance, comparison to cases either in the literature or within datasets of previously analyzed cases and parental studies to determine if the change is inherited or *de novo*.[28]

This concern over identification of a copy number change of unknown clinical significance has lead to many groups offering prenatal microarray to choose either different reporting criteria for a genomic aberration in the prenatal period versus the postnatal period (when the phenotype of the patient is more defined) and/or using a microarray platform that is more targeted to regions of the genome that are well understood in regards to their clinical consequence when unbalanced. The alteration in reporting criteria is often based upon an increased threshold in the size of the abnormality as the larger abnormalities are more likely to have included a haplosensitive or triplosensitive gene. Still, even with the increased size threshold, genomic microarray technology can still identify imbalances not visible by a standard chromosome study. In addition, many labs offering prenatal microarray analysis place a high emphasis on rapid availability of parental DNA so that an identified abnormality can be rapidly characterized as inherited or *de novo*, as an inherited alteration from a normal parent is also less likely to result in a clinical consequence in the fetus. A further complication to the identification of a copy number change is reduced penetrance and variable expressivity as has been demonstrated for numerous microdeletions/duplications associated with autism.[29–31] In these circumstances, parental studies may be useful for counseling for recurrent risk, but will be less useful in determining the consequence of a deletion in these regions for the current pregnancy.

Another consideration with prenatal microarray technology is the potential for the identification of adult onset conditions, such as detection of a deletion of the PMP22 gene which would be predicted to result in Hereditary Neuropathy with Liability to Pressure Palsies (HNPP), a condition that is characterized by recurrent sensory and motor neuropathy in a single nerve and first manifests in usually the second or third decade.[32] As there is little that can be done to prevent the condition, and the symptoms are generally mild and do not significantly impact quality of life, the identification of such condition in the prenatal period may have little value. However, a duplication of this same region is predicted to result in Charcot-Marie-Tooth neuropathy type 1 (CMT1), a demyelinating peripheral neuropathy characterized by distal muscle weakness and atrophy, sensory loss, and slow nerve conduction velocity that presents between age five and 25.[33] As this condition is generally more severe than HNPP, its detection in the prenatal period may be warranted. However, this condition does not affect intelligence or life span. Issues such as these concerning PMP22 and many other genes leads to concerns about whether or not microarray platforms used in the prenatal population should be blinded in regards to adult onset conditions without extensive pre-test genetic counseling.

3.4.4 *Review of published prospective studies*

A review of recently published literature on the experience of laboratories offering prenatal genomic microarray is of value, as it can highlight the benefits, as well as the extent of the limitations of this technology.

The first published study to prospectively analyze genomic microarray in the prenatal population used an array targeted for known microdeletion/microduplication syndromes with a relatively less dense whole genome backbone, and analyzed 56 amniotic fluid and 42 chorionic villus samples.[34] Traditional G-banded chromosome studies were also performed on all 98 cases. Clinically significant abnormalities were identified in five of the 98 cases, four cases with trisomy 21, and one case with an inherited unbalanced translocation. All five of these abnormalities were also visible by the cytogenetic analysis. Within these 98 cases, copy number changes known to be clinically benign were detected in 31 cases, whereas a copy number change of initial uncertain significance was detected in 12 cases. For these 12 cases, parental studies showed that nine of these 12 copy number changes were inherited leaving only three cases with uncertain clinical significance.

The first prospective study to analyze the prenatal population by microarray looking only for abnormalities that were not detected by a standard G-banded chromosome analysis was reported by Shaffer *et al.*[35] This study included 132 amniotic fluid samples and 19 chorionic villus samples. A clinically significant abnormality missed by the chromosome study was detected in two of the 151 cases. Copy number changes recognized as clinically benign were detected in 7.9% of the cases, and a copy number change of uncertain clinically significance in 0.7% of cases (1/151). The reduction in the category of copy number change of uncertain clinical significance identified in this study, as compared to the previous, the authors felt was due to additional experience that time had provided with using this technology as well as the application of this technology on tens of thousands of postnatal cases.

The largest published study to date analyzed 254 amniotic fluid and 53 chorionic villus samples.[36] Fifteen clearly clinically significant abnormalities were detected out of the 300 cases, indicating a detection rate of 5%, with two of these abnormalities not detected by the accompanying chromosome study. Four of these 15 cases had a small supernumerary marker chromosome identified by the chromosome analysis, in three of these four cases the marker was mosaic. Further characterization of the marker was achieved through the microarray analysis which allowed for determination of marker chromosome origin and genomic content. Copy number changes likely to be benign were detected in 13% of cases, and in 3% of cases a copy number change of uncertain clinical significance was detected. Therefore, looking at these perspective studies, it is clear that copy number changes of uncertain clinical significance are encountered but perhaps with a reduced frequency than of initial concern.

If the experience of these initial studies holds true, depending upon the design of the array platform, the knowledge gained from the use of genomic microarray in the larger postnatal population and the availability of parental samples, the category of copy number change of uncertain clinical significance will likely be currently around 1–3% and will decrease as our understanding of the genome increases. Although, if higher density platforms are utilized with less conservative reporting standards, the number of reported copy number changes of uncertain clinical significance could also increase.

3.4.5 *Clinical indications for a prenatal genomic microarray*

The ideal population for prenatal genomic microarray is also a topic of debate. The clinical indication most common for a standard chromosome study is advanced maternal age or an abnormal serum screen. With improved screening, the number of women undergoing an amniocentesis or CVS procedure will likely decrease. For those that undergo the procedure due to an increased risk for trisomy 13, 18, or 21, rapid aneuploidy detection using FISH, MLPA, or QF-PCR would resolve the identified concern.[23] Some may argue that since the invasive amniocentesis or CVS procedure has already been performed, a chromosome analysis should also be performed to identify any other chromosome defect. However, the risk of a non-trisomy, poor prognosis chromosome defect being identified by a standard chromosome analysis is estimated at 1:1600 whereas the possibility of identifying an abnormality of uncertain significance such as a mosaic finding or a small supernumerary marker is twice this prevalence.[23] With this reasoning, the UK National Screening Committee and the London Genetics Commissioners no longer require a standard chromosome analysis to follow a normal QF-PCR result in the absence of a more specific indication such as an abnormal ultrasound.[23]

The next logical argument may be that the amniotic fluid or CVS material remaining after a normal rapid aneuploidy test should be analyzed by genomic microarray as it will have an increased detection for a disability-causing imbalance.[23] As the possibility of detection of a copy number change of uncertain clinical significance remains, and the phenotype of the fetus is usually uncharacterized in these situations, a targeted array for well-characterized regions of the genome, coupled with pre- and post-test genetic counseling[37] is warranted for this situation. Furthermore, larger studies are needed to identify the true detection rate of disabling genomic imbalances in this relatively unscreened population with genomic microarray and the accompanying psychological and social impact of high-density whole genome analyses in the prenatal period.

Another common indication for a prenatal chromosome study is an abnormal ultrasound. It is possible that if genomic microarray is applied to this more targeted population, the detection of clinically significant genomic imbalances would increase. Still, determining which ultrasound findings may be the best indicators for a prenatal microarray is difficult as many of the currently understood microdeletion/microduplication syndromes seen in the postnatal population do not have specific prenatal ultrasound findings.

A third potential application for prenatal genomic microarray is further characterization of a chromosome abnormality detected by traditional chromosome analysis. The identified abnormalities may be either an apparently balanced translocation or inversion or a supernumerary marker chromosome of unknown origin.

Until recently, a *de novo* and apparently balanced translocation or inversion detected through a standard prenatal chromosome study was associated with a 6.7% risk of congenital anomaly.[38] This is slightly more than a two-fold increase above the general population risk. This increased risk is generally thought to be due to disruption of dosage sensitive genes or regulatory elements at the break-points. However, numerous studies examining apparently balanced translocations and inversions have shown that in 30–40% of these cases, there is an imbalance detectable by genomic microarray analysis with the imbalance occurring at either one of the breakpoints or as a cryptic imbalance elsewhere in the genome.[39–41] Therefore, it is likely that if a genomic microarray were performed subsequent to the identification of a *de novo* and apparently balanced rearrangement in a prenatal sample, this would allow for better characterization of the potential clinical consequence as the aberration could be more appropriately characterized as balanced or unbalanced.

De novo supernumerary marker chromosomes are also seen in approximately 1/2500 prenatal cases[38] and represent an additional challenge for interpretation. Due to their small size, it can be often difficult to determine the origin of these chromosomes. Yet without the determination of their origin and genetic content, the likelihood of a clinical consequence due to the marker is relatively unknown. However, these supernumerary marker chromosomes are often mosaic and the characterization of a mosaic finding by genomic microarray is limited based on the level of mosaicism in the tissue studied. Furthermore, the level of mosaicism may vary across different tissues, further complicating the prediction of the clinical consequence. Still, in the Van de Veyver *et al.* study,[36] three mosaic and one non-mosaic supernumerary marker chromosomes were successfully characterized by the genomic microarray platform utilized.

When considering the different options for detection of a genomic imbalance in the prenatal population, it is worth considering the indication for the analysis in each individual situation. It is currently common for a full chromosome analysis from either amniocytes or chorionic villi to be performed for indications such as advanced maternal age, an abnormal ultrasound, a family history of a chromosome imbalance, or an abnormal maternal serum screen showing an increased risk of trisomy 18 or 21, as well as parental anxiety. When the clinical indication is an increased risk for the common aneuploidies due to advanced maternal age or an abnormal serum screen, then a rapid aneuploidy test through FISH, QF-PCR or MLPA may be sufficient to rule out the identified concern. A full chromosome analysis subsequent to a normal FISH, QF-PCR or MLPA result may detect a clinically significant unbalanced chromosome abnormality, but this would likely be a rare event as there was no previous indication for such a finding.

For the indication of an abnormal ultrasound showing multiple structural malformations consistent with a chromosome imbalance, a genomic microarray analysis is likely to detect more clinically significant chromosome imbalances than either a standard chromosome analysis or any of the targeted rapid aneuploidy detection technologies. However, many of the microdeletion/microduplication syndromes identified in the postnatal population may not have any obvious ultrasound findings, or the findings may be transitory.

If the indication is family history of a previously identified chromosome abnormality, then a standard chromosome study should be sufficient, as it is clear that the aberration can be detected with this technology. If the clinical indication is parental anxiety, then careful genetic counseling should proceed any testing as the various technologies have different clinical utilities and sensitivities.

3.5 Conclusion

Genomic imbalances have been detected in prenatal specimens since the late 1960s. Recent advances in prenatal genomic diagnosis have included an improved detection rate for fetal aneuploidy using first and second trimester maternal serum screening and ultrasound, as well as rapid and sensitive detection of genomic imbalances by molecular diagnostic methods including microarray. In the future, maternal serum screening may include direct analysis of fetal nucleic acids in addition to or instead of the currently used fetal protein markers.

References

1. Milunsky A. (2004) *Genetic Disorders and the Fetus: Diagnosis, Prevention, and Treatment.* Johns Hopkins University Press, Baltimore.
2. Nicolaides KH, Azar G, Byrne D, Mansur C, Marks K. (1992) Fetal nuchal translucency: ultrasound screening for chromosomal defects in first trimester of pregnancy. *BMJ* 304: 867–869.
3. Wald NJ, Watt HC, Hackshaw AK. (1999) Integrated screening for Down's syndrome on the basis of tests performed during the first and second trimesters. *N Engl J Med* 341: 461–467.
4. Malone FD, Canick JA, Ball RH, Nyberg DA, Comstock CH, Bukowski R, Berkowitz RL, Gross SJ, Dugoff L, Craigo SD, Timor-Tritsch IE, Carr SR, Wolfe HM, Dukes K, Bianchi DW, Rudnicka AR, Hackshaw AK,

Lambert-Messerlian G, Wald NJ, D'Alton ME. (2005) First-trimester or second-trimester screening, or both, for Down's syndrome. *N Engl J Med* 353: 2001–2011.

5. Wald NJ, Rodeck C, Hackshaw AK, Walters J, Chitty L, Mackinson AM. (2003) First and second trimester antenatal screening for Down's syndrome: the results of the Serum, Urine and Ultrasound Screening Study (SURUSS). *J Med Screen* 10: 56–104.

6. Cuckle HS, Malone FD, Wright D, Porter TF, Nyberg DA, Comstock CH, Saade GR, Berkowitz RL, Ferreira JC, Dugoff L, Craigo SD, Timor IE, Carr SR, Wolfe HM, D'Alton ME. (2008) Contingent screening for Down syndrome — results from the FaSTER trial. *Prenat Diagn* 28: 89–94.

7. Palomaki GE, Neveux LM, Knight GJ, Haddow JE. (2003) Maternal serum-integrated screening for trisomy 18 using both first- and second-trimester markers. *Prenat Diagn* 23: 243–247.

8. Resta RG. (2005) Changing demographics of advanced maternal age (AMA) and the impact on the predicted incidence of Down syndrome in the United States: implications for prenatal screening and genetic counseling. *Am J Med Genet A* 133A: 31–36.

9. ACOG Practice Bulletin No. 77. (2007) screening for fetal chromosomal abnormalities. *Obstet Gynecol* 109: 217–227.

10. Grody WW, Cutting GR, Klinger KW, Richards CS, Watson MS, Desnick RJ. (2001) Laboratory standards and guidelines for population-based cystic fibrosis carrier screening. *Genet Med* 3: 149–154.

11. Gross SJ, Pletcher BA, Monaghan KG. (2008) Carrier screening in individuals of Ashkenazi Jewish descent. *Genet Med* 10: 54–56.

12. Milunsky A. (2004) *Genetic Disorders and the Fetus: Diagnosis, Prevention, and Treatment.* Johns Hopkins University Press, Baltimore.

13. Hook EB. (1977) Exclusion of chromosomal mosaicism: tables of 90%, 95% and 99% confidence limits and comments on use. *Am J Hum Genet* 29: 94–97.

14. Hsu LY, Benn PA. (1999) Revised guidelines for the diagnosis of mosaicism in amniocytes. *Prenat Diagn* 19: 1081–1082.

15. Lewin P, Kleinfinger P, Bazin A, Mossafa H, Szpiro-Tapia S. (2000) Defining the efficiency of fluorescence *in situ* hybridization on uncultured amniocytes on a retrospective cohort of 27407 prenatal diagnoses. *Prenat Diagn* 20: 1–6.

16. Evans MI, Henry GP, Miller WA, Bui TH, Snidjers RJ, Wapner RJ, Miny P, Johnson MP, Peakman D, Johnson A, Nicolaides K, Holzgreve W, Ebrahim SA, Babu R, Jackson L. (1999) International, collaborative assessment of 146,000 prenatal karyotypes: expected limitations if only chromosome-specific probes and fluorescent *in situ* hybridization are used. *Hum Reprod* 14: 1213–1216.

17. Shaffer LG, Bui TH. (2007) Molecular cytogenetic and rapid aneuploidy detection methods in prenatal diagnosis. *Am J Med Genet C Semin Med Genet* 145C: 87–98.

18. Test and Technology Transfer Committee. (2000) Technical and clinical assessment of fluorescence *in situ* hybridization: an ACMG/ASHG position statement. I. Technical considerations. *Genet Med* 2: 356–361.

19. Cirigliano V, Voglino G, Canadas MP, Marongiu A, Ejarque M, Ordonez E, Plaja A, Massobrio M, Todros T, Fuster C, Campogrande M, Egozcue J, Adinolfi M. (2004) Rapid prenatal diagnosis of common chromosome aneuploidies by QF-PCR. Assessment on 18,000 consecutive clinical samples. *Mol Hum Reprod* 10: 839–846.

20. Cirigliano V, Voglino G, Ordonez E, Marongiu A, Paz Canadas M, Ejarque M, Rueda L, Lloveras E, Fuster C, Adinolfi M. (2009) Rapid prenatal diagnosis of common chromosome aneuploidies by QF-PCR, results of 9 years of clinical experience. *Prenat Diagn* 29: 40–49.

21. Hochstenbach R, Meijer J, van de Brug J, Vossebeld-Hoff I, Jansen R, van der Luijt RB, Sinke RJ, Page-Christiaens GC, Ploos van Amstel JK, de Pater JM. (2005) Rapid detection of chromosomal aneuploidies in uncultured amniocytes by multiplex ligation-dependent probe amplification (MLPA). *Prenat Diagn* 25: 1032–1039.

22. Van Opstal D, Boter M, de Jong D, van den Berg C, Bruggenwirth HT, Wildschut HIJ, de Klein A, Galjaard RJH. (2009) Rapid aneuploidy detection with multiplex ligation-dependent probe amplification: a prospective study of 4000 amniotic fluid samples. *Eur J Hum Gene* 17: 112–121.

23. Ogilvie CM, Yaron Y, Beaudet AL. (2009) Current controversies in prenatal diagnosis 3: for prenatal diagnosis, should we offer less or more than metaphase karyotyping? *Prenat Diagn* 29: 11–14.

24. Bejjani BA, Shaffer LG. (2008) Clinical utility of contemporary molecular cytogenetics. *Annu Rev Genomics Hum Genet* 9: 71–86.

25. Stankiewicz P, Beaudet AL. (2007) Use of array CGH in the evaluation of dysmorphology, malformations, developmental delay, and idiopathic mental retardation. *Curr Opin Genet Dev* 17: 182–192.

26. Vermeesch JR, Fiegler H, de Leeuw N, Szuhai K, Schoumans J, Ciccone R, Speleman F, Rauch A, Clayton-Smith J, Van Ravenswaaij C, Sanlaville D, Patsalis PC, Firth H, Devriendt K, Zuffardi O. (2007) Guidelines for molecular karyotyping in constitutional genetic diagnosis. *Eur J Hum Genet* 15: 1105–1114.

27. Aston E, Whitby H, Maxwell T, Glaus N, Cowley B, Lowry D, Zhu XL, Issa B, South ST, Brothman AR. (2008) Comparison of targeted and whole genome analysis of postnatal specimens using a commercially available array based comparative genomic hybridisation (aCGH) microarray platform. *J Med Genet* 45: 268–274.

28. Lee C, Iafrate AJ, Brothman AR. (2007) Copy number variations and clinical cytogenetic diagnosis of constitutional disorders. *Nat Genet* 39: S48–54.

29. Weiss LA, Shen Y, Korn JM, Arking DE, Miller DT, Fossdal R, Saemundsen E, Stefansson H, Ferreira MA, Green T, Platt OS, Ruderfer DM, Walsh CA, Altshuler D, Chakravarti A, Tanzi RE, Stefansson K, Santangelo SL, Gusella JF, Sklar P, Wu BL, Daly MJ. (2008) Association between microdeletion and microduplication at 16p11.2 and autism. *N Engl J Med* 358: 667–675.

30. Mefford HC, Sharp AJ, Baker C, Itsara A, Jiang Z, Buysse K, Huang S, *et al.* (2008) Recurrent rearrangements of chromosome 1q21.1 and variable pediatric phenotypes. *N Engl J Med* 359: 1685–1699.

31. Cai G, Edelmann L, Goldsmith JE, Cohen N, Nakamine A, Reichert JG, Hoffman EJ, Zurawiecki DM, Silverman JM, Hollander E, Soorya L, Anagnostou E, Betancur C, Buxbaum JD. (2008) Multiplex ligation-dependent probe amplification for genetic screening in autism spectrum disorders: efficient identification of known microduplications and identification of a novel microduplication in ASMT. *BMC Med Genomics* 1: 50.

32. Bird TD. (2008) *Hereditary Neuropathy with Liability to Pressure Palsies. GeneReviews.* University of Washington, Seattle. http://www.ncbi.nlm.nih.gov/bookshelf/br.fcgi?book=gene&part=hnpp

33. Bird TD. (2007) *Charcot-Marie-Tooth Hereditary Neuropathy Overview. GeneReviews.* University of Washington, Seattle. http://www.ncbi.nlm.nih.gov/bookshelf/br.fcgi?book=gene&part=cmt1

34. Sahoo T, Cheung SW, Ward P, Darilek S, Patel A, del Gaudio D, Kang SH, Lalani SR, Li J, McAdoo S, Burke A, Shaw CA, Stankiewicz P, Chinault AC, Van den Veyver IB, Roa BB, Beaudet AL, Eng CM. (2006) Prenatal diagnosis of chromosomal abnormalities using array-based comparative genomic hybridization. *Genet Med* 8: 719–727.

35. Shaffer B, Tran S, Norton M, Malabed K, Pena S, Caughey A. (2008) Amniocenetisis based on the potential for significant chromosomal abnormalities: a decision analysis. *Am J Obste Gynecol* 199: DOI 10.1016/j.ajog. 2008.1009.1674|1644.

36. Van den Veyver IB, Patel A, Shaw CA, Pursley AN, Kang SHL, Simovich MJ, Ward PA, Darilek S, Johnson A, Neill SE, Bi W, White LD, Eng CM, Lupski JR, Cheung SW, Beaudet AL. (2009) Clinical use of array comparative genomic hybridization (aCGH) for prenatal diagnosis in 300 cases. *Prenat Diagn* 29: 29–39.

37. Darilek S, Ward P, Pursley A, Plunkett K, Furman P, Magoulas P, Patel A, Cheung SW, Eng CM. (2008) Pre- and postnatal genetic testing by array-comparative genomic hybridization: genetic counseling perspectives. *Genet Med* 10: 13–18.

38. Warburton D. (1991) *De novo* balanced chromosome rearrangements and extra marker chromosomes identified at prenatal diagnosis: clinical significance and distribution of breakpoints. *Am J Hum Genet* 49: 995–1013.

39. De Gregori M, Ciccone R, Magini P, Pramparo T, Gimelli S, Messa J, Novara F, *et al.* (2007) Cryptic deletions are a common finding in "balanced" reciprocal and complex chromosome rearrangements: a study of 59 patients. *J Med Genet* 44: 750–762.

40. Gribble SM, Prigmore E, Burford DC, Porter KM, Ng BL, Douglas EJ, Fiegler H, Carr P, Kalaitzopoulos D, Clegg S, Sandstrom R, Temple IK, Youings SA, Thomas NS, Dennis NR, Jacobs PA, Crolla JA, Carter NP. (2005) The complex nature of constitutional *de novo* apparently balanced translocations in patients presenting with abnormal phenotypes. *J Med Genet* 42: 8–16.

41. Higgins AW, Alkuraya FS, Bosco AF, Brown KK, Bruns GA, Donovan DJ, Eisenman R, *et al.* (2008) Characterization of apparently balanced chromosomal rearrangements from the developmental genome anatomy project. *Am J Hum Genet* 82: 712–722.

Chapter 4

Fetal Imaging in Detection of Congenital Heart Disease

Olivera Kontic-Vucinic* and Joshua A. Copel[†]

4.1 The Significance of Congenital Heart Disease

4.1.1 *The incidence of congenital heart diseases*

In the majority of the developed countries, prenatal ultrasound for detection of fetal anomalies is a standard part of pregnancy management. Fetal heart examination is a critical part of the fetal anatomic scan, for several reasons. Congenital heart diseases (CHD) are the most prevalent major congenital anomalies, with an estimated incidence between 4 and 13/1000 live births.[1,2] More than 32,000 neonates are born with some form of CHD each year in the US.[3] Moderate to severe forms of CHD is found in about 6/1000 live births, with 3 or 4/1000 live neonates who will probably require some kind of medical or surgical treatment.[4,5]

The overall incidence of aneuploidy in fetal heart disease is estimated to be 33%.[6] Different studies have found chromosomal abnormalities in 5% to 13% of live births with CHD and the incidence has ranged from 15% to 50% in prenatal series.[7,8] Additionally, between 8% and 42% of patients with CHD also have other associated non-cardiac anomalies,

*Associate Professor, Obstetrics and Gynecology, University of Belgrade School of Medicine.
†Professor, Obstetrics, Gynecology and Reproductive Science, and Pediatrics, Yale University School of Medicine.

while non-chromosomal syndromes and associations comprise 1% to 5% of patients with CHD.[7] Importantly, more than 50% of all fetuses with abnormal karyotype have cardiac anomalies. Therefore, it seems prudent to recommend a comprehensive and detailed anatomy/anomaly scan for all fetuses diagnosed with a cardiac defect. Chromosomal study may also be indicated depending on the type of cardiac anomaly.[6,9,10]

The incidence of cardiac defects observed during the first and second trimesters is noticeably different compared to the incidence of the same defects at term. Apart from the fact that many ventricular septal defects may dramatically decrease and even close spontaneously before birth, a noteworthy proportion of CHD associated with chromosome abnormalities or extracardiac anomalies may end in spontaneous or induced fetal demise. This will affect the overall incidence, as well as the relative frequencies of particular anomalies. On the other hand, some forms of CHD probably have a higher incidence at term than during the earlier stages of gestation, due to their natural history. There are several examples of CHD that evolve dramatically during the course of pregnancy, from first trimester to term.[11,12] Mild aortic or pulmonary valve stenosis could be examples of such evolution. Additionally, some important entities, including ductal constriction or closure of the foramen ovale, fetal dysrhythmias, valvular regurgitation, myocardial dysfunction, and congestive heart failure may not emerge until late in gestation.[12,13]

4.1.2 *The morbidity and mortality associated with CHD*

CHD is associated with significant infant morbidity and mortality, due both to its complexity and high incidence. About 25% of total infant deaths are due to congenital malformations, with approximately one third of those related to CHD. According to the World Health Organization, between 1950 and 1994, as much as 42% of infant deaths were attributable to cardiac defects. Among an estimated one million babies with CHD born each year worldwide, 280,000 will die annually in the neonatal period.[14] The real significance and magnitude of this problem can be recognized from the outcomes following the natural history of frequent congenital cardiac anomalies. Patients with large atrial septal defects have a risk of mortality of 5–15% before the age of 30 years. The presence of a patent ductus arteriosus carries a 30% mortality risk during the first year of life. For the same period, risk of death among children born with tetralogy of Fallot with pulmonary stenosis is 25%, and increases up to 95% by the age of 40. During the first year of life, mortality rate for transposition of the great arteries is 90%. Hypoplastic left heart syndrome results in the mortality of the majority of the neonates within the first two weeks of birth.[14]

4.2 The Importance of Prenatal Diagnosis of CHD

4.2.1 *What do we achieve with prenatal diagnosis? The place and impact of fetal echocardiography*

Fetal echocardiography is recognized and accepted as a useful and valuable technique for prenatal diagnosis of CHD. This imaging modality has affected both the fetus and the neonate with CHD in a variety of extremely important ways.

Screening for CHD has increased the percentage of cases that are detected prenatally. Wide application of this technique along with advances in imaging technology have resulted in more exact and, importantly, earlier identification of fetal cardiac defects. Consequently, the timely and accurate prenatal diagnosis of cardiac defects can guide prenatal management and monitoring, may influence the location, timing, and mode of delivery, provide anticipation of necessary immediate postnatal care, influence postnatal management in terms of reduced surgical delays, shorter intensive care unit stays, and avoidance of severe, sometimes life-threatening hemodynamic compromise and ultimately may improve the outcome of fetuses with particular types of cardiac lesions.[13,15–18]

Fetal echocardiography allows for the precise diagnosis of fetal arrhythmias and makes it possible to follow up on the effectiveness of medication started *in utero*. Also, a few congenital cardiac abnormalities may require prenatal intervention, and fetal echocardiography is used to identify candidates for *in utero* intervention, to guide these procedures, and to monitor post-interventional cardiac status.[18–22]

The timely prenatal diagnosis of CHD allows for reassurance of families when the scan is normal, and may improve maternal psychological status in both normal and abnormal scans. It also provides a better counseling of parents regarding the anticipated course of the affected fetus for the remainder of the pregnancy, the expected pre- and postnatal interventions and other management options that may be required, as well as pre- and postnatal prognosis.[23] Timely diagnosed CHD also provides for additional counseling on the risks of chromosomal abnormalities and genetic syndromes associated with CHD. This imaging modality can also serve for the evaluation and management of some non-cardiac abnormalities with consequential impact on the cardiovascular system, such as congenital cystic adenomatoid malformation, congenital diaphragmatic hernia, and twin–twin transfusion syndrome.

4.2.2 *Prenatal insight — in utero evolution of CHD*

One of the most important accomplishments of fetal echocardiography has been remarkable improvement of our knowledge and understanding of the morphology and the pathophysiology of CHD before birth, including the timing and mechanisms of formation, as well as their development and evolution *in utero*.

Heart development is first seen in embryos of 18 or 19 days, and cardiac embryogenesis occurs in the first six or seven weeks of the pregnancy. From that point to term, heart disease can evolve in various distinct ways. Serial observations throughout pregnancy have shown that some of the major structural abnormalities like abnormalities of situs, defects of septation, conotruncal lesions, ventricular looping abnormalities, and transposition of the great arteries develop during a period of embryogenesis, and many of those lesions continue to progress during the pregnancy, partially but importantly as a consequence of the fetal circulation.[12] Some subtle anomalies may develop or become evident latter — in the second or even third trimester.[12,24] Many cardiac lesions will fully develop only after hemodynamic modifications take place after birth.

As already mentioned, for a variety of lesions, the range of severity seen in the neonate depends on the timing of the altered circulation that occurred *in utero*. Some forms of cardiac lesions are progressive in nature, and this is the most obviously seen in the obstructive lesions which can vary in severity and ultimately cause a critically reduced rate of growth of chambers or arteries, as a consequence of reduced blood flow to these structures. This is particularly true if the obstruction occurs prior to 20 weeks, because although the process of fetal growth is constant throughout gestation, the greatest proportion of cardiac growth happens in the first 20 weeks of pregnancy. Aortic and pulmonary valve stenoses are examples of lesions generating severe secondary pathology when onset occurs early in gestation.[25,26] Early detected left heart obstructive lesion may gradually cause hypoplastic left heart syndrome (Fig. 4.1).[27,28] Worsening stenosis of the pulmonary valve may progress to pulmonary atresia with right ventricular hypoplasia (Fig. 4.2).[29,30] A similar mechanism of progression, due to insufficient growth of the pulmonary arteries, may be implied for ventricular outflow tract obstruction in fetuses with tetralogy of Fallot.[31] Other conotruncal lesions, including double-outlet right ventricle, and interrupted aortic arch type b, are commonly associated with obstruction to one of the outflow tracts and a ventricular septal defect. Progression of the obstruction may arise in more serious condition by term. Early detected discrete coarctation of the aorta may progress to the more complex lesion with severe aortic arch hypoplasia.

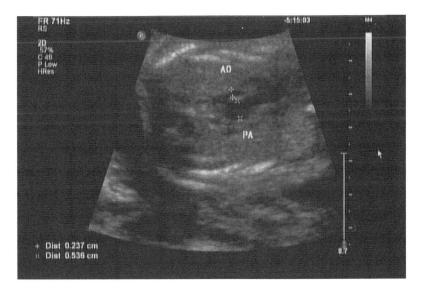

Fig. 4.1.   Hypoplastic left heart (Ao — aorta; PA — pulmonary artery).

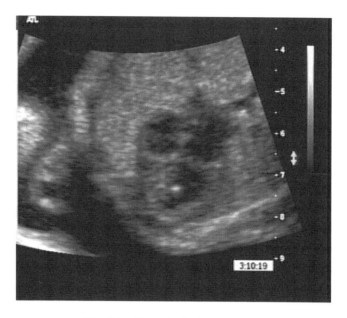

Fig. 4.2.   Hypoplastic right ventricle.

Significant semilunar and AV valve regurgitation, either occurring as an isolated lesion or as part of a complex cardiac disease, is poorly tolerated by fetal circulation. The different forms of tricuspid valve disease best illustrate this. Progression of tricuspid insufficiency may include progressive cardiomegaly, incompetence of the right ventricle, progressive anatomic/functional obstruction to right ventricular outflow (including pulmonary stenosis, pulmonary atresia or functional pulmonary atresia), damaged diastolic function of the left ventricle, resulting in severe cardiovascular compromise and eventually death.

Although the postnatal course for the majority of neonates born with transposition of the great arteries tends to be relatively favorable, some children with intact ventricular septum are born severely oxygen deprived, due to progressive foramen ovale restriction and ductus arteriosus constriction during the late third trimester.[13] In some other more complex forms of diseases there may be progressive outflow tract obstruction and significant diminution of ventricular septal defect, which may alter the prognosis for those infants.[12]

Although most cardiac defects tend to progress towards a more severe form, some lesions evolve to a less severe form. Evaluation of natural history of muscular ventricular septal defects diagnosed *in utero* revealed that about one-third of these defects spontaneously close *in utero*.[32]

Finally, some severe forms of CHD lead to congestive heart failure and intrauterine demise.[30] Fetal congestive heart failure occurs as adverse outcome in the course of progression of lesions with significant atrioventricular valvular insufficiency, biventricular systolic and diastolic dysfunction, and dysrhythmias. Given the dismal prognosis of most affected fetuses, this condition should be considered during the planning of perinatal management. Primary cardiomyopathies (dilated and hypertrophic) are conditions with variable timing of development during the second or third trimester. Since the fetal and neonatal circulations usually tolerate cardiomyopathies poorly, the prognosis, particularly for dilated cardiomyopathy, is gloomy, with a few exceptions. Close monitoring and serial assessment of pregnancies at risk for fetal cardiomyopathy is required.

Some intracardiac tumors may also progress in the second and third trimester.[33,34] Although rhabdomyomas may expand in size, causing inflow or outflow tract obstruction and occasionally cardiovascular compromise in the mid-trimester, they typically undergo spontaneous regression in the third trimester and after birth. In contrast, fibromas and hemangiomas may continue to increase in the late gestation and postnatally. It has been observed that teratomas may cause progressive pericardial effusion.

4.3 Examination of Fetal Heart

4.3.1 *What affects the detection rate?*

Currently, screening for fetal heart defects is one of the most demanding tasks of fetal ultrasonography. At the same time, it is one of the least successful aspects.[4,35] Given the global significance of CHD, the most important concern is the fact that despite efforts to improve prenatal detection of these anomalies, they continue to remain among the most frequently missed abnormalities by fetal ultrasonography.[4,36–38] Recently published results are appropriate illustration of this problem. Among neonates with critical heart disease admitted to a tertiary care center, diagnosis was established prenatally in 53%, in the newborn nursery in 38%, and after newborn hospital discharge in 8% of cases.[39]

Due to the challenges inherent with screening the fetus for CHD, reported prenatal detection rates have varied widely between the centers.[36,40–43] Among the various possible causes, examiners experience and competence is by far the most important one. Fetal echocardiography is highly operator dependent, and low sensitivity has been reported for screening for CHD by inexperienced examiners, while skilled investigators achieved significantly better detection rates, with a high degree of diagnostic precision.[44] Improvements in this particular field will ultimately optimize all the other results regarding CHD.

Some of the observed variations can also be attributed to objective obstacles, such as quality of ultrasound equipment, maternal obesity, abdominal scars, gestational age, inadequate amniotic fluid volume, and unfavorable fetal position. However, it is necessary to emphasize that not all fetal cardiac problems can be detected, and moreover a normal screening ultrasound does not completely eliminate the possibility of a heart defect.[36] Nevertheless, the proportion of congenital heart anomalies detected prenatally has increased over time, in particular for more severe malformations.[41,45]

4.3.2 *Timing for fetal echocardiography*

In general, ultrasound examination of the fetal heart can be performed at any time during the second trimester when detailed cardiac anatomy can be properly visualized.[46] Considering previously mentioned issues regarding the development of CHD, the proposed timing is a compromise between scanning at adequate period of gestation not to miss late-developing lesions, and at the same time delivering the diagnosis to parents as early as possible, so they have enough time for necessary additional testing, counseling and considering the options for pregnancy management.[47]

Currently, the fetal heart can be visualized transvaginally by nine weeks of gestation, and abdominally by 11 weeks.[48] Certain anomalies may be identified during the late first and early second trimester of pregnancy, particularly in the presence of increased nuchal translucency (NT).[49,50] It has been shown that increased nuchal translucency thickness represents an important risk factor for major cardiac defects, in particular left-sided obstructive lesions.[51–53] In fetuses at risk of CHD, for many cases, distinction between a normal and abnormal cardiac morphology can be recognized at or even before 16 weeks of pregnancy.[54] However, apart from the fact that the earlier scan is less accurate than the second trimester scan, we have to keep in mind that some forms of cardiac defects do not become apparent in the early stage of pregnancy.

As a consequence some of those late-developing lesions, which consequently evolve in relation to fetal blood flow, may go undetected in the course of an early scan.[11,47] That is the main reason why the fetal cardiac examination is optimally performed between 18 and 22 weeks of gestation in areas where the permissible limit of termination of pregnancy is 24 weeks. Nevertheless, the earlier scan may be offered to the patients at significantly increased risk of congenital heart anomalies, accompanied by a follow-up scan at 20–22 weeks.[47,48] As a rule, if a CHD is suspected at any scan, the fetus should be reexamined promptly, regardless of gestational age.

Patients at a slightly increased risk for CHD should be scheduled for a comprehensive fetal cardiac scan between 18 and 22 weeks of gestation. Apart from this, evaluation of detection rates for different CHD screening programs by Stoll has shown that the best results are achieved in countries where every woman has access to three ultrasound scans — at 12 weeks for NT, around the 22nd week for a detailed anatomic scan, and at 32 weeks for growth check and revalidation of the morphology.[55]

4.3.3 *Who should be examined?*

Examination of fetal heart is performed either as part of a screening fetal sonography for a low-risk population, or as a fetal echocardiography — comprehensive diagnostic scan for patients at high risk for CHD.

Identified risk factors increase the probability of CHD beyond the expected rate for a low-risk population. Many risk factors have been recognized and categorized as maternal or fetal in origin.[9,52,56,57]

Among the maternal factors, family history, e.g. first-degree relative or proband (mother or father) with CHD is the most obvious. The risk to the next generation is higher if the mother is affected (6%), than if the father is affected (2%). One prior child with CHD born to mother and/or father carries the recurrence risk of 2% for any subsequent pregnancy. With two affected children, the risk increases to 10%. Maternal pre-existing metabolic disease like type 1 diabetes (2% risk of CHD) and phenylketonuria are also associated with increased risk for CHD. Early pregnancy exposure to teratogens including lithium, phenytoin, carba-mazepine, warfarin, alcohol, paroxitene, and isotretinoin, are reported to be associated with an increased risk of heart malformations. Precise risks vary with the medication and the duration of exposure and dosing. One of the most recently recognized factors is *in vitro* fertilization. Over 134,000 assisted reproductive technology (ART) procedures were performed in the USA in 2005 and more than 52,000 infants were live-born as a result of these procedures, representing 1% of all US births.[58] The most recent population-based, multicenter, case-control study of birth defects has shown that ART was significantly associated with some septal heart defects, in particular atrial septal defects secundum/not otherwise speci-fied defects and ventricular septal defects plus atrial septal defects, among singleton births. The mechanism is not clear.[59]

A number of major extracardiac anomalies are frequently associated with heart disease. Increased nuchal translucency thickness in the first trimester represents an important risk factor for major cardiac defects. As expected, the same applies for abnormal fetal karyotype. Assumed low-risk pregnancies with an abnormal four-chamber view or outflow tracts naturally raise the risk for CHD. The risk is also increased in cases of observed abnormal visceral/cardiac situs, and persistent bradycardia or tachycardia. Nonimmune fetal hydrops can be due to CHD in up to 25% of cases. Risk is also increased in intrauterine growth restriction, polyhydramnios, fetal pericardial/pleural effusion and ascites. Finally, monochorionic twin pregnancies raise higher concerns for CHD. The inci-dence of structural heart disease in monochorionic twins is significantly increased, which justifies referral of these pregnancies for fetal echocar-diography as a standard part of their assessment. If one twin is affected, the risk to the other twin is increased further.[60]

Importantly, not all risk factors for fetal heart anomalies are equal. Some of them comprise significantly increased risks, while the others are associated with only moderately increased risk. Moreover, the majority of cases of prenatally diagnosed CHD occur in patients with no identifiable risk factors.[53,61] Consequently, most cases are currently assumed to be idiopathic or sporadically attributable to known genetic syndromes. Therefore, prenatal screening for CHD based exclusively on the existence of risk factors is not particularly effective, which makes routine screening of all pregnancies necessary.[62] The aim of the screening is to identify which fetuses should undergo further comprehensive evaluation with fetal echocardiography. This makes the rate of detection of CHD largely dependant on the sensitivity of the prenatal screening ultrasound. Therefore, effective screening for CHD in low-risk pregnancies remains immensely important for increasing the percentage of cases diagnosed prenatally.[45,63]

4.3.4 *Screening for CHD*

Screening for CHD should be performed for evaluation of fetuses in low-risk pregnancies as part of a routine prenatal care.[64,65] The first trials for fetal cardiac screening used the four-chamber view alone (Fig. 4.3).[66,67] Despite the well-documented utility of a four-chamber view, this approach has later proved insufficient and inadequate for identification of anomalies of the ventricular outflow tracts and great arteries. The overall detection rate of CHD in screening programs utilizing this view was only 15–20%.[10,24,68] As many defects can have normal-appearing four-chamber view, it has been suggested that the screening examination should, besides the four-chamber view, include the views for situs determination, assessment of the ventricular outflow tracts and great arteries.[69–71] International Society of Ultrasound in Obs/Gyn recommended guidelines for two levels screening for heart anomalies in low-risk fetuses.[35] Suggested screening comprises a basic scan performed by analyzing a four-chamber view of the fetal heart, and additional extended-basic scan which evaluates the proportion and relationships of both arterial outflow tracts. These two complementary examinations are designed to optimize the detection rate of heart defects during a routine second-trimester scan.[72] In experienced hands, a detection rate of CHD of 55% using only the four-chamber view, increases to 80% when the outflow tracts are included.[10,44,61] Assessment of outflow tract views along with the four-chamber view for the low-risk fetal cardiac screening has been widely promoted.[68,73] Detected or suspected heart anomalies should be referred for more detailed analysis using fetal echocardiography.

The basic cardiac screening examination relies on a four-chamber view of the fetal heart (Fig. 4.3), and involves a careful evaluation of specific entities.[35,72] General observation should reveal normal cardiac situs, axis and position, with a majority of the normally sized heart in the left chest (Fig. 4.4), presence of four cardiac chambers, and absence of pericardial effusion or cardiac hypertrophy. Evaluation of atria should find uniform size of atria, foramen ovale flap in the left atrium, and present atrial septum primum. Assessment of ventricles allows us to observe: approximately equal size of ventricles, no signs of cardia hypertrophy, presence of moderator band at the right ventricular apex and intact ventricular septum (apex to crux) (Fig. 4.5). Both atrioventricular valves should open and move freely, and the tricuspid valve leaflet insertion on the ventricular septum

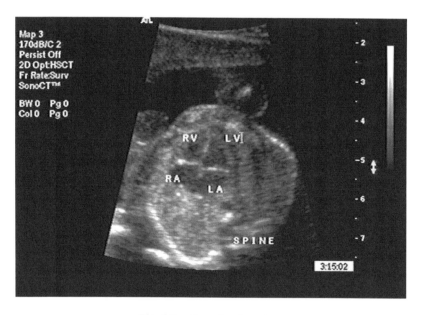

Fig. 4.3. Four-chamber view.

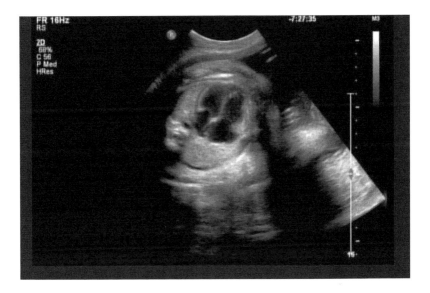

Fig. 4.4.   Cardiomegaly and edema.

should be slightly more apical than the septal leaflet of the mitral valve. Finally, cardiac rate and regular rhythm should be confirmed, and clinically significant bradycardia, tachycardia and dysrhythmias must be noted.[74]

Most studies have shown that if an adequate four-chamber view can be obtained, competent evaluation of the outflow tracts is usually achievable, resulting in improved detection rates for major cardiac malformations.[10,75] Additional outflow tract views are more likely to detect ventricular septal defects and conotruncal anomalies such as tetralogy of Fallot, transposition of the great arteries, double outlet right ventricle, and truncus arteriosus. Examination of outflow tracts should at least confirm that the great vessels are similar in size and that they cross each other at appropriate angles as they originate from their respective ventricles. Apart from confirming the crossing nature of outflow tracts to arterial trunks, left and right ventricular outflow tract views should assess the patency of the outflow tracts and semilunar valves, as well as septal integrity. Failure to verify these findings requires additional evaluation.

The additional three-vessel view is described to assess the sizes and relationships of the pulmonary artery, ascending aorta, and superior vena

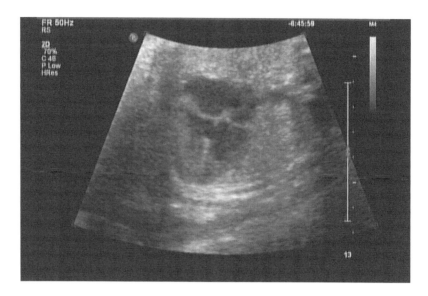

Fig. 4.5.   Ventricular septal defect.

cava, and can also be used to estimate vascular relationships to the fetal trachea.[76,77]

4.3.5 *Fetal echocardiography*

Patients with recognized increased risk or with suspected fetal cardiac anomalies should be offered a more detailed scan, considering higher detection rate of CHD with fetal echocardiography than with screening scans.[46] It has been shown that complete agreement between the prenatal and postnatal diagnosis in fetuses with complex CHD is as high as 96% when performed by experienced examiners.[78,79]

The basic goal for a fetal echocardiography is to verify the existence or absence of CHD. An abnormal scan necessitates further characterization of the anomaly along with the differential diagnoses. It should also identify fetuses that will require prompt postnatal medical or surgical intervention, particularly those with ductal-dependent lesions.[15,46,80,81]

Regardless of the nature of the anomaly, which may to some extent require the individualization of the examination, for the purpose of the complete anatomical assessment, fetal echocardiography includes a meticulous evaluation of the transverse view of the upper abdomen, the four-chamber view, both ventricular outflow tract views, three-vessel and trachea view, basal short-axis view, and aortic arch view.[70,77,82] Using this methodological approach, three segments of the heart (the atria, the ventricles, and the great arteries), and two connectors (the atrioventricular and the ventriculoarterial connections) can be assessed.[82,83] The final goal of this examination is to assess and confirm anatomical relationships and functional flow characteristics of the fetal heart, through a consistent analysis of the following (Figs. 4.6–4.10):

(1) cardiac axis and situs,
(2) ventricular morphology,
(3) pericardial effusions,
(4) venous-atrial, atrioventricular and ventriculoarterial connections of the heart,
(5) size and relationships of the left and right ventricular outflow tracts,

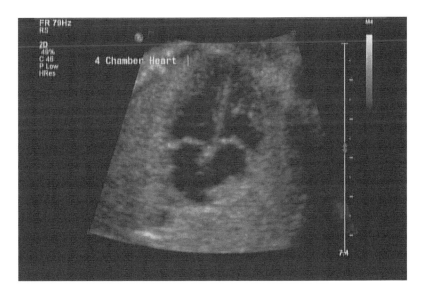

Fig. 4.6. Four-chamber view.

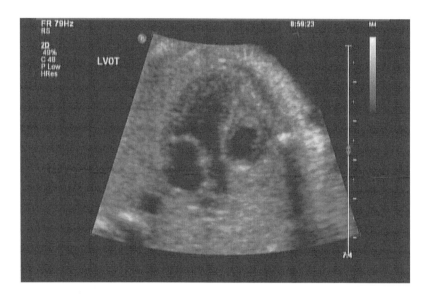

Fig. 4.7. Left ventricular outflow tract view.

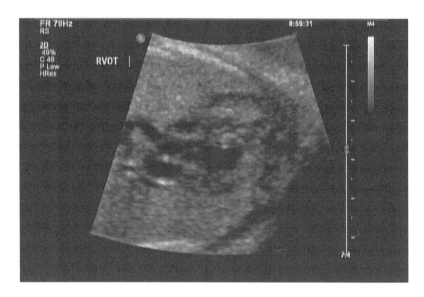

Fig. 4.8. Right ventricular outflow tract view.

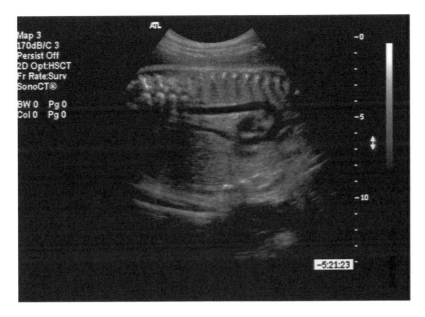

Fig. 4.9.   Aortic arch view of fetal heart.

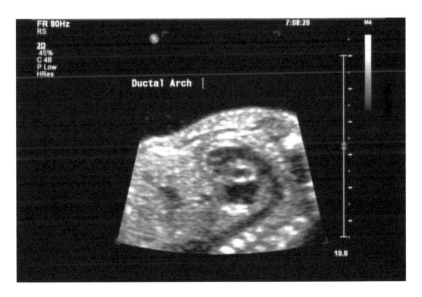

Fig. 4.10.   Ductal arch view of fetal heart.

(6) ductal and aortic arches,
(7) interventricular septum,
(8) atrial septum, atrial chamber size, and foramen ovale,
(9) atrioventricular and semilunar valves,
(10) flow across each heart connection, as seen with Doppler flow mapping.

4.4 Imaging Modalities

The fetal cardiac examination can be performed using various imaging modalities, ranging from two-dimensional (2D) to four-dimensional (4D) ultrasonography with spatiotemporal image correlation (STIC). The evaluation of specific lesions can be individualized, but a high-resolution ultrasound system with color and power Doppler, pulsed wave spectral Doppler and M-mode capabilities are generally required. The vast majority of fetal echocardiography is obtained with real-time gray-scale imaging of the cardiac and major vascular structures (Fig. 4.11) with a complementary color Doppler evaluation (Fig. 4.12) of the vascular inlets and outflow

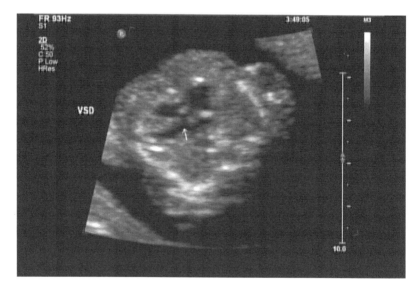

Fig. 4.11. Ventricular septal defect.

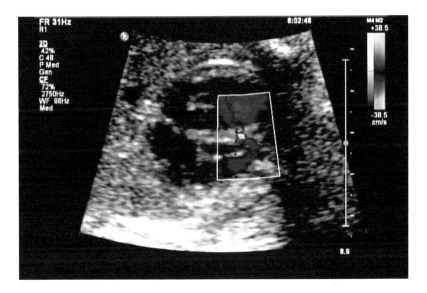

Fig. 4.12. Doppler image of ventricular septal defect.

tracts, as well as the great arteries. The power Doppler technique, additionally facilitates recognition and analysis of the vascular anatomy. Both Doppler ultrasonography and M-mode echocardiography are also powerful tools for the study of fetal cardiac dysrhythmias.

Doppler ultrasonography provides indispensable information about fetal cardiac lesions. Several studies have proved the value of color flow and Doppler sonography for the analysis and interpretation of fetal venous and intracardiac blood flow.[84,85] Spectral Doppler ultrasonography can be used to further distinguish the character and severity of suspected flow disturbances. Continuous-wave Doppler sonography is occasionally useful in cases of valvular disease, to measure very high velocity flow across stenotic or incompetent valves. If required, these techniques may also be employed to assess fetal cardiac function using different parameters such as ventricular ejection fraction, stroke volume, cardiac output, mechanical PR intervals, Tei index, and ventricular strain parameters.[86,87]

Venous Doppler flow measurement is an additional resource which provides advanced study of the fetal circulation (Figs. 4.13 and 4.14). Abnormal ductus venosus (DV) waveforms are found in a variety of

CHD. Abnormalities in the DV waveform such as reduced, absent, or reversed flow during atrial systole, could be the signs of early cardiac dysfunction. Moreover, measurement of the DV pulsatility is an useful additional parameter for predicting the risk for cardiac failure and death in fetuses with isolated structural CHD. Second- and third-trimester DV pulsatility measurements can provide important prognostic value regarding adverse perinatal outcomes regardless of karyotype and type of cardiac lesion, and also independent of the gestational age of affected fetuses. During this period of gestation, abnormal DV waveforms are detectable in 64% of fetuses with CHD, although predominantly seen in relationship with defects affecting the right ventricular function. Therefore, DV Doppler studies are clinically applicable and relevant for monitoring cardiac function in fetuses with CHD.[88,89]

Volume images acquired with three-dimensional (3D) and four-dimensional (4D) ultrasonography allow a supplemental, sophisticated approach for analyzing complex cardiac lesions, with an intention to further increase accurate evaluation of the anomaly.[90–93] Contemporary technology allows real-time 3D or 4D ultrasound for immediate acquisition of the

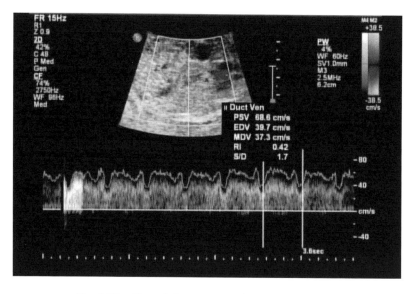

Fig. 4.13.   Normal ductus venosus Doppler wave form.

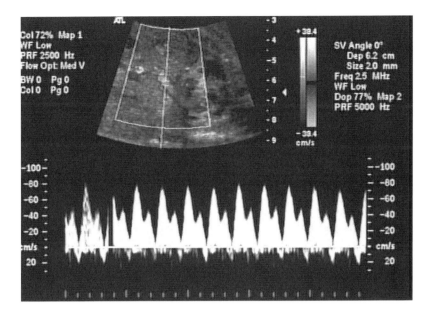

Fig. 4.14.   Abnormal ductus venosus Doppler wave form.

volume data of the entire heart. Following the collection of the volume data set, which can be obtained within seconds, subsequent interactive review may be performed any time. The image reconstruction enables the analyst to evaluate the sequences of two-dimensional images in diverse views, to assess intracardiac anatomy details at different depth planes, and importantly, to recreate casts of blood flow of the chambers and great vessels. Some investigators have suggested that this approach may facilitate and enhance the analysis of both the four chambers and the outflow tracts.[94,95] However, other authors still have concerns regarding suboptimal image resolution with 3D imaging and substantial expertise required to analyze volume data sets.[96]

4.5 Counseling

Following the diagnosis of a cardiac malformation, the counselor must address the available information and attempt to provide a realistic picture of what we know about the different aspects of the prognosis.[97] The interpretation of some cardiac abnormalities can be challenging, and accurate prenatal diagnosis is particularly important, although diagnostic limitations of fetal echocardiography must be emphasized. Only an accurate differential diagnosis will result in appropriate prenatal counseling, because even subtle differences can considerably modify the therapeutic approach and overall prognosis.[24] The counselor should be competent to provide the parents with comprehensive information about the problem, including an exact description of the anatomy of the defect or the mechanism of the arrhythmia, nature and severity of the anomaly, possible association with extracardiac and chromosomal anomalies, anticipated prenatal evolution, clinical management and follow up, recommended center for delivery, possible need for *in utero* medical treatment, information regarding the necessity for surgical intervention and the type of intervention available for the condition pre- and postnatally, the number of anticipated procedures along with associated mortality and morbidity, short- and long-term results of treatment including implications for quality of life, when available. Another important piece of information that should also be given to the couple is about recurrence risks in subsequent pregnancies.[56] Obviously, this kind of prenatal counseling requires a multidisciplinary approach and collaboration.

Many factors will influence the decision of the couple to continue the pregnancy or to terminate it. By far, the most important is the type of anomaly and its prognosis. Generally, cardiac defects can be essentially divided into several major groups, for purposes of counseling. First are cardiac lesions that are warning signs of chromosomal anomalies, syndromes, and associations. Given the global incidence of 33% for chromosomal anomalies found in association with CHD, the counseling should cover this aspect. These anomalies usually belong to two subgroups, i.e., atrioventricular septal defects and conotruncal anomalies. For example, counseling for prenatally diagnosed atrioventricular septal defect (Fig. 4.16) should include the 58% risk of aneuploidy and 50% risk of trisomy 21.[98] Fluorescent *in situ* hybridization testing for the chromosome 22q11 deletion might be requested in the case of conotruncal anomalies. Another group is comprised of complex anomalies that will become critical at birth. In general, in these types of CHD, which are well tolerated prenatally due to the presence of fetal shunts, the karyotype and

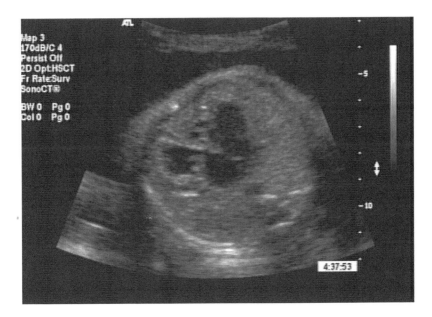

Fig. 4.15. Hypoplastic right heart.

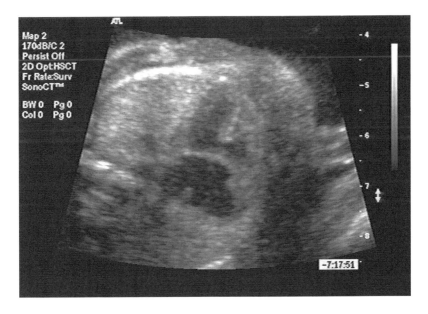

Fig. 4.16. AV canal.

morphological assessment are normal. Thus, the second group includes all forms of single ventricle physiology (Fig. 4.15), with the hypoplasic left heart as the most frequently prenatally established diagnosis. The third group comprises two ventricle hearts with critical shunts, while all the other CHD could be categorized in the fourth group. Accurate diagnosis is essential to consider the prognosis and organize proper care at birth.

4.6 The Impact of Fetal Echocardiography — Changing the Prognosis

4.6.1 *Impact of fetal echocardiography on structural cardiac disease*

As mentioned before, fetal echocardiography has impacted the fetus with CHD in many ways. Fetal echocardiography has allowed for earlier and increased recognition of CHD prenatally. Although it seems plausible that early prenatal diagnosis of CHD leads to a better outcome for the majority of lesions, surprisingly, only recently have studies shown an improvement in postnatal outcome with the prenatal diagnosis of CHD. The favorable impact on the perinatal course is particularly apparent in the preoperative condition of neonates with severe cardiac defects.[15–17,99–101] These benefits include reduced preoperative morbidity, less metabolic acidosis, and better end-organ perfusion. It appears that patients diagnosed only postnatally had worse metabolic acidosis and multi-organ dysfunction compared to those diagnosed prenatally. Prenatal detection of CHD allows for planned delivery at a center with appropriate neonatal intensive care unit, accessible prostaglandin and mechanical ventilation, and congenital heart surgery facilities easily available, if needed.[17,23,30]

In ductal-dependent lesions, such as critical left heart obstructive lesions, and pulmonary atresia, as well as with transposition of the great arteries, the crucial advantage of prenatal diagnosis seems to be avoidance of severe hemodynamic compromise prior to effective intervention. Specific effects of prenatally diagnosed critical left heart obstructive lesions compared with those diagnosed postnatally include all the previously mentioned benefits, i.e. timely transfer to the proposed site of delivery, decreased postnatal morbidity due to the avoidance of hemodynamic decompensation and non-cardiac organ failure, shorter presurgical intensive care unit stays and consequently decreased surgical delays.[99] Although the majority of the studies have found similar surgical results and hospital mortality between prenatally and postnatally diagnosed patients, some investigators have shown that the group of prenatally diagnosed patients with hypoplastic left heart syndrome had an increased survival rate following surgery compared with postnatally diagnosed patients, probably by improving their preoperative status.[16,17,99,102] Importantly, improved preoperative condition and decreased surgical delays in the first group may positively influence long-term neurodevelopmental outcomes.

Evaluation of some other major structural heart anomalies like transposition of the great arteries, pulmonary atresia with intact ventricular septum, diagnosed pre- and postnatally, has revealed a similar impact.[30,100] Prenatal diagnosis of transposition of the great arteries, compared with postnatal diagnosis, results in decreased morbidity as well as both preoperative and postoperative mortality.[15] Also, prenatal identification of the subgroup of high-risk patients with d-transposition of the great arteries and functionally intact ventricular septum, with abnormal features of the foramen ovale and ductus arteriosus, may improve postnatal course and outcome.[13] Although no advantages were found regarding survival rate of patients with prenatally diagnosed univentricular hearts, better survival was reported for prenatally detected patients undergoing biventricular repair compared with those diagnosed postnatally.[103] Franklin reported that a prenatal diagnosis of severe coarctation of the aorta results in less cardiovascular collapse and death as well as increased survival rate and better preoperative clinical condition than in those without a prenatal diagnosis.[17]

Overall, it appears that prenatal diagnosis of structural cardiac disease results in reduced preoperative morbidity, improves postnatal outcome, and may allow better long-term neurodevelopmental outcome. However, due to a lack of sufficient number of patients, caused by termination of some pregnancies, home deaths of some neonates and variation in surgical techniques and results, conclusive assessment of the impact of prenatal diagnosis is yet unavailable.[16,23] It is reasonable to expect that the improved effect of fetal echocardiography on structural cardiac disease may enhance as advances in interventional techniques evolve.

4.6.2 *Impact of fetal echocardiography on functional cardiac disease*

Advanced ultrasound modalities, such as Doppler tissue imaging and the myocardial performance index (Tei Index), allow reliable and reproducible assessment of the intrauterine fetal cardiac function. Fetal echocardiography is extremely valuable for assessing and monitoring the cardiac function and response to medical treatment in patients with decreased cardiac function or heart failure. The Tei Index has been reported to be an useful, noninvasive, Doppler-derived myocardial performance index that serves as a combined index of global myocardial (systolic and diastolic) function.[104] This index is used increasingly to evaluate fetal ventricular function. Application of newer assessment techniques may yield better insight into fetal cardiac function.

4.6.3 *Impact of fetal echocardiography on fetal arrhythmias*

Evaluation of rate and variability of the fetal heartbeat presents an important and indispensable part of the fetal heart scan. One of the greatest impacts of fetal echocardiography is that it allows accurate identification of different types of arrhythmias, detection of possibly associated cardiac anomalies, assessment of the ventricular function, and monitoring of the fetal response to the medical therapy if required.[105]

Dysrhythmias can appear and progress throughout gestation either in isolation or in the presence of structural heart anomaly or primary myocardial disease. Employment of improved and new diagnostic modalities has significantly increased prenatal diagnosis of rhythm disturbances and our understanding of the electrophysiological events and mechanisms involved in it.[106] Correct description of the type of arrhythmia can be achieved using either M-mode, applied at the level of the four-chamber view, or pulsed Doppler sampling directed to the flow in the left ventricular inflow-outflow tract area, fetal superior vena cava-ascending aorta, the inferior vena cava-descending aorta and pulmonary artery and vein.[107] Regardless of which modality is used, analysis of cardiac rhythm is based on the capability to record atrial and ventricular contractions simultaneously.

Fetal M-mode imaging and pulse-wave Doppler echocardiography have become the most routinely used and useful modalities. Other sophisticated approaches to evaluating fetal arrhythmias have also been developed, such as fetal electrocardiography, magnetocardiography, or tissue Doppler velocity imaging which provides a fetal kinetocardiogram.[108–110]

Tissue Doppler velocity imaging is a relatively recently developed ultrasound-based technique, which uses high-frame-rate, four-chamber-view images for sampling atrial and ventricular wall motion. The tissue velocity data generates velocity curves that are used to analyze the temporal relationship between atrial and ventricular contractions.[109] All of these modalities can be used for evaluation of the atrioventricular (AV) interval, which is a surrogate for the PR interval on the ECG. Furthermore, evaluating fetuses at risk of fetal heart block, assessment of the AV interval during sinus rhythm is the only way to diagnose first-degree AV block. During tachycardia, measurement of AV and ventriculo-atrial (VA) intervals, and their temporal relationship, gives insight into the mechanisms of tachycardia.[107,111,112] Although each technique has advantages and limitations, they all give us a novel insight into the detection, identification and understanding of fetal arrhythmias, and offer additional assistance for studying the action and effects of antiarrhythmic drugs.

Fetal dysrhythmia, which can be present as an abnormality in rate (sustained tachy- or bradycardia), variability (irregular beats or extrasystoles), or as a combination of these, must be detected, evaluated and sometimes treated. Irregularities of fetal cardiac rhythm are common, but most of them are intermittent extrasystoles, which are clinically irrelevant.[74] Isolated ectopic beats, regardless of being atrial or ventricular, conducted or not, do not require any kind of treatment due to their self-limiting nature and spontaneous resolution. Isolated extrasystoles are not associated with fetal compromise, so these irregularities do not represent an indication for delivery, with a generally favorable prenatal and postnatal course.[113] Once the final diagnosis of fetal isolated ectopics is established, it allows for reassurance of families that the rhythm is benign, and subsequent follow-up can be done through routine care.[74] Nevertheless, there is a 1–2% risk of a tachyarrhythmia that might require fetal intervention, making evaluation of fetuses with cardiac dysrhythmias still worthwhile.[113]

Fetal echocardiography has provided additional characterization and specification of the natural course of both tachyarrhythmias and bradyarrhythmias. Less than 10% of observed dysrhythmias are due to sustained tachy- or bradyarrhythmias, which include supraventricular tachycardia (SVT), ventricular tachycardia, atrial flutter and complete atrioventricular (AV) block.[106] Some of those entities can be life-threatening, and the fact that they are potentially treatable means that precise prenatal diagnosis is essential for the selection of treatment. *In utero* medication of sustained fetal arrhythmias, which untreated can ultimately cause fetal hydrops and death, remains the main area of implementation of prenatal diagnosis. The effectiveness of prenatal treatment in conversion to sinus rhythm along with improved survival rate has been demonstrated, particularly in hydropic fetuses.[114] Required intrauterine anti-arrhythmic drugs are usually delivered to the fetus transplacentally, by giving the mother oral or intravenous treatment. In hydropic fetuses, ultrasound guidance has allowed different routes for direct fetal injection (e.g. intramuscular or intravenous into the umbilical cord).

Persistent fetal bradycardia requires further echocardiography evaluation and precise categorization regarding prognosis and possible treatment options. The differential diagnosis includes sinus bradycardia, atrial bradycardia, blocked atrial bigeminy, atrial flutter with high-degree block, and complete heart block.

Sinus bradycardia can be a manifestation of a fetal distress, even a preterminal fetus, and sinus node dysfunction. Rarely, this disturbance might be the single sign of long-QT syndrome, which raises the risk for ventricular tachycardia in affected fetuses and neonates.[115] Atrial bradycardia emerges evaluation for the cardiac and abdominal abnormalities commonly seen with polysplenia, while blocked atrial bigeminy requires only close observation.

Fetal AV block may develop at any period of gestation, when associated with structural heart disease. AV block is characterized by normal atrial activity and a disturbance of electrical conduction between atria and ventricles. Second- and third-degree AV block should be differentiated from blocked atrial bigeminy as management and prognosis differ. Although complete AV block is rare, it presents the most distinguishing marker of unfavorable fetal outcome. In most cases, progression to complete block is rapid and requires close monitoring, due to risk of cardiovascular compromise leading to hydrops fetalis or intrauterine death.[106] Evaluation of fetuses with complete atrioventricular block diagnosed prenatally showed that 50% of cases arise in the presence of complex structural heart abnormalities.[116] Most of these patients have a rather poor prognosis, with a significant mortality rate in the fetal or neonatal periods. Demises are related to the presence of structural heart defects, progressive heart failure and hydrops. Prenatal diagnosis of isolated complete congenital atrioventricular block is also associated with significant intrauterine mortality.[117] Isolated complete congenital atrioventricular block, as an acquired consequence of damaged fetal AV conduction tissue caused by transplacental passage of maternal anti-Ro or anti-La antibodies, makes up another 50% of cases. Given the high probability that this kind of damage requires a fetal immune response, this might predispose fetus for treatment with steroids or other methods of modifying the fetal immune response.[118,119]

Currently used prenatal therapy for bradycardia due to heart block is empirical. Although most of the attempts to reverse an already established block with transplacental steroid treatment have failed, one author has reported that treatment with fluorinated steroids has been associated with improved survival to one year of age, potentially as a consequence of a lesser risk of other immune-mediated complications.[120] Possible benefits are yet to be assessed over the side effects.[121] There is also some evidence of a favorable effect of therapy with beta-agonists in cases with very low heart rates although these agents do not reestablish a normal atrioventricular contraction sequence.[122] Further important consideration should include improved identification of fetuses suitable for prophylactic steroid treatment, with the purpose of preventing the generation of heart block. This could be achieved through measurement of atrioventricular conduction times using Doppler.[123] Although experience is limited, *in utero* ventricular pacing has not been beneficial for selected fetuses with complete atrioventricular block.[124]

Fetal echocardiography is a powerful tool for the assessment of cardiac structure and function when tachyarrhythmias are detected. *In utero* tachycardia requires prompt and detailed cardiac and obstetric evaluation. Without treatment, sustained fetal tachycardia causes serious morbidity leading to fetal heart failure, hydrops and finally fetal demise. In cases without obvious signs of heart failure, mortality risk is 0–4%, significantly increasing up to 27% in presence of hydrops fetalis.[114] Precise diagnosis of fetal tachycardia is a crucial prerequisite for successful treatment.[97,125] Following the establishment of the correct diagnosis, fetal echocardiography provides necessary information regarding the selection of appropriate *in utero* medical treatment, allows fetal monitoring and assessment of the efficacy of administered medications, can have an impact on delivery and provides for counseling of families regarding the expected pre- and postnatal course and long-term prognosis.

The vast majority of tachyarrhythmias are atrioventricular nodal re-entrant tachycardias. Atrial flutter is the second most common, and alternative types include sinus tachycardia, ventricular tachycardia and atrial fibrillation. Echocardiography and measurement of AV and VA time intervals is the conventional way by which the diagnosis and differential diagnosis are made. The timely detection and treatment of atrial flutter and supraventricular tachycardia have been shown to help prevent the occurrence of adverse outcomes in certain cases. Generally, there are three possible management approaches: (1) close monitoring without either medical therapy or prompt delivery, (2) anti-arrhythmic pharmacological therapy, and (3) immediate delivery. Expectant, close monitoring management can be considered for fetuses with intermittent tachycardia and no signs of hemodynamic compromise. Although not all fetuses will require the initiation of anti-arrhythmic drugs, or preterm delivery, this approach allows for it, if necessary. In cases of threatened congestive heart failure and consecutive fetal demise, the choice between immediate delivery or drug therapy should be based on factors like gestational age and lung maturity, the extent of fetal circulatory compromise, and available neonatal facilities for postnatal treatment.[106] Prenatal treatment decreases fetal mortality to 5–10%, with apparently reasonably low neurological sequelae.[114,126] For hydropic fetuses the rate of favorable perinatal outcome is directly related to prompt commencement of therapy and delivery close to term.

The selection of medication varies regarding the type and mechanism of the tachycardia, drug availability and experience with its use. The preferred route for drug administration is transplacental. The direct fetal route is a final resort reserved for the severe cases of tachycardia, accompanied with severe hydrops and placental edema. Although no preferences have been proved for any anti-arrhythmic drug, several agents are considered effective and relatively safe. Among these, digoxin has been frequently used as first-line therapy. Given to the mother, it will usually convert a reentry tachycardia or flutter. Sotalol may be more efficient in ectopic atrial tachycardia.[125,127] In the presence of fetal hydrops, digoxin is less effective because of diminished transplacental passage, and sotalol is commonly used instead. Other commonly used agents include flecainide and beta-blockers. It is important to inform the parents about possible risks and benefits of chosen treatment.

4.7 The Impact of Fetal Echocardiography — Delivery

In cases of major structural lesion, those with fetal heart failure, complete heart block and therapy non-responsive tachyarrhythmias, delivery should be planned at a tertiary care center, where required postnatal treatment can be achieved.[97] Minor problems, for example small muscular ventricular septal defects, can be delivered at the referring hospital.

Preterm delivery is almost never indicated in congenital heart disease. Exceptions could be therapy-resistant tachyarrhythmia with signs of progressive heart failure or heart block with heart failure. Even in those cases, cautious estimation must be undertaken regarding anticipated advantage of treating the neonate directly versus the disadvantage of preterm delivery. With few exceptions, vaginal delivery should remain the primary option in fetal congenital heart disease, as most babies are unlikely to experience problems until after delivery.[97] Exact timing of delivery is now less critical in ductal-dependent heart anomalies, which can be managed with prostaglandin infusions for the days before surgery.

Cesarean section could be indicated in some cases of fetal brady- or tachyarrhythmias, due to difficulties with intrapartum fetal heart rate monitoring. Considering the exact timing of delivery, elective Cesarean section may be advantageous in cases where immediate postnatal cardiac surgical or catheter interventions are required. One of the examples is total anomalous pulmonary venous return with severe obstruction to pulmonary venous flow, where heart surgery within hours of birth may be the sole option. In transposition of the great arteries with restrictive foramen ovale, and low saturations, prompt postnatal atrioseptostomy is important. But since the catheterization laboratory is not a prerequisite for this procedure, Cesarean birth is unnecessary for planning in advance.

4.8 The Impact of Fetal Echocardiography — What Can We Do for Affected Fetus/Neonates?

4.8.1 *Improvement of quality of care*

Dramatic evolution of congenital and pediatric cardiac surgery over the last decades is a result of improved understanding of the anatomy and physiology of the different cardiac anomalies, important advances in diagnostic modalities, significantly improved perioperative care, and improvement of perfusion, monitoring techniques and equipment. Significant technological improvements, the development of the heart-lung machine and the advances of surgical techniques have resulted in the capability to correct the substantial proportion of congenital cardiac anomalies with significantly improved outcomes. Over the years, the results have steadily improved, and patients previously facing either death or extremely decreased quality of life as a consequence of unrepaired congenital cardiac defect, now have a much better chance for a life of a satisfactory quality.

There is no doubt that prenatal diagnosis of congenital heart defects has deeply impacted obstetric and neonatal management of high-risk neonates, especially those in need of the immediate postnatal management. In neonates with ductal-dependent systemic circulation, it allows for prevention of postnatal shock from hypoxia or pulmonary overcirculation due to closure of the ductus arteriosus. Simultaneously, established prenatal diagnosis has allowed for better preoperative preparations of those patients. For example, pulmonary vascular resistance is responsive to both oxygen and carbon dioxide concentrations. Advanced ventilatory manipulation of pulmonary vascular resistance allows for a neonate not to require intubation to achieve the desired clinical parameters. Control of pulmonary blood flow has allowed optimal preparation of neonates before surgery.[128,129] Intraoperative improvements in attenuation of inflammatory response, myocardial protection, pH management, and postoperative advances regarding use of inhaled nitric oxide, extracorporal membrane oxygenation, as well as improvements in low cardiac output management also allow for better results.[129] Those simultaneous advances in a variety of medical subspecialties in the developed world has resulted in a decreased rate of overall mortality for pediatric congenital cardiac surgery to approximately 4%, which means that 96% of the children born with these challenging conditions are now surviving.[14,130]

4.8.2 *Impact on pediatric cardiology and cardiac surgery*

As already mentioned, there has been notable improvement in the short- and long-term outcomes of surgery for congenital heart diseases in neonates, due to the advances in pre-, intra- and postoperative care and techniques. Although our capabilities to treat most forms of CHD *in utero* are still limited, the majority of the heart defects can be treated postnatally by surgery or catheter intervention, with very low and constantly improving early mortality rates.[97] Reported data have shown that overall operative risks in specialized institutions have significantly decreased to 1.5–3%, and are still decreasing, reaching lower rates.[97,131] Reduced morbidity rate is also achieved. This trend is applicable even to serious forms of CHD, including the hypoplastic left heart syndrome, where contemporary developments in surgical treatment have resulted in a much more favorable early survival rate.[132,133] Although early mortality rates are of interest to parents counseled for CHD, the long term prognosis regarding late morbidity and mortality, need for re-operations or re-interventions, neurodevelopment, and anticipated quality of life may actually be even more important. With measurable improvements in postnatal care, long-term normal psychomotor development is an achievable reality in a substantial proportion of patients.

Despite the global reduction in required re-operations, specific rates depend on the type of the defect. Although diagnosed, some anomalies do not require any intervention, for example small ventricular septal defects. Transposition of the great arteries or pulmonary valve stenosis usually require only one surgical or catheter procedure. Even though technically demanding, the operation for transposition of the great arteries includes operative risk less than 10%, with excellent short-term and long-term results.[134] Examples of the defects that often require repeated re-operations are truncus arteriosus communis, and pulmonary atresia with ventricular septal defect. Management of aortic valve disease in children is still palliative, and commonly requires multiple re-operations, because of the lack of an ideal valve substitute. The Ross operation and its modifications, due to improved operative technical details, have satisfactory early results with operative risk less than 2%, but long-term results are not yet reassuring. Despite the newly applied improvements intended for prevention of unfavorable outcomes, whatever therapy is elected for those patients, the challenges to early and late optimal results are still noteworthy.[135] Although even recently pulmonary atresia with ventricular septal defect was frequently fatal, currently employed surgical technique allows some patients to have biventricular repair with physiologic normal circulation. As for long-term results this procedure is yet to be assessed. Good long-term treatment results can be achieved in most cases of isolated heart defects after a biventricular repair, even though some of those cases would later need re-operations.

The presence of one or two useful ventricles is the most critical anatomical factor influencing prognosis in congenital cardiac surgery. Most lesions with two adequate ventricles will now achieve satisfactory biventricular repair. Anomalies with only one well-developed ventricle (Figs. 4.17 and 4.18), such as tricuspid or pulmonary atresia or hypoplastic left heart syndrome, cannot be repaired to a biventricular circulation. Surgical treatment options for patients with hypoplastic left heart syndrome are limited to heart transplantation and staged reconstruction. The much more common staged reconstruction is comprised of a sequence of palliative operations leading to a Fontan circulation, providing long-term survival for nearly all forms of single-ventricle. Nevertheless, this palliative surgery requires multiple operations and, despite the improvements, still carries noticeable morbidity and even mortality. Due to the modification of the surgical technique, previously high operative mortality rate for staged reconstruction (Norwood procedure) decreased to less than 10%. The other two stages of reconstruction, the bidirectional Glenn and the Fontan procedures have a very low mortality rate.[129,136] Although short-term results are fairly good, long-term follow-up after the Fontan

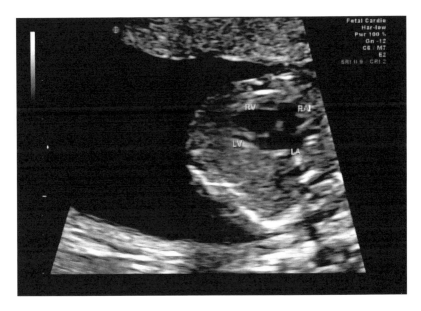

Fig. 4.17. Hypoplastic left heart.

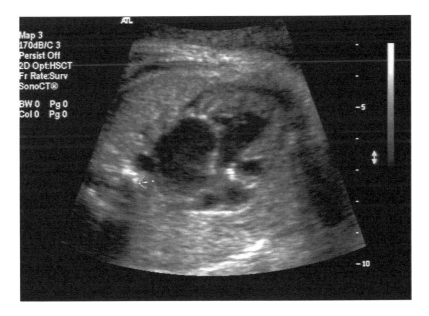

Fig. 4.18. Hypoplastic right ventricle.

operation has shown an appreciable rate of late complications and mortality and significantly compromised quality of life.[137] Long-term prognosis for pulmonary atresia with intact ventricular septum varies from an excellent two-ventricle repair to single-ventricle palliation. Some encouraging results have been published regarding the overall quality of life in children with pulmonary atresia and intact ventricular septum in both univentricular and a biventricular repair.[138]

Over the last 25 years, interventional procedures in neonates with congenital heart disease, used either as a supplemental or an alternative approach to surgical treatment have evolved dramatically. Although currently available procedures are in different stages of progress and achieve various rates of success, further improvements in both the instrumentation and techniques will eventually increase the proportion of favorable results. This includes interventions like dilatation of critical pulmonary and aortic valve stenosis, dilatation of postoperative aortic coarctation, atrial septostomy, coiling of aortopulmonary collaterals, endomyocardial biopsy, and pericardial drainage. The primary goal for these procedures is to provide stabilization and better condition of the neonates with complex heart disease before undergoing surgical repair, thus optimizing the outcome, decreasing the mortality rate of surgical procedures, and finally reducing the necessity for early surgery.

4.8.3 *Impact on fetal cardiac intervention*

The prenatal treatment options for fetal cardiac disease are still limited, and can be subdivided into the treatment of fetal tachyarrhythmias, fetal complete heart block and prenatal catheter interventions. Apart from prenatal detection of CHD, fetal echocardiography serves as a key tool in the identification of optimal candidates for *in utero* intervention and to guide the procedures.[19]

The natural course of some heart defects is to progress during pregnancy. In some cases of fetal valvular aortic stenosis, growth of left heart structures may be substantially impaired, resulting in the delivery of a neonate with hypoplastic left heart syndrome.[27,28] This can make postnatal biventricular repair impossible, and lead to the univentricular repair or heart transplantation as the only available options. Similarly, fetal pulmonary valve stenosis may advance during the course of pregnancy, to the degree of pulmonary atresia.[29,30] With the intent to prevent impaired ventricular growth and thus avoid postnatal univentricular surgical repair and consequently enable a probability of a biventricular repair, attempts have been made to balloon dilate the aortic or pulmonary valve in the fetus.[18,19,139,140] Although it was shown that timely and successful aortic valve dilation may result in normal ventricular anatomy and function at birth, the worldwide results of prenatal treatment with ultrasound-guided, transuterine, transthoracic balloon valvuloplasty of critical aortic stenosis were initially disappointing.[18,19] Despite some encouraging results achieved in very few selected cases with right heart obstructive lesions, those procedures require immense improvement in order to validate their feasibility and beneficial effect on increasing the chances of a biventricular repair in left or right heart obstructive disease.[139]

Apart from technical challenges inherent to this approach, considering the fact that these interventions carry a substantial maternal and fetal risk, the benefit/risk ratio must be carefully balanced. Improving results of the modified Norwood procedure makes these prenatal procedures even harder to justify. Timely identification of high-risk fetuses and anticipation of a progressive course of disease before significant hypoplasia of the affected ventricle occurs, remains one of the most critical issues. It appears that prenatal catheter intervention could also be used in a restrictive foramen ovale in fetal hypoplastic left heart syndrome.[141] While waiting for further improvement in patient selection, advances in fetoscopic systems, and in transcatheter techniques, another option is a careful anticipation of delivery with immediate postnatal intervention.[97,142,143] Still, if a two-ventricle outcome can be achieved, there may eventually be a benefit to prenatal interventions in selected cases.

4.9 Overall Effects of Fetal Echocardiography on CHD — Can We Do Better?

Fetal echocardiography may have diverse effects on both the birth incidence and the survival of CHD. Despite the fact that this imaging modality has allowed for recognition of different CHD prenatally, it may also result in a decrease in the birth incidence of particular types of severe congenital heart malformations. Namely, not all of the diagnosed fetuses will survive to term, because of two key reasons, i.e., natural development of the disease resulting in fetal demise and elective termination of pregnancy because of anticipated poor prognoses and currently limited treatment options.[30] Reported overall spontaneous intrauterine death rate in continuing pregnancies, after the diagnosis of a cardiac defect was 6–10%.[144] This risk is low in cases of isolated cardiac malformations, with sinus rhythm, good myocardial function and in the absence of noteworthy atrioventricular valve regurgitation. The risk of intrauterine demise significantly increases in the presence of associated malformations and chromosomal anomalies, myocardial dysfunction, severe atrioventricular valve regurgitation, concomitant brady- or tachyarrhythmia or fetal complete heart block.[116,127]

The rate of termination after a prenatal diagnosis of CHD varies between different countries and centers.[145] Gestational age at diagnosis and the coexistence of associated chromosomal and extracardiac anomalies are the most influential decision making factors.[6,54] The overall termination rate is around 50% after the diagnosis of a CHD before the gestational age limit for termination, with a higher rate in cases with early diagnosis of more severe types of defects and imminent risk of intrauterine progression.[63,144–146] Hypoplastic left heart syndrome and pulmonary atresia with intact ventricular septum are examples of decreased incidence at birth due to prenatal diagnosis.[30,63] A review of the EUROCAT database found that the average termination rate for hypoplastic left heart syndrome was 85% when diagnosed before 24 weeks of gestation, compared with 37% when diagnosed after 24 weeks of gestation, which is the legal termination limit for most of the countries.[145] Unfortunately, for some fully treatable heart anomalies with anticipated good long-term prognosis such as a transposition of the great arteries, the termination rate is also high.[145] As a consequence, multiple studies have confirmed the decline in the number of infants born with certain types of cardiac defects, particularly in those that essentially alter the four-chamber view projection. A choice to interrupt pregnancy may be additionally influenced by several different factors including current legislation, family structure and social and economical status, religion, different approaches to the counseling process and importantly, the results of treatment at the particular center. It appears that the effect of prenatally established diagnosis on birth incidence may differ in different settings.[41] For example, improved preoperative preparation of the critically ill neonates in the US is at least partially the consequence of achieved prenatal diagnosis.[129]

We have shown that prenatally diagnosed cases of CHD, with planned referral center delivery and anticipated prompt postnatal treatment, results in a superior survival chance than a comparable case with postnatally established diagnosis. But, despite this logical premise, the advantage of prenatal diagnosis has been surprisingly difficult to prove. A number of studies in prenatal series has proved a better neonatal preoperative status but, with respect to survival rates, similar or even a higher mortality rate was observed compared with postnatally diagnosed cases.[30,41,99,100] Several factors can affect these results. First, as the indications for fetal echocardiography include extracardiac malformations, chromosome defects and complex cardiac anomalies, the spectrum of CHD in prenatal series is substantially different than postnatal series. Another potentially important consideration is the tendency to a lower gestational age and weight at birth in prenatal diagnosis series, due to the planned induction of labor.[103] Additionally, most series with only postnatal diagnosis suffer selection bias by not including cases of intrauterine demises, neonates who died with or without established CHD diagnosis before reaching the referral center, and neonates considered unsuitable for cardiac surgery, thus providing improved mortality and morbidity rates.[105]

Nevertheless, the survival rate in more recent fetal series was significantly better, probably as a result of better postnatal management and increased recognition of less severe cases.[62,63] Importantly, studies specifically designed to identify the previously mentioned type of occult mortality have shown a favorable impact of prenatal diagnosis in mortality and morbidity in particular groups of CHD, such as hypoplastic left heart, transposition of the great arteries, and coarctation of the aorta.[15–17] The advantage of prenatal diagnosis is that it allows immediate cardiac assessment of the neonate and thus avoids late diagnosis after an infant has already developed severe circulatory compromise. Prenatal echocardiography has the remarkable potential to improve postnatal survival in ductal-dependent pulmonary or systemic circulation heart defects. With prenatally established diagnosis, life-saving prostaglandin therapy can be started in time, thereby avoiding the possibility of circulatory collapse and resuscitation when the arterial duct constricts within hours or days after birth. Prenatal diagnosis reduces the risk of death and neurological damages which can occur in neonates discharged home from the maternity ward undiagnosed.[15–17] Some previously untreatable prenatal cases now survive to term as a consequence of enhancement of prenatal treatment. Sustained supraventricular tachycardia is a good example for such severe abnormalities responsive to prenatal treatment.

With a constantly rising rate of early prenatal diagnosis of complex CHD, more and more of the complex forms of CHD, which are currently diagnosed and treated after birth, will just be seen *in utero*.[105] On the other hand, it is also possible that, over time, with improved treatment options and outcomes regarding long-term survival rates, neurologic development, and anticipated quality of life, the termination rate may go down, and the birth incidence may increase.

References

1. Ferencz C, Rubin JD, McCarter RJ, *et al.* (1985) Congenital heart disease: prevalence at livebirth. The Baltimore–Washington infant study. *Am J Epidemiol* 121: 31–36.
2. Centers for Disease Control and Prevention. (1998) Trends in infant mortality attributable to birth defects — United States, 1980–1995. *MMWR Morb Mortal Wkly Rep* 47: 773.
3. March of Dimes. (2001) Congenital Heart Defects. White Plains, NY: March of Dimes; Available at: http://www. marchofdimes.com/professionals/681_1212.asp.
4. Allan L, Benacerraf B, Copel JA, *et al.* (2001) Isolated major congenital heart disease. *Ultrasound Obstet Gynecol* 17: 370.
5. Hoffman JI, Kaplan S. (2002) The incidence of congenital heart disease. *J Am Coll Cardiol* 39: 1890.
6. Wimalasundera RC, Gardiner HM. (2004) Congenital heart disease and aneuploidy. *Prenat Diagn* 24: 1116–1122.
7. Grech V, Gatt M. (1999) Syndromes and malformations associated with congenital heart disease in population-based study. *Int J Cardiol* 68: 151.

8. Moore JW, Binder GA, Berry R. (2004) Prenatal diagnosis of aneuploidy and deletion 22q11.2 in fetuses with ultrasound detection of cardiac defects. *Am J Obstet Gynecol* 191: 2069.

9. Copel JA, Pilu G, Kleinman CS. (1986) Congenital heart disease and extracardiac anomalies; associations and indications for fetal echocardiography. *Am J Obstet Gynecol* 154: 1121.

10. Bromley B, Estroff JA, Sanders SP, *et al.* (1992) Fetal echocardiography: Accuracy and limitations in a population at high and low risk for heart defects. *Am J Obstet Gynecol* 166: 1473.

11. Smrcek JM, Berg C, Geipel A, *et al.* (2006). Detection rate of early fetal echocardiography and *in utero* development of congenital heart defects. *J Ultrasound Med* 25: 187.

12. Trines J, Hornberger LK. (2004) Evolution of heart disease *in utero. Pediatr Cardiol* 25: 287.

13. Maeno YV, Kamenir SA, Sinclair B, *et al.* (1999) Prenatal features of ductus arteriosus constriction and restrictive foramen ovale in d-transposition of the great arteries. *Circulation* 99: 1209–1214.

14. Tchervenkov CI, Jacobs JP, Bernier PL. (2008) The improvement of care for paediatric and congenital cardiac disease across the World: a challenge for the World Society for Pediatric and Congenital Heart Surgery. *Cardiol Young* 18: 63–69.

15. Bonnet D, Coltri A, Butera G, *et al.* (1999) Detection of transposition of the great arteries in fetuses reduces neonatal morbidity and mortality. *Circulation* 99: 916–918.

16. Tworetzky W, McElhinney DB, Reddy VM, *et al.* (2001) Improved surgical outcome after fetal diagnosis of hypoplastic left heart syndrome. *Circulation* 103: 1269–1273.

17. Franklin O, Burch M, Manning N, *et al.* (2002) Prenatal diagnosis of coarctation of the aorta improves survival and reduces morbidity. *Heart* 87: 67–69.

18. Tworetzky W, Wilkins-Haug L, Jennings RW, *et al.* (2004) Balloon dilation of severe aortic stenosis in the fetus: potential for prevention of hypoplastic left heart syndrome: candidate selection, technique, and results of successful intervention. *Circulation* 110: 2125.

19. Kohl T, Sharland G, Allan LD, *et al.* (2000) World experience of percutaneous ultrasound-guided balloon valvuloplasty in human fetuses with severe aortic valve obstruction. *Am J Cardiol* 85: 1230–1233.

20. Jaeggi ET, Fouron JC, Silverman ED, *et al.* (2004a) Transplacental fetal treatment improves the outcome of prenatally diagnosed complete atrioventricular block without structural heart disease. *Circulation* 110: 1542.

21. Makikallio K, McElhinney DB, Levine JC, *et al.* (2006) Fetal aortic valve stenosis and the evolution of hypoplastic left heart syndrome: patient selection for fetal intervention. *Circulation* 113: 1401.

22. Galindo A, Gutierrez-Larraya F, Velasco JM, *et al.* (2006) Pulmonary balloon valvuloplasty in a fetus with critical pulmonary stenosis/atresia with intact ventricular septum and heart failure. *Fetal Diagn Ther* 21: 100.

23. Kovalchin JP, Silverman NH. (2004) The impact of fetal echocardiography. *Pediatr Cardiol* 25: 299–306.

24. Yagel S, Weissman A, Rotstein Z, *et al.* (1997) Congenital heart defects: natural course and *in utero* development. *Circulation* 96: 550–555.

25. Allan LD, Sharland GK, Tynan MJ. (1989) The natural history of the hypoplastic left heart syndrome. *Int J Cardiol* 25: 343–346.

26. Hornberger LK, Benacerraf BR, Bromley BS, *et al.* (1991) Prenatal detection of severe right ventricular outflow tract obstruction: pulmonary stenosis and pulmonary atresia. *J Ultrasound Med* 13: 743–750.

27. Hornberger LK, Sanders SP, Rein AJ, *et al.* (1995a) Left heart obstructive lesions and left ventricular growth in the midtrimester fetus. A longitudinal study. *Circulation* 92: 1531–1538.

28. Simpson JM, Sharland GK. (1997) Natural history and outcome of aortic stenosis diagnosed prenatally. *Heart* 77: 205–210.

29. Todros T, Paladini D, Chiappa E, *et al.* (2003) Pulmonary stenosis and atresia with intact ventricular septum during prenatal life. *Ultrasound Obstet Gynecol* 21: 228–233.

30. Daubeney PE, Sharland GK, Cook AC, *et al.* (1998) Pulmonary atresia with intact ventricular septum: impact of fetal echocardiography on incidence at birth and postnatal outcome. UK and Eire Collaborative Study of Pulmonary Atresia with Intact Ventricular Septum. *Circulation* 98: 562–566.

31. Hornberger LK, Sanders SP, Sahn DJ, *et al.* (1995b) *In utero* pulmonary artery and aortic growth and potential for progression of pulmonary outflow tract obstruction in tetralogy of Fallot. *J Am Coll Cardiol* 25: 739–745.

32. Paladini D, Palmieri S, Lamberti A, *et al.* (2000) Characterization and natural history of ventricular septal defects in the fetus. *Ultrasound Obstet Gynecol* 16: 118–122.

33. Weber H, Kleinman C, Hellenbrand W, *et al.* (1988) Development of a benign intrapericardial tumor between 20 and 40 weeks of gestation. *Pediatr Cardiol* 9: 153.

34. Nir A, Ekstein S, Nadjari M, *et al.* (2001) Rhabdomyoma in the fetus: illustration of tumor growth during the second half of gestation. *Pediatr Cardiol* 22: 515–518.

35. International Society of Ultrasound in Obs/Gyn. (2006) Cardiac screening examination of the fetus: Guidelines for performing the "basic" and the "extend basic" cardiac scan. *Ultrasound Obstet Gynecol* 27: 107–113.

36. Garne E, Stoll C, Clementi M. (2001) Euroscan group evaluation of prenatal diagnosis of congenital heart disease by ultrasound: experience from 20 European registries. *Ultrasound Obstet Gynecol* 17: 386.

37. Heide H, Thomson J, Wharton G, *et al.* (2004) Poor sensitivity of routine fetal anomaly ultrasound screening for antenatal detection of atrioventricular septal defect. *Heart* 90: 916.

38. Tegnander E, Eik-Nes S. (2006) The examiner's ultrasound experience has a significant impact on the detection rate of congenital heart defects at the second-trimester fetal examination. *Ultrasound Obstet Gynecol* 28: 8.

39. Dorfman AT, Marino BS, Wernovsky G, *et al.* (2008) Critical heart disease in the neonate: presentation and outcome at a tertiary care center. *Pediatr Crit Care Med* 9(2): 193–202.

40. Crane JP, LeFevre ML, Winborn RC, *et al.* (1994) A randomized trial of prenatal ultrasonographic screening: impact on the detection, management, and outcome of anomalous fetuses. The RADIUS Study Group. *Am J Obstet Gynecol* 171: 392–399.

41. Montana E, Khoury MJ, Cragan JD, *et al.* (1996) Trends and outcomes after prenatal diagnosis of congenital cardiac malformations by fetal echocardiography in a well defined birth population, Atlanta, Georgia, 1990–1994. *J Am Coll Cardiol* 28: 1805.

42. Todros T, Faggiano F, Chiappa E, *et al.* (1997) Accuracy of routine ultrasonography in screening heart disease prenatally. Gruppo Piemontese for Prenatal Screening of Congenital Heart Disease. *Prenatal Diagn* 17: 901–906.

43. Jaeggi ET, Sholler GF, Jones OD, *et al.* (2001) Comparative analysis of pattern, management and outcome of pre- versus postnatally diagnosed major congenital heart disease: a population-based study. *Ultrasound Obstet Gynecol* 17: 380.

44. DeVore GR. (1998) Influence of prenatal diagnosis on congenital heart defects. *Ann NY Acad* 847: 46–52.

45. Todros T. (2000) Prenatal diagnosis and management of fetal cardiovascular malformations. *Curr Opin Obstet Gynecol* 12: 105–109.

46. Lee W, Allan L, Carvalho JS, *et al.* (2008) ISUOG consensus statement: what constitutes a fetal echoradiogram? *Ultrasound Obstet Gynecol* 32: 239–242.

47. Allan LD. (2003) Cardiac anatomy screening: when is the best time for screening in pregnancy? *Curr Opin Obstet Gynecol* 15: 143.

48. Souka AP, Pilalis A, Kavalakis I, *et al.* (2006) Screening for major structural abnormalities at the 11- to 14-week ultrasound scan. *Am J Obstet Gynecol* 194: 393.

49. Carvalho JS. (2004a) Fetal heart scanning in the first trimester. *Prenat Diagn* 24: 1060–1067.

50. Huggon IC, Ghi T, Cook AC, *et al.* (2002) Fetal cardiac abnormalities identified prior to 14 weeks' gestation. *Ultrasound Obstet Gynecol* 20: 22–29.

51. Hyett JA, Perdu M, Sharland GK, *et al.* (1997) Increased nuchal translucency at 10–14 weeks of gestation as a marker for major cardiac defects. *Ultrasound Obstet Gynecol* 10: 242–246.

52. Hyett J, Perdu M, Sharland G, *et al.* (1999) Using fetal nuchal translucency to screen for major congenital cardiac defects at 10–14 weeks of gestation: population based cohort study. *BMJ* 318: 81.

53. Devine PC, Simpson LL. (2000) Nuchal translucency and its relationship to congenital heart disease. *Sem Perinatol* 24: 343–351.

54. Carvalho JS, Moscoso G, Tekay A, *et al.* (2004b) Clinical impact of first and early second trimester fetal echocardiography on high risk pregnancies. *Heart* 90: 921.

55. Stoll C, Dott B, Alembik Y, *et al.* (2002) Evaluation and evolution during time of prenatal diagnosis of congenital heart diseases by routine fetal ultrasonographic examination. *Ann Genet* 45: 21–27.

56. Gill HK, Splitt M, Sharland GK, *et al.* (2003) Patterns of recurrence of congenital heart disease: an analysis of 6640 consecutive pregnancies evaluated by detail fetal echocardiography. *J Am Coll Cardiol* 42: 923.

57. Small M, Copel JA. (2004) Indications for fetal echocardiography. *Pediatr Cardiol* 25: 210.

58. Wright VC, Chang J, Jeng G, *et al.* (2008) Centers for Disease Control and Prevention (CDC). Assisted reproductive technology surveillance — United States, 2005. *MMWR Surveill Summ* 57: 1–23.

59. Reefhuis J, Honein MA, Schieve LA, *et al.* (2009) National Birth Defects Prevention Study. Assisted reproductive technology and major structural birth defects in the United States. *Hum Reprod* 24(2): 360–366.

60. Manning A, Archer N. (2006) A study to determine the incidence of structural congenital heart disease in monochorionic twins. *Prenatal Diagn* 26(11): 1062–1064.

61. Stumpflen I, Stumpflen A, Wimmer M, *et al.* (1996) Effect of detailed fetal echocardiography as part of routine prenatal ultrasonographic screening on detection of congenital heart disease. *Lancet* 348: 854–857.

62. Allan LD. (2000) A practical approach to fetal heart scanning. *Sem Perinatol* 24: 324–330.

63. Allan LD, Sharland GK, Milburn A, *et al.* (1994) Prospective diagnosis of 1006 consecutive cases of congenital heart disease in the fetus. *J Am Coll Cardiol* 23: 1452–1458.

64. American Institute of Ultrasound in Medicine. (2007) Practice guideline for the performance of obstetric ultrasound examinations. Available at: http://www.aium.org/publications/guidelines.aspx.

65. American College of Obstetricians and Gynecologists. (2009) ACOG Practice Bulletin. Ultrasonography in pregnancy. *Obstet Gynecol* 113: 451–461.

66. Allan LD, Crawford DC, Chita SK, *et al.* (1986) Prenatal screening for congenital heart disease. *Br Med J (Clin Res Ed)* 292: 1717.

67. Copel JA, Pilu G, Green J, *et al.* (1987) Fetal echocardiographic screening for congenital heart disease. The importance of the four-chamber view. *Am J Obstet Gynecol* 157: 648.

68. Chaoui R. (2003) The four-chamber view: four reasons why it seems to fail in screening for cardiac abnormalities and suggestions to improve detection rate. *Ultrasound Obstet Gynecol* 22: 3–10.

69. DeVore GR. (1992) The aortic and pulmonary outflow tract screening examination in the human fetus. *J Ultrasound Med* 11: 345.

70. Yagel S, Cohen SM, Achiron R. (2001) Examination of the fetal heart by five short-axis views: a proposed screening method for comprehensive cardiac evaluation. *Ultrasound Obstet Gynecol* 17: 367.

71. Allan L, Dangel J, Fessolva V, *et al.* (2004) Recommendations for the practice of fetal cardiology in Europe. Developed by the Fetal Cardiology Working Group of the Association for European Pediatric Cardiology. *Cardiol Young* 14: 109–114.

72. Lee W. American Institute of Ultrasound in Medicine. (1998) Performance of the basic fetal cardiac ultrasound examination. *J Ultrasound Med* 17: 601–607. Erratum in *J Ultrasound Med* 17: 796.

73. Carvalho JS, Mavrides E, Shinebourne EA, *et al.* (2002) Improving the effectiveness of routine prenatal screening for major congenital heart defects. *Heart* 88: 387–391.

74. Copel JA, Liang RI, Demasio K, *et al.* (2000) The clinical significance of the irregular fetal heart rhythm. *Am J Obstet Gynecol* 182: 813–817.

75. Yoo S-J, Lee Y-H, Kim ES, *et al.* (1997) Three-vessel view of the fetal upper mediastinum: an easy means of detecting abnormalities of the ventricular outflow tracts and great arteries during obstetric screening. *Ultrasound Obstet Gynecol* 173–182.

76. Yoo S-J, Lee Y-H, Cho KS. (1999a) Abnormal three-vessel view on sonography: a clue to the diagnosis of congenital heart disease in the fetus. *AJR Am J Roentgenol* 172: 825–830.

77. Yagel S, Arbel R, Anteby EY, *et al.* (2002) The three vessels and trachea view (3VT) in fetal cardiac scanning. *Ultrasound Obstet Gynecol* 20: 340–345.

78. Meyer-Wittkopf M, Cooper S, Sholler G. (2001) Correlation between fetal cardiac diagnosis by obstetric and pediatric cardiologist sonographers and comparison with postnatal findings. *Ultrasound Obstet Gynecol* 17: 392–397.

79. Berkley EM, Goens MB, Karr S, *et al.* (2009) Utility of fetal echocardiography in postnatal management of infants with prenataly diagnosed congenital heart disease. *Prenatal Diagn* DOI: 10.1002/pd.2260.

80. Vinals F, Tapia J, Giuliano A. (2002) Prenatal detection of ductal-dependent congenital heart disease: how can things be made easier? *Ultrasound Obstet Gynecol* 19: 246–249.

81. Starikov RS, Bsat FA, Knee A, *et al.* (2009) Utility of fetal echocardiography after normal cardiac imaging findings on detailed fetal anatomic ultrasonography. *J Ultrasound Med* 28: 603–608.

82. Carvalho JS, Ho SY, Shinebourne EA. (2005) Sequential segmental analysis in complex fetal cardiac abnormalities: a logical approach to diagnosis. *Ultrasound Obstet Gynecol* 26: 105–111.

83. Yoo SJ, Lee YH, Cho KS, *et al.* (1999b) Sequential segmental approach to fetal congenital heart disease. *Cardiol Young* 9: 430.

84. Axt-Fliedner R, Diler S, Georg T, *et al.* (2004a) Reference values of ductus venosus blood flow velocities and waveform indices from 10 to 20 weeks' gestation. *Arch Gynecol Obstet* 269: 199–204.

85. Axt-Fliedner R, Wiegank U, Fetsch C, *et al.* (2004b) Reference values of fetal ductus venosus, inferior vena cava and hepatic vein blood flow velocities and waveform indices during the second and third trimester of pregnancy. *Arch Gynecol Obstet* 270: 46–55.

86. DeVore GR. (2005) Assessing fetal cardiac ventricular function. *Semin Fetal Neonatal Med* 10: 515–541.

87. Larsen LU, Petersen OB, Norrild K, *et al.* (2006) Strain rate derived for color Doppler myocardial imaging for assessment of fetal cardiac function. *Ultrasound Obstet Gynecol* 27: 210–213.

88. Baez E, Steinhard J, Huber A, *et al.* (2005) Ductus venosus Blood Flow Velocity Waveforms as a Predictor for Fetal Outcome in Isolated Congenital Heart Disease. *Fetal Diagn Ther* 20: 383–389.

89. Bianco K, Small M, Julien S, *et al.* (2006) Second-trimester ductus venosus measurement and adverse perinatal outcome in fetuses with congenital heart disease. *J Ultrasound Med* 25: 979–982.

90. DeVore GR, Falkensammer P, Sklansky MS, *et al.* (2003) Spatiotemporal image correlation (STIC): a new technology for evaluation of the fetal heart. *Ultrasound Obstet Gynecol* 22: 380–387.

91. Goncalves LF, Lee W, Chaiworapongsa T, *et al.* (2003) Four-dimensional ultrasongraphy of the fetal heart with spatiotemporal image correlation. *Am J Obstet Gynecol* 189: 1792–1802.

92. Chaoui R, Hoffmann J, Heling KS. (2004) Three-dimensional (3D) and 4D color Doppler fetal echocardiography using spatio-temporal image correlation (STIC). *Ultrasound Obstet Gynecol* 23: 535.

93. Paladini D, Vassallo M, Sglavo G, *et al.* (2006) The role of spatio-temporal image correlation (STIC) with tomographic ultrasound imaging (TUI) in the sequential analysis of fetal congenital heart disease. *Ultrasound Obstet Gynecol* 27: 555.

94. DeVore GR, Polanco B, Sklansky MS, *et al.* (2004) The "spin" technique: A new method for examination of the fetal outflow tracts using three-dimensional ultrasound. *Ultrasound Obstet Gynecol* 24: 72.

95. Sklansky M, Miller D, DeVore G, *et al.* (2005) Prenatal screening for congenital heart disease using real-time three-dimensional echocardiography

and a novel "sweep volume" acquisition technique. *Ultrasound Obstet Gynecol* 25: 435.

96. Abuhamad A. (2004) Automated multiplanar imaging: a novel approach to ultrasonography. *J Ultrasound Med* 23: 573.

97. Mellander M. (2005) Perinatal management, counselling and outcome of fetuses with congenital heart disease. *Semin Fetal Neonatal Med* 10: 586–593.

98. Delisle MF, Sandor GG, Tessier F, *et al.* (1999) Outcome of fetuses diagnosed with atrioventricular septal defect. *Obstet Gynecol* 94: 763–767.

99. Eapen RS, Rowland DG, Franklin WH. (1998) Effect of prenatal diagnosis of critical left heart obstruction on perinatal morbidity and mortality. *Am J Perinatol* 15: 237–242.

100. Kumar RK, Newburger JW, Gauvreau K, *et al.* (1999) Comparison of outcome when hypoplastic left heart syndrome and transposition of the great arteries are diagnosed prenatally versus when diagnosis of these two conditions is made only postnatally. *Am J Cardiol* 83: 1649–1653.

101. Verheijen PM, Lisowski LA, Stoutenbeek P, *et al.* (2001) Prenatal diagnosis of congenital heart disease affects preoperative acidosis in the newborn patient. *J Thorac Cardiovasc Surg* 121: 798–803.

102. Mahle WT, Clancy RR, McGaurn SP, *et al.* (2001) Impact of prenatal diagnosis on survival and early neurologic morbidity in neonates with the hypoplastic left heart syndrome. *Pediatrics* 107: 1277–1282.

103. Copel JA, Tan AS, Kleinman CS. (1997) Does a prenatal diagnosis of congenital heart disease alter short-term outcome? *Ultrasound Obstet Gynecol* 10: 237–241.

104. Friedman D, Buyon J, Kim M, *et al.* (2003) Fetal cardiac function assessed by Doppler myocardial performance index (Tei Index). *Ultrasound Obstet Gynecol* 21: 33–36.

105. Chiappa E. (2007) The impact of prenatal diagnosis of congenital heart disease on pediatric cardiology and cardiac surgery. *Cardiovasc Med* 8: 12–16.

106. Api O and Carvalho JS. (2008) Fetal dysrhythmias. *Best Prac Res Clin Obstet Gynaecol* 22: 31–48.

107. Carvalho JS, Prefumo F, Ciardelli V, *et al.* (2007) Evaluation of fetal arrhythmias from simultaneous pulsed wave Doppler in pulmonary artery and vein. *Heart* 93: 1448–1453.

108. Quartero HW, Stinstra JG, Golbach EG, *et al.* (2002) Clinical implications of fetal magnetocardiography. *Ultrasound Obstet Gynecol* 20: 142–153.

109. Rein A, O'Donnell C, Geva T, *et al.* (2002) Use of tissue velocity imaging in the diagnosis of fetal cardiac arrhythmias. *Circulation* 106: 1827–1833.

110. Taylor MJ, Smith MJ, Thomas M, *et al.* (2003) Non-invasive fetal electrocardiography in singleton and multiple pregnancies. *Br J Obstet Gynaecol* 110: 668–678.

111. Glickstein JS, Buyon J, Friedman D. (2000) Pulsed Doppler echocardiographic assessment of the fetal PR interval. *Am J Cardiol* 86: 236–239.

112. Fouron JC, Fournier A, Proulx F, *et al.* (2003) Management of fetal tachyarrhythmia based on superior vena cava/aorta Doppler flow recordings. *Heart* 89: 1211–1216.

113. Simpson JL, Yates RW, Sharland GK. (1996) Irregular heart rate in the fetus: not always benign. *Cardiol Young* 6: 28–31.

114. Simpson JM, Sharland GK. (1998) Fetal tachycardia: management and outcome of 127 consecutive cases. *Heart* 79: 576–581.

115. Beinder E, Grancay T, Menendez T, *et al.* (2001) Fetal sinus bradycardia and the long QT syndrome. *Am J Obstet Gynecol* 185: 743–747.

116. Schmidt KG, Ulmer HE, Silverman NH, *et al.* (1991) Perinatal outcome of fetal complete atrioventricular block: a multicenter experience. *J Am Coll Cardiol* 17: 1360–1366.

117. Jaeggi ET, Hamilton RM, Silverman ED, *et al.* (2002) Outcome of children with fetal, neonatal or childhood diagnosis of isolated congenital atrioventricular block. A single institution's experience of 30 years. *J Am Coll Cardio* 39: 130–137.

118. Groves AM, Allan LD, Rosenthal E. (1995) Therapeutic trial of sympathomimetics in three cases of complete heart block in the fetus. *Circulation* 92: 3394–3396.

119. Groves AM, Allan LD, Rosenthal E. (1996) Outcome of isolated congenital complete heart block diagnosed *in utero*. *Heart* 75: 190–194.

120. Jaeggi ET, Silverman ED, Yoo SJ, *et al.* (2004b) Is immunemediated complete fetal atrioventricular block reversible by transplacental dexamethasone therapy? *Ultrasound Obstet Gynecol* 23: 602–605.

121. Costedoat-Chalumeau N, Amoura Z, Le Thi Hong D, *et al.* (2003) Questions about dexamethasone use for the prevention of anti-SSA related congenital heart block. *Ann Rheum Dis* 62: 1010–1012.

122. Robinson BV, Ettedgui JA, Sherman FS. (2001) Use of terbutaline in the treatment of complete heart block in the fetus. *Cardiol Young* 11: 683–686.

123. Sonesson SE, Salomonsson S, Jacobsson LA, *et al.* (2004) Signs of first-degree heart block occur in one-third of fetuses of pregnant women with anti-SSA/Ro 52-kd antibodies. *Arthritis Rheum* 50: 1253–1261.

124. Carpenter Jr RJ, Strasburger JF, Garson Jr A, *et al.* (1986) Fetal ventricular pacing for hydrops secondary to complete atrioventricular block. *J Am Coll Cardiol* 8: 1434–1436.

125. Fouron JC. (2004) Fetal arrhythmias: the Saint-Justine hospital experience. *Prenat Diagn* 24: 1068–1080.

126. Oudijk MA, Gooskens RH, Stoutenbeek P, *et al.* (2004) Neurological outcome of children who were treated for fetal tachycardia complicated by hydrops. *Ultrasound Obstet Gynecol* 24: 154–158.

127. Krapp M, Kohl T, Simpson JM, *et al.* (2003) Review of diagnosis, treatment, and outcome of fetal atrial flutter compared with supraventricular tachycardia. *Heart* 89: 913–917.

128. Day RS, Tani LY, Minich LL, *et al.* (1995) Congenital heart disease with ductal-dependent systemic perfusion: doppler ultrasonography flow velocities are altered by changes in the fraction of inspired oxygen. *J Heart Lung Transplant* 14: 718–725.

129. el-Zein C, Ilbawi MN. (2008) Recent advances in neonatal cardiac surgery. *World J Surg* 32: 340–345.

130. Jacobs JP, Wernovsky G, Elliott MJ. (2007) Analysis of outcomes for congenital cardiac disease: can we do better? *Cardiol Young* 17: 145–158.

131. Lundstrom NR, Berggren H, Bjorkhem G, *et al.* (2000) Centralization of pediatric heart surgery in Sweden. *Pediatr Cardiol* 21: 353–357.

132. Mair R, Tulzer G, Sames E, *et al.* (2003) Right ventricular to pulmonary artery conduit instead of modified Blalock-Taussig shunt improves postoperative hemodynamics in newborns after the Norwood operation. *J Thorac Cardiovasc Surg* 126: 1378–1384.

133. Pizarro C, Malec E, Maher KO, *et al.* (2003) Right ventricle to pulmonary artery conduit improves outcome after stage I Norwood for hypoplastic left heart syndrome. *Circulation* 108: II155–160.

134. Rehnstrom P, Gilljam T, Sudow G, *et al.* (2003) Excellent survival and low complication rate in medium-term follow-up after arterial switch operation for complete transposition. *Scand Cardiovasc J* 37: 104–106.

135. Mavroudis C, Backer CL, Kaushal S. (2009) Aortic stenosis and aortic insufficiency in children: impact of valvuloplasty and modified Ross-Konno procedure. *Semin Thorac Cardiovasc Surg Pediatr Card Surg Annu* 76–86.

136. Tweddell JS, Hoffman GM, Fedderly RT, *et al.* (2000) Patients at risk for low systemic oxygen delivery after the Norwood procedure. *Ann Thorac Surg* 69: 1893–1899.

137. van den Bosch AE, Roos-Hesselink JW, Van Domburg R, *et al.* (2004) Long-term outcome and quality of life in adult patients after the Fontan operation. *Am J Cardiol* 93: 1141–1145.

138. Ekman-Joelsson BM, Berntsson L, Sunnegardh J. (2004) Quality of life in children with pulmonary atresia and intact ventricular septum. *Cardiol Young* 14: 615–621.

139. Tulzer G, Arzt W, Franklin RC, *et al.* (2002) Fetal pulmonary valvuloplasty for critical pulmonary stenosis or atresia with intact septum. *Lancet* 360: 1567–1568.

140. Arzt W, Tulzer G, Aigner M, *et al.* (2003) Invasive intrauterine treatment of pulmonary atresia/intact ventricular septum with heart failure. *Ultrasound Obstet Gynecol* 21: 186–188.

141. Marshall AC, van der Velde ME, Tworetzky W, *et al.* (2004) Creation of an atrial septal defect in utero for fetuses with hypoplastic left heart syndrome and intact or highly restrictive atrial septum. *Circulation* 110: 253–258.

142. Meyer-Wittkopf M. (2002) Interventional fetal therapy: possible perspective and current shortcomings. *Ultrasound Obstet Gynecol* 20: 527–531.

143. Chiappa E, Bouslenko Z, Todros T, *et al.* (2003) Postnatal management of critical aortic stenosis in the fetus: an alternative to *in utero* treatment. *Cardiol Young* 13: 46.

144. Brick DH, Allan LD. (2002) Outcome of prenatally diagnosed congenital heart disease: an update. *Pediatr Cardiol* 23: 449–453.

145. Garne E, Loane M, Dolk H, *et al.* (2005) Prenatal diagnosis of severe structural congenital malformations in Europe. *Ultrasound Obstet Gynecol* 25: 6–11.

146. Bull C, on behalf of the British Pediatric Cardiac Association. (1999) Current and potential impact of fetal diagnosis on the prevalence and spectrum of serious congenital heart disease at term. *Lancet* 354: 1242–1247.

Chapter 5

Imaging the Newborn Brain

Christopher T. Whitlow* and T. Michael O'Shea[†]

Ultrasound is the most frequently used method for imaging the brain of neonates. Unlike computerized tomography and magnetic resonance imaging, ultrasonography does not require moving the infant out of the neonatal intensive care unit. Important clinical uses of ultrasound include screening, diagnosis, and prognosis. In the first week of life, ultrasound can be used to detect intraventricular hemorrhage in preterm infants. After an intraventricular hemorrhage is diagnosed, ultrasound can be used to monitor changes in ventricular size over time.[1] Close to the time of discharge from neonatal intensive care, ultrasound can provide prognostic information useful for parents, neonatologists, and rehabilitative specialists. The sensitivity of ultrasound for detection of brain lesions other than intraventricular hemorrhage and ventricular enlargement is lower than that of magnetic resonance imaging.[2–4] In this chapter, we will review the clinical utility of both cranial ultrasound and magnetic resonance imaging, with a focus on the care of neonates. We will not discuss computerized tomography, which is used less frequently than either ultrasound or magnetic resonance imaging.

---

*Department of Radiology (Neuroradiology), Wake Forest University School of Medicine.
[†]Department of Pediatrics (Neonatology), Wake Forest University School of Medicine.

5.1 Ultrasound

5.1.1 *Historical aspects*

Brain ultrasound was first described in the medical literature during the 1960s,[5] but the first reports involving preterm neonates appeared in the late 1970s, when Pape[6] and Slovis[7] reported on the use of real-time linear array and sector scanning to detect intraventricular and parenchymal hemorrhage, and ventricular enlargement. Within a few years of these initial descriptions, ultrasonography became a routine procedure for very low birth weight neonates and other high risk groups. The rationale is that the prevalence of abnormalities among certain groups of neonates (e.g. very low birth weight infants) is substantial, even in the absence of symptoms suggestive of intracranial hemorrhage.[8–10] Further, ultrasonography is portable and noninvasive and involves no radiation exposure.

In the 1980s, an increasing number of longitudinal follow-up studies of very low birth weight and very preterm infants included brain ultrasound findings as a risk factor of interest,[11,12] and cohort studies were initiated to relate ultrasound findings to neurodevelopmental outcome.[13–19] Among the most influential reports was that by Papile and her colleagues who described four grades of cerebral intraventricular hemorrhage,[8] and an association between increasing grade of hemorrhage and increasing probability of an adverse neurodevelopmental outcome.[20] Of particular significance was Papile grade 4 intraventricular hemorrhage, referring to echodensity in the brain parenchyma superolateral to the lateral ventricles. Studies of infants with this lesion have consistently identified a high risk of adverse outcome.[21–26] By the late 1980s, it was apparent that even more predictive of neurodevelopmental impairment was echolucency in the brain parenchyma,[27] a marker of cerebral white matter damage[28,29] that tends to appear later in life than echodensities.[19,28,30] Serial ultrasonography of preterm infants revealed that parenchymal echodensity can be a transient finding.[31–34] These observations led to a change in clinical practice and research prototcols whereby ultrasounds were obtained not only in the first two weeks of life, when almost all cases of intraventricular hemorrhage can be diagnosed, but also after the first two weeks, when echolucency might be detected for the first time.[19,35–37]

Also during the 1980s, it was recognized that ventricular enlargement could result either from obstruction to cerebrospinal fluid flow after intraventricular hemorrhage (i.e. post-hemorrhage hydrocephalus) or from white matter necrosis.[38] Thus ventricular enlargement, in addition to periventricular (parenchymal) echolucency, was identified as a brain ultrasound indicator of white matter damage.[38,39]

Once the prognostic importance of brain ultrasound abnormalities was recognized, applications of ultrasonography broadened beyond solely clinical uses. Over the past two decades, brain ultrasound has been used extensively in epidemiological studies of neonatal brain injury[11,26,40–54] and clinical trials.[55–58] For some trials, ultrasound abnormalities were the outcomes of primary interest.[59–62] Despite the advent of magnetic resonance imaging, brain ultrasound remains an essential component of medical care in neonatal intensive care unit.

Prior to the development of brain ultrasound, prediction of infant developmental outcome was based primarily on neonatal morbidities and indicators of social and environmental risk. Within a few years after the first description of neonatal brain ultrasonography, this procedure became an important source of prognostic information that has been used to prioritize and guide efforts to optimize infant developmental outcome.[1,63]

5.1.2 *Technical aspects of neonatal brain ultrasound*

In neonates, ultrasound images are collected through the open fontanelles (i.e. the "acoustic windows") using high frequency sound (5–10 MHz). The ultrasound probe detects sound that is reflected by tissues and takes advantage of differences in *acoustic impedance* — analogous to "acoustic density" — between tissues. Differences in "echogenicity" or "echodensity" between tissues make possible the detection of anatomic structures, hemorrhage and fluid collections, such as the cerebral ventricles. For example, cerebrospinal fluid is hypoechoic and appears black on ultrasound images, whereas bone is hyperechoic and appears white (Fig. 5.1). An important clinical use of ultrasound is the assessment of ventricular size, as discussed later (Section 5.1.6).

The anterior fontanelle is the most widely used acoustic window for routine ultrasound screening and provides good visualization of the head

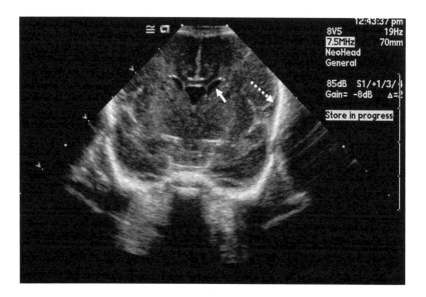

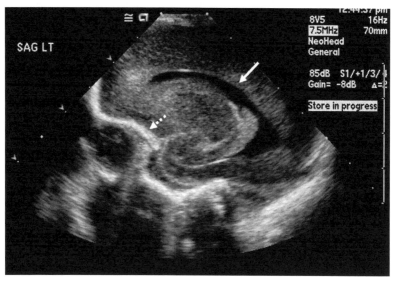

Fig. 5.1. The top picture is a coronal projection, and the bottom picture is a sagittal projection. In both pictures, the dashed arrow points to bone, which is hyperechoic, or echodense, and the solid arrow points to ventricles filled with cerebrospinal fluid, which is hypoechoic, or echolucent.

of the caudate nucleus where germinal matrix hemorrhage occurs, the lateral ventricles, and the periventricular white matter. However, the brainstem and posterior fossa are better seen through the mastoid fontanelle (MF).[64–67] The recent recognition of the prognostic significance of cerebellar hemorrhage, which is more readily distinguishable through the mastoid fontanelle, suggests that images should be obtained through both anterior and mastoid fontanelles. The trigone and occipital horn of the lateral ventricles are best visualized through the posterior fontanelle (PF), improving detection of subtle intraventricular hemorrhages.[68]

5.1.3 *Describing and classifying brain ultrasound abnormalities*

Several methods of classifying intraventricular hemorrhage have been used for clinical care and research. Probably the most widely used is that described by Papile *et al.*, which was based on computerized tomography performed between three and 10 days of age.[8] Brain hemorrhage was classified as grade 1 if present only in the germinal matrix region but not in the ventricles, grade 2 if present in the non-distended ventricles, grade 3 if present in distended ventricles, and grade 4 if present in both the ventricles and the brain parenchyma.

Krishnamoorthy and his colleagues modified the Papile classification by referring to grade 1 hemorrhage as either blood confined to the germinal matrix subependymal region or blood in less than one half of one lateral ventricle, grade 2 as blood partially filling both lateral ventricles or filling more than one half of one lateral ventricle, grade 3 as blood completely filling and distending both lateral ventricles, and grade 4 as ventricular and intraparenchymal hemorrhage.[69] In 15 survivors of intraventricular hemorrhage, classified based on computerized tomography, all three with grade 4 hemorrhage, but none of the 12 with grades 1 or 2 hemorrhage, had major neurological abnormalities at follow up.[69]

A considerably larger sample of very low birth weight infants ($n =$ 198) was studied by Papile *et al.* These infants underwent computerized tomography between three and 10 days of life and neurodevelopmental assessments at 12–24 months of corrected age.[20] Based on these assessments, a major handicap was defined as abnormal neuromotor examination, blindness, severe sensorineural hearing loss, seizure disorder, or an abnormally low score on the Bayley Scales of Infant Development. The risk of major handicap increased with increasing grade of hemorrhage. Among infants with no hemorrhage, grade 1 hemorrhage, and grade 2 hemorrhage, the risks of a major handicap were 10%, 9% and 11%, respectively. In contrast, the risks of major handicap after grades 3 and 4 hemorrhage were 36% and 76%, respectively.[20]

Thorburn *et al.* were among the first groups to apply a modification of the Papile classification to brain ultrasound abnormalities in very preterm infants (i.e., < 33 weeks). They performed ultrasound scans daily for the first four days of life, at one week of age, and then once or twice weekly until discharge, and referred to grade 1 hemorrhage as hemorrhage confined to the germinal matrix region or hemorrhage in less than one half of one or both lateral ventricles, grade 2 as intraventricular hemorrhage not distending more than half of one or both lateral ventricles, grade 3 as hemorrhage distending any part of the ventricular system, and grade 4 as hemorrhage in the brain parenchyma. Only 4% of infants with normal ultrasounds and no infants with grade 1 hemorrhage had a major neurodevelopmental handicap, as compared to 100% of infants with grades 2 to 4 hemorrhage. Perhaps most important was the finding that all three infants with either cyst formation at the site of a preexisting grade 4 hemorrhage or ventricular enlargement without rapid head growth (i.e., without hydrocephalus) developed cerebral palsy.[70]

Shankaran and colleagues used a slightly different method to classify brain ultrasound abnormalities. They performed ultrasonography on admission and every three days for the first two weeks of life, and classified infants based on the most severe form of the hemorrhage found in the first two weeks.[71] Hemorrhage was classified as mild if it was confined to the subependymal periventricular region or if it was accompanied by a small amount of blood in a normal sized lateral ventricle. This would correspond closely to grades 1 and 2 of the Papile classification and grade 1 of the Krishnamoorthy classification. Hemorrhage was classified as moderate when there was an intermediate amount of blood in an enlarged lateral ventricle, and severe if it filled the entire lateral ventricle or if there was intracerebral hemorrhage.[71] The latter would correspond closely to grades 3 and 4 of the Papile and Krishnamoorthy classifications. None of the patients with mild hemorrhage had neurological abnormality at follow up as compared to 53% of those with moderate hemorrhage and 60% of those with severe hemorrhage.[71]

While the classification systems used by Papile and Krishnamoorthy distinguish between intraventricular hemorrhage with and without acute dilation of the ventricles (between days three and two weeks of life), serial examination of the brain of infants with ultrasound demonstrated that in some infants with intraventricular hemorrhage, ventricular dilation might not appear for up to 40 days after the diagnosis of intraventricular hemorrhage,[72] and that ventricular dilation can be either transient, persistent but arrested, or progressive.[72,73] In addition, serial ultrasonography lead to the recognition that post-hemorrhagic hydrocephalus is not the only reason for ventricular dilation in infants with intraventricular hemorrhage and that persistent ventricular dilation, with or without intraventricular hemorrhage, is a stronger predictor of adverse neurodevelopmental outcome than is the amount of blood within the ventricles.[17,38,53,54,70,74–77] Serial ultrasonography also revealed that parenchymal echodensity, one of the components of grade 4 hemorrhage in the Papile classification, could be transient[33] or could be replaced by echolucency, referred to as cyst formation,[19,70] and that the prognosis depended more on the appearance of the periventricular white matter on ultrasounds performed late during an infant's hospitalization as compared to the appearance early in life.[19,75] These observations led to methods of classification that separated germinal matrix and intraventricular hemorrhage from parenchymal lesions and ventricular enlargement.

Stewart and her colleagues classified abnormalities found on ultrasounds performed in the first week of life as either small periventricular/intraventricular hemorrhage (little or no distention of the ventricles), large periventricular/intraventricular hemorrhage (marked distention of the ventricles), or parenchymal echodensities, and classified abnormalities on ultrasounds performed at discharge as either uncomplicated periventricular/intraventricular hemorrhage (small or large hemorrhage without parenchymal echodensity, ventricular dilation, or hydrocephalus), ventricular dilation (dilatation of ventricles but not as severe as hydrocephalus), hydrocephalus (ventricular dilation to 5 mm above the 97th centile for this dimension,[78] or cerebral atrophy (cysts or irregular ventricular enlargement without rapid head growth).[75] Eight of nine infants with parenchymal echodensities on early ultrasound had a major neurodevelopmental disorder at follow up, as did 61% of those with cerebral atrophy. Those with uncomplicated periventricular/intraventricular hemorrhage had the same risk of major neurodevelopmental disorder (4%) as those with normal ultrasounds.[75] A similar method of classification was used by Whitaker *et al.* and Pinto-Martin *et al.*, who classified ultrasound abnormalities as simple (germinal matrix hemorrhage alone and/or ventricular hemorrhage), complex (persistent ventricular enlargement and/or persistent parenchymal lesion), or transient (transient ventricular enlargement and/or transient parenchymal lesion).[17] As compared to infants with no ultrasound abnormality, those with simple lesions were at 4.6-fold higher risk of developmental delay at one year adjusted age, whereas those with transient and complex lesions were at 5.6-fold and 30-fold higher risk, respectively.[17] The risk of cerebral palsy was increased 3-fold for infants with a simple lesion and 15-fold for those with a complex lesion.[15]

While increasing grade of intraventricular hemorrhage corresponds to an increasing risk of developmental impairment, the grading system described by Papile *et al*, and used subsequently by many researchers, has several imitations,[39,79] and for at least three reasons, experts suggest that it be abandoned,[39,80] First, a Papile grade 1 intraventricular hemorrhage is not an intraventricular hemorrhage at all, but rather a hemorrhage confined to the germinal matrix located under the ependyma in the area of the ganglionic eminence.[80] Second, some entities which have prognostic significance, such as isolated ventricular enlargement, or parenchymal hemorrhage without intraventricular hemorrhage, are not considered by the Papile system. Third, there is little pathologic support for the concept that echodensity in the brain parenchyma accompanying an intraventricular hemorrhage represents an extension of the intraventricular hemorrhage.[39] In fact, this ultrasound finding does not always represent hemorrhage.[28]

Paneth has described a classification of brain ultrasound findings that takes into account neuropathologic findings and consists of three general categories of abnormalities.[81–84] The first, and probably the most important prognostically, is white matter damage, which can be detected as either multiple small echolucent cysts, large (and often single) porencephalic cysts, ventricular enlargement,[38] or either persistent or transient echodensity.[30] In many infants, white matter damage is not evident on ultrasound.[38,39] A second category of ultrasound lesion, non-parenchymal hemorrhage, includes germinal matrix hemorrhage, which is readily detected with ultrasound as either a subependymal hemorrhage or as hemorrhage extending into the ventricles. In two other non-parenchymal loci, the choroids plexus and the subarachnoid space, hemorrhage is not as easily visualized.[39] As compared to white matter damage, non-parenchymal hemorrhages probably have less impact on developmental outcome. A third category of ultrasound lesion are lesions outside of the white matter other than non-parenchymal hemorrhages. This category includes lesions in the cerebellum, basal ganglia, and brainstem. These lesions are seen often at autopsy of low birth weight infants,[84] but the frequency among survivors is not well characterized. Cerebellar hemorrhage is strongly associated with subsequent developmental impairment,[85] especially when bilateral.[53,54]

5.1.4 *Accuracy of neonatal brain ultrasound*

When using ultrasound as an input to clinical decisions, it is necessary to consider its limitations. The validity of ultrasound has been studied by assessing the level of agreement between ultrasound readers' findings and diagnoses and the gold standard, i.e. postmortem histological examination of the brain. This gold standard is not available from living patients. In such patients, reliability has been studied as an upper bound for the validity of ultrasound interpretations.

5.1.4.1 *The neonatal brain hemorrhage study*

The largest study of agreement between ultrasound diagnosis of germinal matrix/intraventricular hemorrhage and postmortem histological findings is the Central New Jersey Neonatal Brain Hemorrhage Study (NBHS), which involved a population-based sample of 1105 infants with birth weight 501–2000 grams, who were born in the years 1984–1987, in three neonatal intensive care units serving three counties in central New Jersey. Much of what we know about the validity and reliability of ultrasound interpretations is derived from this study.[82,84,86,87] In addition, the NBHS is one of the many large cohort studies that provides information about the positive predictive value of ultrasound for detection of infants who subsequently develop cerebral palsy,[15,63] cognitive impairment,[63,88,89] and behavioral problems.[63,90]

In the NBHS, the specificity of ultrasound detection of germinal matrix/intraventricular hemorrhage was higher than sensitivity. The positive predictive values for germinal matrix hemorrhage and intraventricular hemorrhage were greater than 80%.[82] Ultrasound readers failed to identify germinal matrix/intraventricular hemorrhage in about half of the cases.[82] However, when provided with three scans, collected at four hours, 24 hours, and seven days of life, readers identified over 75% of these non-parenchymal hemorrhages. The sensitivity was greater for larger lesions.[82] When three scans were viewed and the lesion was at least 1 cm, all incidences of germinal matrix/intraventricular hemorrhage were detected.[82]

A number of pathologic abnormalities were found in the hemispheric white matter on postmortem examinations performed on NBHS study participants, including hemorrhagic lesions as well as non-hemorrhagic lesions, such as edema, early liquefaction, or histologic abnormalities of the glial cells or axons.[83] The sensitivity of ultrasound for detecting hemorrhagic white matter damage was 80%. For detecting non-hemorrhagic white matter alterations, the sensitivity was 60%. The specificity of ultrasound detection of white matter abnormalities was greater than 90%.[83]

Large periventricular echodensity ipsilateral to an intraventricular hemorrhage frequently is the ultrasound correlate of hemorrhagic white matter infarction.[21,23–25,83] A conclusion of the NBHS was that if the ventricle is filled with blood (i.e. completely echodense) it may be impossible to distinguish whether white matter damage accompanies an intraventricular hemorrhage.[82]

5.1.4.2 *Other ultrasound validation studies*

In two studies involving a total of 53 newborns, the overall sensitivities for detecting subependymal, intraventricular, and parenchymal hemorrhages, based on autopsy as the gold standard, were 74%, 86%, and 62%, respectively, and the specificities were 81%, 56%, and 99%.[91,92] Studies by Szymonowicz *et al.*[93] and Thorburn *et al.*[94] provide similar conclusions, but these reports do not provide the data needed to pool results with other studies.[94] Trounce *et al.* reported on 20 brain hemispheres with echodensity in the periventricular white matter that was "thought not to be parenchymal extension of intraventricular hemorrhage" and in 85% of these, histological examination confirmed the presence of periventricular leukomalacia.[95] Nwaesei *et al.* described strong correlation between echodense and echolucent lesions in the superolateral angle of the lateral ventricle and the finding of periventricular infarction at autopsy.[28]

To summarize, studies of agreement between ultrasound and autopsy findings suggest that ultrasound is a valid, albeit imperfect, method of diagnosing non-parenchymal hemorrhage and hemorrhagic white matter abnormalities, but detects less than two thirds of instances of non-hemorrhagic white matter abnormality. Additional information about the validity of ultrasound comes from studies of the ability of ultrasound to predict subsequent developmental impairments. The studies of ultrasound-outcome correlations will be discussed in the Sections 5.1.7 and 5.1.8.

5.1.4.3 *Studies of the reliability of ultrasound interpretations*

The validity of ultrasound interpretations cannot be directly studied in living patients because the gold standard (postmortem examination) is not available. Reliability can serve as an upper bound for validity and intra- and inter-reader agreement has been studied for ultrasound findings, as well as diagnoses.[87,96–100] In three studies where efforts were directed towards improving reliability, agreement was good to excellent for the diagnoses of germinal matrix,[87,97] intraventricular hemorrhage,[87,97,98] and parenchymal hemorrhage,[87,97] and for the observation of moderate to severe ventricular enlargement.[87,97,101] In three studies where no efforts to improve reliability were described, inter-reader agreement was poor for germinal matrix hemorrhage and intraventricular hemorrhage without ventricular enlargement, good for intraventricular hemorrhage with ventricular enlargement, good to excellent for intraventricular hemorrhage with parenchymal hemorrhage,[96,99] and fair[96,100] to excellent[99] for ventricular enlargement. The reliability is low for observations about non-hemorrhagic white matter lesions. In two studies in which no efforts were made to improve reliability, the kappa for the observation of periventricular leukomalacia was 0.09 when this lesion was defined as either echodensity or echoluceny,[99] and was only slightly higher when restricted to echolucency.[100] When efforts were made to maximize reliability, the kappa for echodensity was poor, but that for echolucency was good.[101] Unless special efforts are directed to improving reliability, the ascertainment of periventricular cystic lesions, and the diagnosis of periventricular leukomalacia probably is too variable to serve as an outcome of interest for researchers or those involved with continuous quality improvement.[100]

5.1.5   *Ultrasound images as an aid when considering withdrawing or withholding care*

In a small subset of preterm infants, brain ultrasound findings are part of the basis for withdrawing or withholding life support. In a small minority of such cases, this plan of care is based on finding a major congenital anomaly, such as holoprosencephaly or hydranencephaly. Much more often, life support is withdrawn or withheld after finding extensive (intracerebral) intraparenchymal hemorrhage. In one study of neonates withdrawn from life support, intracranial hemorrhage was among the most common reasons for withdrawing support.[102] Presumably, the high risk of adverse outcome leads to the conclusion that the quality of life for the child very likely will be poor.[103] Among preterm infants, the majority of intracranial hemorrhage is diagnosed in the first several days of life.[12,104] Thus, ultrasound scanning of infants at high risk for extensive intracranial hemorrhage can provide information pertinent to decisions about continuing or withdrawing life support for extremely preterm infants.

Brain ultrasonography in the first several days of life is not a part of the neuroimaging practice parameter described later (Section 5.1.9). Based on unpublished data from a cohort study of extremely low gestational age newborns,[101] routine ultrasound is performed in the first one to four days of life in some medical centers, whereas in other centers, ultrasound is performed in the first one to four days only in circumstances when diagnostic suspicion is high, based on risk factors or clinical signs.

This approach might fail to detect all infants with intraparenchymal hemorrhage, as almost one half of all preterm infants with periventricular/intraventricular hemorrhage have no clinical signs.[9] Signs that are predictive of brain hemorrhage include an unexplained fall in hematocrit, failure of the hematocrit to rise after packed red blood cell transfusion, tight anterior fontanelle, decrease in spontaneous activity, decreased tone, abnormal eye signs, and seizures.[9]

Among preterm infants in the first several days of life, the most important brain ultrasound lesion related to prognosis is the periventricular echodensity accompanying large intraventricular hemorrhage. These lesions, referred to variably as Papile grade 4 intraventricular hemorrhage, parenchymal lesion,[105] intraparenchymal echodensity,[23] periventricular echodensity,[24,25] periventricular intraparenchymal cerebral hemorrhage,[106] and periventricular hemorrhage infarction,[21,107] are typically observed ipsilateral to the ventricle with the larger amount of hemorrhage in infants with bilateral intraventricular hemorrhage.[24] Neuropathological correlation indicates that this ultrasound abnormality leads to, or occurs with, necrosis of periventricular tissue.[23] Recent authors have referred to this ultrasound abnormality as periventricular hemorrhagic infarction,[21] and a severity score has been described, with "points" assigned for each of the following; midline shift, bilateral lesions, and presence in more than one territory on parasagittal view, based on ultrasound findings.[108] This score ranges from 0 to 3, and higher severity scores are associated with higher risk of impairment (see Fig. 5.2).[109] In addition to increasing the risk of neurological and neurocognitive impairments, this lesion is strongly associated with epilepsy later in life.[109,110]

Another lesion associated with a very high risk of neurodevelopmental impairment is bilateral cerebellar hemorrhage. In one study of 11 infants with this lesion, 60% developed cerebral palsy[53] and 73% had delayed early cognitive function.[54] In a study of nine infants with this lesion, the mean score on a test of early cognitive function was more than three standard deviations below normal.[85]

A recent school-age follow up suggests the need for caution when basing the decision to withdraw life support from an infant on an ultrasound image obtained in the first week of life.[22] Roze *et al.* evaluated 21 children, at a mean age of 8.7 years, who had experienced neonatal

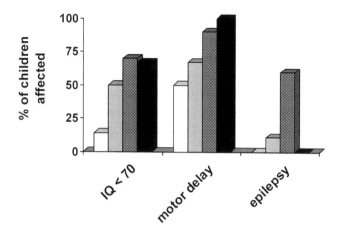

Fig. 5.2.   Risk of adverse neurological and cognitive outcomes as a function of severity of periventricular hemorrhagic infarction. Data reported in Hassan B *et al.* (2007) *Pediatrics* 120(4): 785–792. White bars correspond to severity level = 0; gray bars to level 1; cross hatched bars to level 2; black bars to level 3.

periventricular hemorrhagic infarction. Although 76% had cerebral palsy, in 81% of cases the functional impairment was mild. The median intelligence quotient was 83, and 57% of the children attended normal education classes. The characteristics of the periventricular hemorrhagic infarction were not related to the functional motor outcome, intelligence, visual perception, visual motor integration, and most of the behavioral problems that were assessed.[22]

5.1.6   *Ultrasound for detection and monitoring intraventricular hemorrhage*

Ultrasonography has a limited role in the acute management of preterm infants with intraventricular hemorrhage because there are no evidence-based approaches to the acute management of this disorder.[111–113] However, some infants with intraventricular hemorrhage and coagulopathy, especially when due to thrombocytopenia, might benefit from treatment to improve coagulation, and in these patients earlier identification of the hemorrhage is a potential benefit of ultrasound. The platelet count at which transfusion of platelets is indicated is not known.[114]

If, in the future, an effective treatment for acute intraventricular hemorrhage is identified, more frequent and earlier ultrasound scanning of preterm infants at high risk for this disorder would be warranted. One approach that is being investigated involves placing ventricular catheters through which tissue plasminogen activator is infused and the products of fibrinolysis removed.[115] In a randomized controlled trial, this procedure did not decrease the need for shunt surgery.[116] Neurodevelopmental follow up of study participants is ongoing.

Currently, the clinical utility of a brain ultrasound in the first one to two weeks of life is to identify infants with intraventricular hemorrhage so that these infants can be scheduled for serial ultrasonography to monitor changes in ventricular size. Post-hemorrhagic hydrocephalus is a complication of intraventricular hemorrhage that is predictive of an increased risk of neurodevelopmental impairment. Ultrasonographically detected ventricular dilation can precede rapid increase in head circumference by days to weeks,[117–120] and clinical signs are even slower to develop.[121] Thus, serial ultrasonography after an intraventricular hemorrhage can identify infants with post-hemorrhagic ventricular dilation sooner than serial measurements of head circumference. Today ultrasound is typically performed with a one- to two-week interval between successive scans until the ventricular size has been stable for at least two successive scans. It should be noted that in a small percentage of cases, preterm infants with arrested and resolved post-hemorrhagic hydrocephalus can develop progressive ventricular enlargement. Thus, infants with intraventricular hemorrhage need continued monitoring of head size throughout the first year of life.[122]

A variety of methods have been described for quantifying cerebral ventricular size. One approach is to measure the ventricular index, the distance between the midline and the lateral extent of the lateral ventricle on a coronal scan.[78] Johnson *et al.* described the lateral ventricular ratio, referring to the ratio of the ventricular index to the brain hemispheric width, and reported excellent agreement between the lateral ventricular ratio as measured with ultrasound and computerized tomography.[123] Brann *et al.* found only modest correlation between ventricular index and ventricular volume estimated by manually tracing the outline of the ventricles on digitized images,[124] and Grasby *et al.* found that the ventricular index correlated poorly with expert opinion.[125] Ventricular height in a parasagittal plane, measured at the level of the apex of the thalamus, just posterior to the foramen of Monro,[126] and the diagonal width of the frontal horn, at right angles to the longest dimension, at the widest point, in a coronal plane,[127] correlated well with each other and with expert opinion.[125]

In one longitudinal follow-up study from the early 1980s, of 409 infants with subependymal or intraventricular hemorrhage, 13% developed progressive ventricular enlargement. In two thirds of these cases, ventricular enlargement arrested before it was severe, as assessed with ultrasound or computerized tomography. In one third of those with arrested dilation, a spontaneous decrease in ventricular size was noted and in two thirds the ventricles remained dilated, but not severely. Only 11% of the infants with severe ventricular enlargement were symptomatic.[128] In a more recent multi-center study of 1527 extremely low birth weight infants with intraventricular hemorrhage, a ventriculoperitoneal shunt was placed in 15% of infants for post-hemorrhagic hydrocephalus. Only 1% of infants with a Papile grade 2 hemorrhage underwent shunt placement, as compared to 18% of infants with grade 3, and 29% with grade 4 hemorrhage. Interestingly, 1% of 1003 infants with grade 1 hemorrhage underwent shunt placement, perhaps because intraventricular hemorrhage was not detected with ultrasound screening.[129] Thus, the overall risk of post-hemorrhagic hydrocephalus is low with grades 1 and 2 hemorrhage, but is substantial with grades 3 and 4.

Since only a minority of infants with post-hemorrhagic ventricular dilatation develop severe enlargement and clinical signs of increased intracranial pressure and because all interventions for this disorder have potential complications, it is not surprising that there are no widely accepted criteria for when to intervene for post-hemorrhagic ventricular dilatation. Randomized trials of medical interventions to decrease cerebrospinal fluid flow, serial lumbar puncture to drain cerebrospinal fluid, and instillation of an agent to promote fibrinolysis have not identified benefits, so in many neonatal intensive care units these approaches are not used at all. Observational studies by de Vries and her colleagues[130,131] suggest an association between intervening earlier, by draining cerebrospinal fluid, and improvement of neurodevelopmental outcome, but a moderate sized randomized trial did not detect a benefit of this approach.[111]

To summarize, it is clear that timely detection of intraventricular hemorrhage and ventricular enlargement due to intraventricular hemorrhage depends on ultrasonography, but it is not clear what the treatment implications are for infants who are found to have these disorders.

5.1.7 *Ultrasound for predicting preschool neurodevelopmental outcome*

We have described earlier how one ultrasound finding — periventricular echodensity (also referred to as intraparenchymal echodensity, grade IV hemorrhage, and periventricular hemorrhagic infarction) is highly predictive of subsequent neurodevelopmental impairment and how this prognostic information might be of interest to clinicians and parents in the life of a preterm infant. Close to the time of discharge from neonatal intensive care, ultrasound can once again provide useful prognostic information. This information can help parents anticipate the challenges their infant might encounter and guide rehabilitative specialists in their efforts to promote the infant's neuromotor, cognitive, and adaptive development.

In early reports relating to ultrasound abnormalities and prognosis, the focus was on germinal matrix and intraventricular hemorrhage,[132] classified using the Papile grading system (*vide supra*). In a study based on ultrasounds performed in the early 1980s, similar rates of neurodevelopmental disorders, such as cerebral palsy or developmental delay, were found among infants with normal ultrasounds and infants with germinal matrix/intraventricular hemorrhage, unless the latter infants' "late" ultrasound (i.e., those obtained close to when the infant was discharged from the hospital) showed evidence of ventricular enlargement, cystic changes in the white matter, or hydrocephalus.[75] Most studies indicate that infants with grade 1 or grade 2 germinal matrix/intraventricular hemorrhage, when not complicated by hydrocephalus or white matter damage, are not at increased risk for neurodevelopmental impairments, although in separate studies, "uncomplicated" germinal matrix/intraventricular hemorrhage was associated with a decrease in cortical volume, at about 40 weeks postmenstrual age,[133] worse scores on the Bayley Scales of

Infant Development,[134] and an increased risk of cerebral palsy.[15,19] In some studies in which infants with germinal matrix/intraventricular hemorrhage did not always have a "late" ultrasound, effects attributed to germinal matrix/intraventricular hemorrhage might have been caused by lesions in the periventricular white matter since germinal matrix/intraventricular hemorrhage is associated with white matter damage[135] and such damage may not be detected by scans performed in the first 1–2 weeks of life.[19,30] Nonetheless, in 10 studies performed in the 1980s, the prevalence of cerebral palsy among 378 preterm infants with "isolated" germinal matrix/intraventricular hemorrhage was 4.8%,[63] identical to the prevalence among 1008 very low birth weight or very premature infants (described in five studies), whose neonatal ultrasound was normal.[13,14,19,75,134] Uncomplicated intraventricular hemorrhage has been associated with reduced cortical volume at near-term age, so further study of this lesion in larger cohorts is warranted.[135]

While infants with isolated germinal matrix hemorrhage and intraventricular hemorrhage without ventricular enlargement usually remain free from neurodevelopmental impairment, a favorable prognosis is less likely with two other ultrasound findings detectable in the first two weeks of life. High risk brain lesions include large periventricular echodensity ipsilateral to an intraventricular hemorrhage (i.e. periventricular hemorrhagic infarction),[15,23,53,109] and large intraventricular hemorrhage with ventricular dilation.[129] Among surviving infants with periventricular hemorrhagic infarction, a critical determinant of neurodevelopmental outcome is whether periventricular echolucency develops, which typically occurs several weeks after the diagnosis is made of periventricular hemorrhagic infarction.[136] In a recent multicenter study of over 1000 extremely low gestational age newborns, those with parenchymal echolucency were 75% more likely than those with parenchymal echodensity to develop cerebral palsy,[53] and 50% more likely to have delayed mental development at 24 months adjusted age.[54]

While more than 90% of infants with a periventricular hemorrhagic infarction severity score (as described by Bassan *et al.*[108] of two or three will develop a neuromotor abnormality, and two thirds will have cognitive impairment, only slightly more than half of infants with a severity score of 0 or 1 will develop neuromotor abnormality and less than one half will have cognitive impairment.[109] A favorable outcome is seen in more than one half of infants with focal echodensity.[109] The form of cerebral palsy most strongly associated with periventricular hemorrhagic infarction is hemiplegia.[53] One report suggests that this is the neonatal brain lesion that accounts for a majority of preterm infants with epilepsy.[110]

Ultrasounds performed after the first month of life provide more valid information about prognosis than scans performed earlier[30,75,136] because the former are more sensitive for detection of non-hemorrhagic white matter damage. As discussed earlier, the most important ultrasound indicators of white matter damage are echolucency (i.e., hypoechoic lesions) and persistent ventricular enlargement (i.e., ventriculomegaly).[137] In a large study of weekly ultrasound scanning, 46% of infants with white matter echolucency were identified only after 28 days of life, and 14% of infants with these abnormalities were not identified until 40 weeks postmenstrual age.[30] Multiple periventricular echolucencies, which can be either unilateral or bilateral, and appear after the first two weeks of life, usually indicate macroscopic cavities in the periventricular white matter[83] and have been referred to as periventricular leukomalacia by ultrasonographers.[29]

In a review of studies completed in the 1980s,[63] the pooled prevalences of cerebral palsy for infants with ventricular enlargement, white matter echodensity, and white matter echolucency, were respectively, 48% (of 392 infants), 59% (of 135 infants), and 59% (of 358 infants). These prevalences are 16–20 times higher than very preterm infants with normal ultrasounds or uncomplicated germinal matrix/intraventricular hemorrhage.[30,138] Based on a review of 15 studies of parenchymal echolucency, this lesion is associated more strongly with cerebral palsy than mental retardation, and the risk of both of these outcomes relates to the extent of white matter damage, quantified in terms of whether unilateral or bilateral, and the size of the echolucencies, and the rostrocaudal location (frontal, parietal, occipital).[138] About one half of infants with echolucency involving the frontal, parietal, and occipital regions, and about one quarter of those with echolucency limited to either the parietal or occipital regions, develop mental retardation.[138]

Based on a multicenter study of over 1000 infants born before 28 weeks gestation, infants with unilateral ventricular enlargement are three times more likely to develop hemiplegia as compared to quadriplegia, while those with bilateral ventricular enlargement are almost four times more likely to develop quadriplegia than hemiplegia.[53] Ventricular enlargement on a "late" ultrasound (i.e. one performed after two weeks of life) is a better predictor of cerebral palsy than ventricular enlargement detected earlier in life. Among infants with this finding on a "late" ultrasound, the risk of cerebral palsy is 50%.[53] Among infants with unilateral echolucency, quadriplegia and hemiplegia are equally likely, occurring in about one sixth of infants with this lesion. In contrast, among infants with bilateral echolucency, quadriplegia is much more likely.[53] Ultrasound indicators of white matter damage are more strongly associated with delayed psychomotor development than delayed mental development during infancy. The risk of delayed mental and psychomotor development increases as the extent of echolucency increases, but the same is not true for echodensity.[54]

Unlike echolucency, echodensity frequently is transient, and the association between transient echodensity and subsequent developmental impairments depends on the duration of the echodensity. Among infants whose echodensity were not persistent, the prevalence of cerebral palsy was 10%.[63] It has been suggested that echodensity present for less than seven days be classified as brief, for 7–13 days be classified as intermediate, and for more than 13 days be classified as prolonged flare.[33] It should be emphasized that small echolucencies inferior to the ventricle, in the region where germinal matrix hemorrhage is often found, are not associated with an increased risk of developmental impairments.

In summary, ultrasound scans obtained close to discharge from neonatal intensive care identifies infants with white matter damage, who are at greatly increased risk of cerebral palsy and, to a lesser extent, mental retardation (Fig. 5.3). In such cases, parents can be better prepared to care for their child by acquiring information for themselves and developmental services for their child. Other parents can be reassured if their infant is found to have no white matter abnormalities. Since the sensitivity of ultrasound for detecting white matter abnormalities is not perfect, parents should be informed that an infant with a normal neonatal ultrasound may develop cerebral palsy or another developmental impairment, even though the probability is low. However, in view of the potential for plasticity in the developing brain, parents of infants with an ultrasound indicator of white matter damage should be informed that not all infants with this

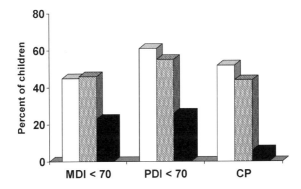

Fig. 5.3. Risk of adverse neurological and cognitive outcomes as a function of ultrasound findings. Data reported in O'Shea *et al.* (2008); *Pediatrics* 122(3): e662–e669 and Kuban *et al.* (2009) *J Child Neurol* 24(1): 63–72. White bars correspond to echolucency; gray bars to ventriculomegaly; black bars to normal ultrasound.

lesion develop cerebral palsy or mental retardation. When describing brain damage identified on ultrasound, we recommend that clinicians avoid the Papile grading system for hemorrhage and instead report on ultrasounds using descriptive terms, such as echodensity or echolucency, rather than diagnostic labels, such as "periventricular leukomalacia", or terms that assume knowledge of etiology, such as "ischemic lesions".

5.1.8 *Ultrasound for predicting school-age neurodevelopmental outcome*

Studies of ultrasound — outcome associations in the first two years of life indicate a strong association with motor impairments[15,30,48,52,54] but relatively modest associations with cognitive impairments.[54] Fewer studies have related ultrasound lesions to school-age outcomes, such as mental retardation, attention deficit, learning disabilities, and school achievement. In general, studies of school-age children, like studies during infancy, indicate that neonatal brain ultrasound lesions are associated more strongly with neuromotor impairments, as compared to neurocognitive impairments and that children with uncomplicated germinal matrix or intraventricular hemorrhage have intelligence test scores similar to infants without ultrasound abnormalities.[139–141]

Studies of school age children consistently have found an association between severe brain ultrasound lesions, such as post-hemorrhagic hydrocephalus, ventricular enlargement and periventricular echolucency, and mental retardation,[77,141,142] with reported odds ratios ranging from 4 for post-hemorrhagic hydrocephalus,[143] to 5 for Papile grade 3–4 IVH or persistent ventricular enlargement[141] and 66 for ventricular enlargement or parenchymal echolucency.[89] Severe brain ultrasound abnormalities are also associated with impairments of neurocognitive functions, including perceptual organization, distractibility, processing speed, and executive function, as well as academic achievement tests.[139] The increased risk of mental retardation among infants with periventricular echolucency or ventricular enlargement was not found when infants with major motor or cognitive disability were excluded, but these infants did have worse motor abilities at six, nine, and 16 years of age,[88,144] as well as more oral motor problems and a slightly lower intelligence quotient at 16 years of age.[144]

Less severe brain ultrasound abnormalities have not been consistently associated with adverse neurocognitive outcomes at school age. In the Neonatal Brain Hemorrhage cohort, germinal matrix/intraventricular hemorrhage was associated with an increased risk of mental retardation,[89] but after excluding children with severe cognitive and motor disability (i.e. disabling cerebral palsy or intelligence quotient more than three standard deviations below the mean), germinal matrix/intraventricular hemorrhage was not associated with lower intelligence quotient. However, even in the absence of severe disability, germinal matrix/intraventricular hemorrhage was associated with worse oral motor function.[144] Similarly, Vollmer *et al.* found that infants with uncomplicated germinal matrix and/or intraventricular hemorrhage did worse than infants without such lesions on a test of motor function, but did not have lower intelligence test scores.[140] While D'Angio *et al.* reported a five-point decrement in intelligence quotient for each one-level increase in grade of intraventricular hemorrhage (using the Papile grading system),[145] this finding assumes a linear relationship between grade and intelligence, an assumption for which there is little support in the literature.

5.1.9 *Routine ultrasound scanning of preterm neonates*

A committee consisting of neonatologists, neurologists, perinatal epidemiologists, and neonatal radiologists, sponsored by the American Academy of Neurology and the Child Neurology Society (AAN/CNS) has reviewed published literature related to neuroimaging of neonates. This committee's recommendation for imaging for the preterm neonates is that, "Routine screening cranial ultrasonography should be performed on all infants of <30 weeks' gestation once between seven and 14 days of age and should be optimally repeated between 36 and 40 weeks' postmenstrual age. This strategy detects lesions such as intraventricular hemorrhage, which influences clinical care, and those such as periventricular leukomalacia and low-pressure ventriculomegaly, which provide information about long-term neurodevelopmental outcome. There is insufficient evidence for routine MRI of all very low birth weight preterm infants with abnormal results on cranial US."

The rationale for this committee's recommendation included their judgment that ultrasound is sufficiently accurate for detecting brain lesions, that knowledge of these brain lesions can influence clinical care, and that the prevalence of these lesions is sufficiently high. The rationale for the recommended timing of ultrasound scans on infants of <30 weeks gestation is that the earlier scan will detect nearly all infants with intraventricular hemorrhage, so that these infants can be monitored for the development of post-hemorrhagic hydrocephalus, and that the later scan will detect infants with ventricular enlargement or periventricular echolucency (leukomalacia) so that these infants can be monitored for the development of cerebral palsy. The committee concluded that although brain MRI detects more white matter abnormalities, more hemorrhages, and more cystic lesions, the current level of evidence is insufficient to conclude that this additional information adds to the prognostic information provided by ultrasound. However, at the time of this writing, the AAN/CNS Committee's report is seven years old, and a future practice parameter from this committee might draw different conclusions with respect to MRI imaging of the preterm brain.

The practice parameter described above is a guideline that can be used along with clinical judgment and consideration of data from one's own institution. For example, based on a retrospective review of data, one group of neonatologists has suggested that in addition to the two scans recommended by the AAN/CNS Committee, an initial scan be performed at 3–5 days of life for infants with birth weight < 1000 grams.[146] Another group has presented data indicating that if two negative scans are obtained at least a week apart, there is a very low probability of finding a significant abnormality on a subsequent scan, unless the infant has a clinical deterioration after the two normal scans. Hence an ultrasound at 36 to 40 weeks postmenstrual age might not always be warranted.[147] And a third group concluded after a review of data on 486 infants born at 3–33 weeks of gestation, that the cut off for routine scanning should be 30 weeks, not 29 weeks, of gestation.[148] Using the screening routine suggested by the AAN/CNS practice guideline,[38] one can expect that an ultrasound indicator of white matter damage (ventricular enlargement or periventricular echolucency) will be found in only slightly more than one half of affected very low birth weight infants[15,149] or extremely low gestational age infants.[53] This indicates that the sensitivity of ultrasound for detecting white matter damage is not as high as clinicians would like. One approach to increase the sensitivity of ultrasound screening is to perform scans more often. Thus de Vries and her colleagues performed ultrasounds weekly until discharge and identified an abnormality in the white matter in 70 of 76 cases (92%).[30]

5.1.10 *Limitations of ultrasound*

Despite the safety, ease of use, and portability of ultrasound, there are limitations to its sensitivity which have been alluded to above. First, readers not infrequently disagreeing about the presence of abnormalities, implying imperfect validity.[87,97,98] Second, a substantial proportion of infants with white matter damage are not identified with ultrasound, at least when the schedule suggested by the AAN/CNS practice guideline.[38] Third, the peripheral cortex, cerebellum, basal ganglia, and brainstem are not well visualized with routine scanning procedures. Thus, magnetic resonance imaging may offer advantages over ultrasound when the goal is a comprehensive identification of brain abnormalities. The predictive value of magnetic resonance has been studied primarily using images obtained near the term equivalent age, or "due date".

Brain magnetic resonance imaging has been used to assess the stage of myelination, and a correlation has been found between brain ultrasound findings in the neonatal period and stage of myelination at 44 weeks. In very preterm infants, increasing delay in myelination is associated with increasing risk of neurodevelopmental impairment at three years of age.[150] Using ultrasound, indicators of white matter damage are found in less than 20% of extremely premature newborns.[101] By comparison, magnetic resonance imaging detects white matter abnormality in at least two thirds of very preterm infants.[151,152] The higher sensitivity for detecting white matter abnormality is reflected in a higher sensitivity for identifying infants who will develop cerebral palsy.[153,154] Of particular importance as a prognostic sign is T1 hyperintensity or cysts in the corona radiate above the posterior limb of the internal capsule on coronal sections. In the absence of this finding, children with T1 hyperintensity are at low risk of cerebral palsy, whereas children with this finding usually develop cerebral palsy.[155] White matter abnormalities on magnetic resonance imaging, but not gray matter abnormalities, are predictive of abnormal general movements at one month of age, an early predictor of cerebral palsy.[156] In the absence of overt brain lesions, an elevated apparent diffusion coefficient, which is indicator of abnormal myelination, correlates with scores on a test of early development.[157] White matter abnormalities seen on magnetic resonance imaging may prove to be more predictive than ultrasound abnormalities of higher neurocognitive functions, such as executive function.[158]

In addition to identifying brain lesions and abnormal myelination, magnetic resonance imaging can estimate overall and regional brain volumes, which might increase its value for predicting specific neurocognitive functions. For example, hippocampal volumes, assessed at term equivalent age in a cohort of very preterm infants, correlated with later working memory deficits,[159] and smaller inferior occipital region brain tissue volume predicted visual motor impairment.[160]

5.2 Magnetic Resonance Imaging

Although ultrasound remains the primary modality for neonatal neuroimaging, magnetic resonance imaging (MRI) has begun to assume an important role, especially given the wide availability of high field strength MRI systems and dedicated pediatric head coils that provide exquisitely detailed multiplanar anatomical images of the developing brain.[3,161–170] The lack of ionizing radiation makes MRI a relatively safe imaging modality for neonates, however, the imaging environment and imaging procedure can be difficult for an infant to endure, and can be dangerous for those infants that are gravely ill or clinically unstable.[171] In this section, we will discuss MRI imaging of the neonatal brain with a focus on term infants.

5.2.1　*History of neonatal brain MRI*

In the early 1980s, Levene and his colleagues were among the first to use MRI to study the neonatal brain.[172] In the late 1980s, Van de Bor used MRI to study myelination in 33 infants born before 30 weeks gestation, some with periventricular leukomalacia and some with periventricular-intraventricular hemorrhage,[173] and in a subsequent study compared the value of neonatal brain ultrasound findings and MRI assessments of myelination as predictors of cerebral palsy.[150] Over the past 20 years, MRI at term equivalent age has been used with increasing frequency for research studies of preterm neonates.[174]

5.2.2　*Technical aspects of neonatal brain MRI*

5.2.2.1　*Patient preparation and monitoring*

MRI of neonates requires a team approach, with considerable coordinated participation and active communication among well trained experienced neonatal intensive care unit (NICU) personnel to ensure patient safety and vital continuous patient monitoring. In particular, neonates are very sensitive to small changes in a variety of physiological measures, such as blood glucose level, temperature, ventilation, and blood pressure that require especially vigilant attention and maintenance. To this end, standard tubes and lines must be organized, appropriately extended, and connected to MR-compatible equipment (e.g. pulse oximeter, ECG, infusion pump), so that patient monitoring and delivery of supportive medications and fluids continues while the patient is in the strong magnetic field of the MR environment. Commercially available MR compatible NICU incubators are presently available that improve the safety and efficiency of this labor intensive process.[175,176] Since patient motion degrades the resolution of MR images, neonates are commonly swaddled and may be placed in commercially available vacuum cushions prior to imaging. Adherence to strict safety guidelines in the MR environment related to ferromagnetic items and ear protection is always crucial for every patient imaged. Ferromagnetic items, such as Searle arterial lines, electronic name tags and metal poppers on clothes, must be removed as they may become deadly projectiles in the strong magnetic field.[3] Ear protection is necessary to attenuate the significant noise generated by the vibration of the gradient coils as electric current through the coils is switched on and off (often greater than 100 dB). Common ear protection includes a combination of silicone based putty (President Putty, Coltene/Whaledent, New Jersey, USA) and commercially available neonatal ear muffs (Natus MiniMuffs, Natus Medical, San Carlos, CA, USA).[3]

5.2.2.2 *MRI technique*

MR scanners with field strengths of 1.5T and 3T are readily available and commonly used for neonatal imaging. Higher field strengths have the advantage of providing a better signal-to-noise ratio (SNR) and shorter the scan time. Good image quality also requires an appropriately fitted head coil. In particular, SNR is degraded if a conventional adult head coil is used for imaging the neonatal brain because a smaller field of view is necessary for imaging. As such, a dedicated neonatal head coil or adult knee joint coil with relatively smaller diameter can be used to properly optimize SNR. Our specific MRI protocol includes isotropic high resolution (2 mm) axial T1-weighted SPGR, motion insensitive PROPELLER axial T2, sagittal and coronal T1, blood/calcium sensitive MPGR, diffusion, as well as pulsed arterial spin labeling (PASL) perfusion sequences. As the neonatal brain has higher water content and lower protein and lipid content than the adult brain, T1 and T2 relaxation times are longer, which requires echo times (TE) and repetition times (TR) to be different for neonatal compared to conventional adult MR imaging.[164,167,177] At our institution, TR ranges from 375–550 ms for T1-weighted sequences, and 3500–5000 ms for T2-weighted sequences.

Diffusion weighted imaging (DWI) is also influenced by the relatively high extracellular space water content and associated rapid molecular diffusion. Apparent diffusion coefficient (ADC) is higher in neonates (maximum at approximately 28 weeks gestational age), but declines with increasing relative anisotropy of white matter during brain maturation and myelination as a result of extracellular water exclusion.[178,179] As a result, a maximum b value of 750–800 s/mm^2 is often used for neonatal imaging, which is less than that used for adults.

5.2.3 *Accuracy of neonatal brain MRI*

MRI has been demonstrated to provide useful information regarding changes of both normal development and diffuse damage in the neonatal brain.[2,180–185] MRI is thought to be particularly accurate for identifying the precise location and global extent of abnormalities, for detecting diffuse and/or subtle abnormalities, and for evaluating sequelae of cerebral maturation, such as the progression of myelination.[151,170,185–188] Many investigations comparing the accuracy of MRI to ultrasound (US) have demonstrated MRI to be superior for the detection of specific types of neonatal brain injury, including more recent studies using the most advanced US and MRI systems.[181,184,186,188–194] For example, several investigations have shown MRI to be more accurate than US for the detection of punctate white matter lesions and diffuse excessive high signal intensity foci that are considered to represent diffuse or subtle white matter (WM) injury.[184,186,188,191,192] In addition, MRI has been shown to provide more anatomical detail than US, which facilitates visualization of the whole brain, as well as deeper and more peripheral cerebral structures, and may partially explain why MRI appears superior to US for the identification of subtle intraventricular hemorrhage (IVH), subarachnoid cysts, subdural hemorrhage, and deep grey matter abnormalities.[181,186,189,190,193,194] MRI has also been shown to be more accurate than US in determining the time course of cerebral hemorrhagic injuries, and can detect these injuries over a longer time interval than US, with persistent changes on MRI even after the associated US abnormalities have resolved.[181,186] Although both US and MRI can demonstrate ventricular dilatation, MRI has been shown to detect additional cases not seen with US, suggesting that mild ventricular dilatation may be more accurately visualized with MRI.[188]

Despite the apparent sensitivity and accuracy of MRI, some clinical entities remain better detected by US. For example, some studies have demonstrated MRI to be less accurate than US for the detection of lenticulostriate vasculopathy, germinolytic cysts, and choroid plexus cysts.[186,188,193] MRI has also been shown to be less accurate than US for identifying calcifications, despite the inclusion of MR susceptibility sequences that are generally more sensitive to the presence of calcification than conventional MR sequences.[186,188,193]

5.2.4 *MRI appearance of normal neonatal brain*

In general MRI can visualize posterior fossa anatomy better than US due to poor acoustic windows to this area. MRI is also the modality of choice for evaluating myelination, sulcation and migration that can be disrupted during maturation.

5.2.4.1 *Myelination*

Brain myelination is generally best visualized on T1-weighted sequences, and appears as areas of increased signal intensity. The progression of myelination during development has been described in very basic terms as proceeding from caudal to rostral, posterior to anterior and central to peripheral.[195,196] The specific neuroanatomical distribution of myelination during early maturation has also been well described. At approximately 25 weeks, myelination can be identified in gracile nuclei, cuneate nuclei, cerebellar vermis, and vestibular nuclei.[163] At approximately 25–28 weeks, myelination is seen in cerebellar peduncles, dentate nucleus, medial longitudinal fasiculus, medial geniculate bodies, subthalamic nuclei of the thalamus, ventrolateral nuclei of the thalamus, inferior colliculi, medial lemnisci, and lateral lemnisci.[163] After approximately 36 weeks, new areas of myelination can be identified in posterior limb of the internal capsule, corona radiate, and lateral geniculate bodies.[163,197]

Although, in general, T1-weighted sequences optimally visualize myelination, T2-weighted sequences may show myelin relatively earlier than T1-weighted images in gray matter structures such as the vestibular nuclei, medial geniculate bodies, lateral geniculate bodies, inferior olivary nuclei, and inferior colliculi.[163]

5.2.4.2 Migrational milestones

Due to the lack of myelination and increased water content in the neonatal brain, periventricular WM demonstrates low signal intensity on T1-weighted sequences and high signal intensity on T2-weighted sequences.[198] During normal brain maturation, three bands of alternating signal intensity on T2-weighted sequences produce a laminated appearance in the region of the centrum semiovale.[198–200] These areas appear as frontal horn "caps" anteriorly and periventricular "arrowheads" posteriorly, and have been termed "white matter crossroads".[198] The white matter crossroads represent dense regions of extracellular matrix and axonal guidance molecules where microglia modify association-commissural and projection fibers prior to reaching their appropriate target destinations.[198,201]

5.2.4.3 Cortical sulcation

Numerous qualitative post-mortem and MRI studies over the last several decades have demonstrated intense cortical development in fetuses and premature neonates to progress temporally in a regionally specific manner.[202–204] In general, previous observational studies have demonstrated morphological differentiation of sulci to originate in the central cortical region and progresses in an occipito-rostral direction, with the medial cortical surface folding before the lateral surface.[204–206] This pattern of sulcation follows a similar temporal course between fetuses and neonates born prematurely, with a slight delay in premature neonates compared to fetuses of the same gestational age. One recent quantitative MRI analysis of premature neonatal cortical development in 35 neonates between 26 and 36 weeks of age based on gestation demonstrated sulci to appear along a temporal course, as follows: superior and inferior temporal sulci at 27–32 weeks; collateral sulcus at 29–30 weeks; post-central sulcus, intraparietal and parieto-occipital sulci at 27–31 weeks; pre-central sulcus at 29–30 weeks; uncinate sulcus at 30–31 weeks; and olfactive sulcus at 32 weeks.[206] These most recent quantitative results are generally concordant with previous observational evaluations of neonates using MRI.[161,207] It is particularly interesting that occipital and parietal regions appear to mature faster than prefrontal regions, as such a time course of development parallels the relatively rapid maturation of visual and motor functions compared to the slower maturation of executive functions of the prefrontal cortex.[208] Furthermore, this regional pattern of temporal progression in cortical development generally coincides with the temporal and morphological sequence of myelination described previously.[208]

5.2.5 *Developmental outcome in infancy and early childhood*

MRI is beginning to play an important role in the prognostication of developmental outcomes in preterm and term neonates. In particular, the visualization of extensive white matter injury and intraventricular hemorrhage, with accompanying ventricular dilatation, appears to be predictive of poor outcomes.[209] The majority of studies investigating the prognostic value of MRI in neonates have focused on developmental outcomes in the first two years of life. For example, abnormal myelination of the posterior limb of the internal capsule associated with IVH and unilateral parenchymal hemorrhage at birth has been shown to be associated with hemiplegia 12 to 24 months after delivery.[210] Similarly, neonatal MRI demonstrating the extent and severity of white matter lesions has been shown to predict the severity of associated motor and visual deficits at 18 months of age.[211,212] Interestingly, many of the lesions identified on MRI in this study were not seen on US, suggesting the keen sensitivity of MRI for detecting changes associated with long-term developmental outcomes.

Although both gray and WM lesions are seen on neonatal MRI, WM lesions are thought to be more associated with long term developmental sequelae as compared to gray matter. For example, moderate to severe white matter abnormalities on MRI 48 hours after birth strongly predict cognitive and psychomotor delay, cerebral palsy, and neurosensory impairment at two years of age.[151] Although gray matter abnormalities were also correlated with cognitive delay, motor impairment, and cerebral palsy in this study, these outcomes were not as statistically robust. This study also demonstrated the superior sensitivity of MRI for detecting neurodevelopmentally significant CNS lesions not apparent on US.[151] One prospective cohort study performing serial MRI scans on preterm infants, with subsequent evaluation of neurodevelopmental outcome measures 12–18 months after birth, demonstrated significant correlations between degree of white matter injury, ventriculomegaly, as well as IVH and severity of neurodevelopmental outcome.[213] Interestingly, early MRI findings prior to term-equivalent age were better predictors of outcome than were MRI findings at term-equivalent age, suggesting that delaying imaging evaluation until term-equivalent age may not be necessary to generate high yield prognostic data.[213]

Very few neonatal MRI studies investigating neurodevelopmental outcomes associated with CNS lesions have been conducted at endpoints later in childhood. In one longitudinal study, lower developmental quotients at 18 to 36 months were correlated with a pattern of diffuse WM signal hyperintensity and post-hemorrhagic ventricular dilation on MRI, but not findings of punctate white matter lesions or hemorrhage alone.[185] In another relatively recent longitudinal study of neuromotor outcomes three to five years after term-equivalent MRI, the severity of motor impairment was highly correlated with severity of T1 hyperintense lesions or cysts in the corona radiata and corticospinal tract near the posterior limb of the internal capsule. Children with periventricular WM lesions, with sparing of this portion of the corona radiate, demonstrated normal motor development.[155]

Taken together, these data suggest that MRI is a viable neonatal neuroimaging method that can guide the clinical management of infants with CNS damage by providing critical information regarding long-term neurodevelopmental outcomes. It should be noted that in several of these prognostic outcomes investigations, MRI was superior to US in detecting the extent and severity of CNS disease. This apparent advantage in sensitivity of MRI may be crucial for identifying patients destined to have poor outcomes and for pinpointing precise neurodevelopmental deficits associated with specific topographic patterns of brain pathology. Future studies may provide additional detailed information about distributed networks of

CNS damage that could guide more targeted intervention based upon specific sequelae of related developmental impairment.

5.2.6 *MRI in term and near-term newborns*

5.2.6.1 *Hypoxic-ischemic injury*

Hypoxic-ischemic injury (HII) in the brain is the result of decreased blood flow (ischemia) and diminished oxygenation (hypoxemia) that affects the brain in a heterogeneous fashion, with some brain areas being more vulnerable than others.[214] HII, when found in preterm neonates, has a different imaging appearance on MRI compared to HII in term neonates due to the immaturity of the preterm neonatal brain.[214] The imaging manifestations of HII can be subdivided based upon the severity of injury into severe versus mild to moderate forms of disease.

5.2.6.2 *Severe asphyxia in preterm neonates*

Severe asphyxia results in injury to the thalami, anterior vermis, and dorsal brainstem most frequently, but also affects the basal ganglia, hippocampi, cerebellum, and corticospinal tracts as well.[214,215] Basal ganglia involvement, however, is less severe than injury of the thalami.[215] Severe asphyxia may also result in germinal matrix hemorrhages and periventricular white matter injury.

Conventional MRI sequences may demonstrate only subtle signal abnormalities on day one post-injury. Diffusion imaging, however, may show signal abnormalities in the thalami within this early time window, but typically peak approximately 3–5 days after injury.[214] By days 2 and 3 post-injury, conventional MRI may demonstrate prolonged T2 and shortened T1, respectively.[216,217] By day 7, conventional MRI may demonstrate a shortened T2 in the area of injury, as well as shortened T1 that persists chronically.[214,216,217]

5.2.6.3 *Mild to moderate asphyxia in preterm neonates*

Mild to moderate asphyxia may result in IVH and/or periventricular leukomalacia (PVL). IVH generally occurs in the first 24 hours of life, most commonly in lower gestational age and lower birth weight infants, with the lowest birth weight infants at highest risk for hemorrhage. IVHs arise from the germinal matrix in the region of the caudothalamic groove, and are classically subdivided into four categories discussed previously in the US section of this chapter. MRI is generally not necessary for characterizing IVH, which is readily visualized by US.

PVL is most commonly seen in the region of the trigones of the lateral ventricles, and is thought to be the result of damage to oligodendrocyte cells (specifically preoligodendrocytes) in this area that are particularly vulnerable to hypoxia-ischemia.[218–220] The decline in prevalence of PVL after 32 weeks gestation has been postulated to be due to maturation of oligodendrocytes that coincides with this time point.[219] The characteristic four stages of PVL ranging from early congestion to late cavitation and development of porencephalic cysts are generally well seen by US, but can be detected earlier with MRI, especially in the setting of non-cystic PVL.[214,221–223] The temporal manifestations of PVL are first seen by day 3–4, and appear as areas of T1 shortening embedded within larger foci of prolonged T2 signal that progress to areas of mild T2-shortening at 6–7 days.[214,217,224] If hemorrhage is present in conjunction with PVL, there may be additional areas of low T2-signal.[211,214]

5.2.6.4 *Severe asphyxia in term neonates*

Severe asphyxia results in injury to central deep gray structures, including the putamina, ventrolateral thalami, hippocampi, dorsal brainstem, lateral geniculate nuclei, and less frequently the perirolandic cortex.[214,217] The remaining cortex is sometimes affected, however, involvement usually indicates a more severe injury and worse neurologic prognosis.[214,217]

Conventional MRI sequences may demonstrate no or only subtle signal abnormalities day 1 post-injury. Diffusion imaging, however, may show signal abnormalities in the ventrolateral thalami, posterior putamina, perirolandic regions and corticospinal tracts within this early time window, but may underestimate the degree of injury.[214,217,225] By day 2 post-injury, conventional MRI may demonstrate injury-related signal increases on T1 and T2 weighted sequences, as well as signal changes in dorsal brainstem and hippocampi.[214,216,226] HII-related changes in diffusion signal subsequently peak approximately 3–5 days after injury, and may pseudonormalize after one week, but demonstrate persistent decreases in ADC values for up to two weeks.[214,217,225,227–229] By the second week post-injury the thalami and posterior putamina demonstrate T2 shortening.[214,216] Chronic changes associated with HII include signal increases on T2 weighted imaging, especially in the ventrolateral thalami, posterior putamina, and corticospinal tracts.[214,226] Thalamic nuclei, basal ganglia structures and perirolandic cortex may demonstrate persistent T1 shortening for months following injury.[214,226]

Heinz and Provenzale[230] have recently proposed a simplified schema of four major signs on MRI to facilitate the diagnosis of hypoxia in the term neonate, collectively referred to as the "1–2–3–4 sign". The four components of the 1–2–3–4 sign are, as follows: (1) increased signal intensity in the basal ganglia on T1-weighted images, (2) increased signal intensity in the thalamus on T1-weighted images, (3) absent or decreased signal intensity in the posterior limb of the internal capsule on T1-weighted images (i.e. the "absent posterior limb sign"), and (4) restricted water diffusion on diffusion-weighted images.[230]

5.2.6.5 *Mild to moderate asphyxia in term neonates*

Mild to moderate injury in term neonates associated with asphyxia produces a unique pattern of changes in the brain along a continuum related to the duration of insult.[217] For example, relatively short duration asphyxia produces minimal to no evidence of brain injury, whereas relatively longer duration injury may produce sequelae of hypoperfusion involving intervascular boundary (watershed) zones. This is thought to be the result of protective shunting of blood to critical brain structures, such as the brainstem, thalami, basal ganglia, hippocampi, and cerebellum from relatively less metabolically active structures, such as the cerebral cortex and white matter.[214,217,231]

Given the location of injury in cortical and subcortical watershed zones, US is of limited value in the evaluation of mild to moderate HII.[214] As with the other categories of asphyxia-associated injury, diffusion-weighted MRI is most sensitive to early and subtle changes in the first 24 hours, which appear as prominent areas of restricted diffusion along parasagittal watershed zones.[214,216] These diffusion-weighted changes may be extremely subtle or entirely absent due to the normally high T2 signal in the relatively unmyelinated neonatal brain.[214,216] ADC maps associated with diffusion sequences are, therefore, of critical importance to exclude false positive and/or negative interpretations due to normal T2 shine-through. Conventional MRI sequences are usually normal on day 1 post-injury.[225] By day 2 post-injury, the earliest changes on conventional MRI may include subtle parasagittal watershed distribution cortical swelling and loss of gray-white matter differentiation, as well as cortical and subcortical white matter T2 hyperintensity.[227] Unlike severe asphyxia, deep gray structures are typically spared in mild to moderate injury.[214] Chronic changes of mild to moderate HII include cerebral atrophy, cortical thinning and diminished white matter volume in a primarily parasagittal watershed distribution.[214]

5.2.7 *Neonatal stroke*

Stroke in neonates is associated with significant devastating long-term morbidity, and occurs in one in 2300–5000 births, an overall incidence second to that of strokes in the elderly population.[232–234] Indeed, the most common time for stroke to occur during childhood is within 2–3 days of birth, likely associated with the complex hemodynamic changes occurring during this time period.[235–237] Although neonatal infarction is most frequently idiopathic, coagulopathies have also been identified as a common etiology in this age group.[236] MRI is generally used as the modality of choice for evaluating the early effects of ischemia in the brain.[225,237] The most sensitive sequence for detecting changes of ischemia is DWI that demonstrates increases in signal intensity, with corresponding decreases on ADC maps. These changes may become apparent within as little as 20 minutes, but generally within 24 hours, and begin to fade by day 4, with signal intensity becoming less than or equal to that of unaffected cortex by approximately day 12 post-injury.[225,236,238,239] Ischemia-associated changes on conventional T1- and T2-weighted sequences become apparent along a slower time-course, with initial dedifferentiation of the gray-white matter interface of affected tissue by 2–3 days post-infarction.[215]

The combination of vasogenic and cytotoxic edema in the injured cortex increases the overall water content of the tissue, resulting in decreased T1 and increased T2 signal intensity.[239] Due to the paucity of white matter myelination in neonates in combination with the altered signal intensity of the affected cortex, visualization of the cortical ribbon becomes difficult, resulting in the so-called "missing cortex" sign.[217,239] By day 6, however, T1 and T2 signal intensity reverses resulting in cortical highlighting that persists for approximately 1–2 months.[239] MR arteriography and venography are becoming increasingly utilized in conjunction with conventional MR imaging to investigate and pinpoint the underlying causes of arterial and venous infarction in the setting of neonatal stroke.[234]

5.2.8 *Neonatal structural abnormalities*

Abnormal brain development can be the result of a host of underlying etiologies, such as genetic defects, teratogenic exposures and fetal injury that result in serious postnatal consequences, such as developmental delay, mental retardation, and seizures. Although most abnormalities of brain development are diagnosed via prenatal US, postnatal imaging is often performed to confirm and explore the extent of an abnormality.[217,240] MRI can be useful in this regard, especially when high spatial resolution and good gray-white contrast is necessary. Commonly encountered neonatal structural abnormalities include those involving the corpus callosum, posterior fossa, and cerebral cortex.

5.2.8.1 *Corpus callosum abnormalities*

Abnormalities of the corpus callosum can be difficult to identify with US, but are usually well seen with MRI given the high spatial resolution and ability to reconstruct images of the brain into coronal and sagittal planes. MRI has the additional advantage of showing the entire brain, which becomes important in the context of corpus callosal abnormalities given the high association with other CNS anomalies. Indeed, additional CNS abnormalities have been described at autopsy in 85% of children with callosal agenesis, including Chiari II malformation,

Dandy-Walker malformation, gray matter heterotopia, holoprosen-cephaly, schizencephaly, and encephaloceles.[241–244]

5.2.8.2   *Posterior fossa abnormalities*

Common abnormalities of the posterior fossa evaluated with MRI include Dandy–Walker malformation, Dandy–Walker variant, mega cisterna magna, arachnoid cyst, Blake pouch cyst, cerebellar dysplasia, cerebellar hypoplasia, cerebellar hemorrhage, Walker–Warburg syndrome, and Chiari II malformation.[244] Since sonographic visualization of the contents of the posterior fossa is obscured by the skull, MRI plays an important role in the diagnosis of abnormalities in this portion of the brain. For example, MRI can provide information about the size and shape of the cerebellar vermis that can help differentiate between Dandy–Walker variant (abnormal vermis) and a mega cisterna magna (intact vermis).[244] Such characterization is particularly important in the evaluation of Dandy–Walker spectrum abnormalities, as the degree of vermian dysplasia may be predictive of long-term neurodevelopmental outcome.[244–246] As with corpus callosal abnormalities, MRI may also aid in the detection of other abnormalities associated with Dandy–Walker malformation (and other posterior fossa abnormalities), such as agenesis of the corpus callosum, polymicrogyria, neuronal heterotopia, and occipital encephaloceles that may also be related to long-term outcomes.[244,247–249]

5.2.8.3   *Cortical development abnormalities*

Common malformations of cortical development include schizencephaly, lissencephaly, polymicrogyria, and gray matter heterotopias, all of which have been shown to be better visualized with MRI, as compared to US.[244,250] These cortical abnormalities have characteristic appearances on MRI and are described briefly, as follows.[244,251] Subependymal heterotopias are small nodules that appear isointense to the germinal matrix, and are seen along the walls of the ventricles. Schizencephaly is characterized by a gray matter-lined cleft that extends from the subarachnoid space to the ipsilateral ventricle. Polymicrogyria can be focal or diffuse and is characterized by the absence of normal sulcation, with numerous associated abnormal cortical convolutions. Classical lissencephaly appears as a thick band of abnormal cortex without the normal multilayered laminated appearance, paucity or absence of normal sulci, and shallow Sylvian fissures.

References

1. Ment LR, Bada HS, Barnes P, Grant PE, Hirtz D, Papile LA, *et al.* (2002) Practice parameter: neuroimaging of the neonate — report of the Quality Standards Subcommittee of the American Academy of Neurology and the Practice Committee of the Child Neurology Society. *Neurology* 58: 1726–1738.

2. Inder TE, Anderson NJ, Spencer C, Wells S, Volpe JJ. (2003) White matter injury in the premature infant: a comparison between serial cranial sonographic and MR findings at term. *Am J Neuroradiol* 24: 805–809.

3. O'Shea TM, Counsell SJ, Bartels DB, Dammann O. (2005) Magnetic resonance and ultrasound brain imaging in preterm infants. *Early Hum Dev* 81: 263–271.

4. Hintz SR, O'Shea M. (2008) Neuroimaging and neurodevelopmental outcomes in preterm infants. *Semin Perinatol* 32: 11–19.

5. Erba G, Lombroso CT. (1968) Detection of ventricular landmarks by two dimensional ultrasonography. *J Neurol Neurosurg Psychiatry* 31: 244.

6. Pape KE, Cusick G, Houang MTW, Reynolds EOR, Blackwell RJ, Sherwood A, *et al.* (1979) Ultrasound detection of brain-damage in preterm infants. *Lancet* 1: 1261–1264.

7. Slovis TL, Kuhns LR. (1981) Real-time sonography of the brain through the anterior fontanelle. *Am J Roentgenol* 136: 277–286.

8. Papile LA, Burstein J, Burstein R, Koffler H. (1978) Incidence and evolution of subependymal and intra-ventricular hemorrhage — study of infants with birth weights less than 1,500 gm. *J Pediat* 92: 529–534.

9. Lazzara A, Ahmann P, Dykes F, Brann AW, Schwartz J. (1980) Clinical predictability of intra-ventricular hemorrhage in preterm infants. *Pediatrics* 65: 30–34.

10. Burstein J. (1979) New Look at young brains. *Am J Roentgenol* 133: 556–557.

11. Paneth N, Jetton J, Pinto-Martin J, Susser M. (1997) Magnesium sulfate in labor and risk of neonatal brain lesions and cerebral palsy in low birth

weight infants. The Neonatal Brain Hemorrhage Study Analysis Group. *Pediatrics* 99: E1.

12. Paneth N, PintoMartin J, Gardiner J, Wallenstein S, Katsikiotis V, Hegyi T, *et al.* (1993) Incidence and timing of germinal matrix intraventricular hemorrhage in low-birth-weight infants. *Am J Epidemiol* 137: 1167–1176.

13. Van de Bor M, Verloove-Vanhorick SP, Baerts W, Brand R, Ruys JH. (1988) Outcome of periventricular-intraventricular hemorrhage at 2 years of age in 484 very preterm infants admitted to 6 neonatal intensive care units in The Netherlands. *Neuropediatrics* 19: 183–185.

14. Kitchen WH, Ford GW, Murton LJ, Rickards AL, Ryan MM, Lissenden JV, *et al.* (1985) Mortality and two year outcome of infants of birthweight 500–1500 g: relationship with neonatal cerebral ultrasound data. *Aust Paediatr J* 21: 253–259.

15. Pinto-Martin JA, Riolo S, Cnaan A, Holzman C, Susser MW, Paneth N. (1995) Cranial ultrasound prediction of disabling and nondisabling cerebral palsy at age two in a low birth weight population. *Pediatrics* 95: 249–254.

16. Aziz K, Vickar DB, Sauve RS, Etches PC, Pain KS, Robertson CMT. (1995) Province-based study of neurologic disability of children weighing 500 through 1249 grams at birth in relation to neonatal cerebral ultrasound findings. *Pediatrics* 95: 837–844.

17. Whitaker A, Johnson J, Sebris S, Pinto J, Wasserman G, Kairam R, *et al.* (1990) Neonatal cranial ultrasound abnormalities — association with developmental delay at age one in low-birth-weight infants. *J Dev Behav Pediatr* 11: 253–260.

18. Bozynski MEA, Nelson MN, Rosatiskertich C, Genaze D, Odonnell K, Naughton P. (1984) 2 Year longitudinal follow-up of premature-infants weighing less-than-or-equal-to 1200 grams at birth — sequelae of intracranial hemorrhage. *J Dev Behav Pediatr* 5: 346–352.

19. Cooke RWI. (1987) Early and late cranial ultrasonographic appearances and outcome in very low birthweight infants. *Arch Dis Child* 62: 931–937.

20. Papile LA, Munsickbruno G, Schaefer A. (1983). Relationship of cerebral intraventricular hemorrhage and early-childhood neurologic handicaps. *J Pediatr* 103: 273–277.

21. Bassan H, Feldman HA, Limperopoulos C, Benson CB, Ringer SA, Veracruz E, *et al.* (2006) Periventricular hemorrhagic infarction: risk factors and neonatal outcome. *Pediatr Neurol* 35: 85–92.

22. Roze E, Kerstjens JM, Maathuis CGB, ter Horst HJ, Bos AF. (2008) Risk factors for adverse outcome in preterm infants with periventricular hemorrhagic infarction. *Pediatrics* 122: E46–E52.

23. Guzzetta F, Schackelford GD, Volpe S, Perlman JM, Volpe JJ. (1986) Periventricular intraparenchymal echodensities in the premature newborn: critical determinant of neurologic outcome. *Pediatrics* 78: 995–1006.

24. Mcmenamin JB, Shackelford GD, Volpe JJ. (1984) Outcome of neonatal intraventricular hemorrhage with periventricular echodense lesions. *Ann Neurol* 15: 285–290.

25. Pidcock FS, Graziani LJ, Stanley C, Mitchell DG, Merton D. (1990) Neurosonographic features of periventricular echodensities associated with cerebral-palsy in preterm infants. *J Pediatr* 116: 417–422.

26. O'Shea TM, Kothadia JM, Roberts DD, Dillard RG. (1998) Perinatal events and the risk of intraparenchymal echodensity in very-low-birthweight neonates. *Paediatr Perinat Epidemiol* 12: 408–421.

27. Holling EE, Leviton A. (1999) Characteristics of cranial ultrasound white-matter echolucencies that predict disability: a review. *Dev Med Child Neurol* 41: 136–139.

28. Nwaesei CG, Pape KE, Martin DJ, Becker LE, Fitz CR. (1984) Periventricular infarction diagnosed by ultrasound: a postmortem correlation. *J Pediatr* 105: 106–110.

29. Fawer CL, Calame A, Perentes E, Anderegg A. (1985) Periventricular leukomalacia: a correlation study between real-time ultrasound and autopsy findings. Periventricular leukomalacia in the neonate. *Neuroradiology* 27: 292–300.

30. de Vries LS, Van Haastert ILC, Rademaker KJ, Koopman C, Groenedaal F. (2004) Ultrasound abnormalities preceding cerebral palsy in high-risk preterm infants. *J Pediatr* 144: 815–820.

31. Pisani F, Leali L, Moretti S, Turco E, Volante E, Bevilacqua G. (2006) Transient periventricular echodensities in preterms and neurodevelopmental outcome. *J Child Neurol* 21: 230–235.

32. Appleton RE, Lee REJ, Hey EN. (1990) Neurodevelopmental outcome of transient neonatal intracerebral echodensities. *Arch Dis Child* 65: 27–29.

33. Dammann O, Leviton A. (1997) Duration of transient hyperechoic images of white matter in very-low-birthweight infants: a proposed classification. *Dev Med Child Neurol* 39: 2–5.

34. Ringelberg J, Vandebor M. (1993) Outcome of transient periventricular echodensities in preterm infants. *Neuropediatrics* 24: 269–273.

35. Shortland D, Levene MI, Trounce J, Ng Y, Graham M. (1988) The evolution and outcome of cavitating periventricular leukomalacia in infancy — a study of 46 cases. *J Perin Med* 16: 241–247.

36. Tamisari L, Vigi V, Fortini C, Scarpa P. (1986) Neonatal periventricular leukomalacia: diagnosis and evolution evaluated by real-time ultrasound. *Helv Paediat Acta* 41: 399–407.

37. Grant EG, Schellinger D, Smith Y, Uscinski RH. (1986) Periventricular leukomalacia in combination with intraventricular hemorrhage — sonographic features and sequelae. *Am J Neuroradiol* 7: 443–447.

38. Leviton A, Gilles F. (1996) Ventriculomegaly, delayed myelination, white matter hypoplasia, and "periventricular" leukomalacia: how are they related? *Pediatr Neurol* 15: 127–136.

39. Paneth N. (1999) Classifying brain damage in preterm infants. *J Pediatr* 134: 527–529.

40. Leviton A, Paneth N. (1990) White matter damage in preterm newborns — an epidemiologic perspective. *Early Hum Dev* 24: 1–22.

41. Dammann O, Leviton A. (1997) Maternal intrauterine infection, cytokines, and brain damage in the preterm newborn. *Pediatr Res* 42: 1–8.

42. Hansen A, Leviton A, Paneth N, Reuss ML, Susser M, Allred EN, *et al.* (1998) The correlation between placental pathology and intraventricular hemorrhage in the preterm infant. *Pediatr Res* 43: 15–19.

43. Leviton A, Paneth N, Susser M, Reuss ML, Allred EN, Kuban K, *et al.* (1997) Maternal receipt of magnesium sulfate does not seem to reduce the risk of neonatal white matter damage. *Pediatrics* 99: E2.

44. Leviton A, Dammann O, Allred EN. (1999) Antenatal corticosteroids and cranial ultrasound abnormalities. *Am J Obstet Gynecol* 181: 1007–1017.

45. Leviton A, Paneth N, Reuss ML, Susser M, Allred EN, Dammann O, *et al.* (1999) Hypothyroxinemia of prematurity and the risk of cerebral white matter damage. *J Pediatr* 134: 706–711.

46. Perlman JM, Risser R, Broyles RS. (1996) Bilateral cystic periventricular leukomalacia in the premature infant: associated risk factors. *Pediatrics* 97: 822–827.

47. Levene MI, Fawer CL, Lamont RF. (1982) Risk-factors in the development of intraventricular hemorrhage in the preterm neonate. *Arch Dis Child* 57: 410–417.

48. Wood NS, Costeloe K, Gibson AT, Hennessy EM, Marlow N, Wilkinson AR. (2005) The EPICure study: associations and antecedents of neurological and developmental disability at 30 months of age following extremely preterm birth. *Arch Dis Childhood-Fetal* 90: 134–140.

49. Larroque B, Marret S, Ancel PY, Arnaud C, Marpeau L, Supernant K, *et al.* (2003) White matter damage and intraventricular hemorrhage in very preterm infants: the epipage study. *J Pediatr* 143: 477–483.

50. Broitman E, Namasivayam A, Higgins RD, Vohr BR, Das A, Bhaskar B, *et al.* (2007) Clinical data predict neurodevelopmental outcome better than head ultrasound in extremely low birth weight infants. *J Pediatr* 151: 500–505.

51. Laptook AR, O'Shea TM, Shankaran S, Bhaskar B, NICHD Neonatal Network. (2005) Adverse neurodevelopmental outcomes among extremely low birth weight infants with a normal head ultrasound: prevalence and antecedents. *Pediatrics* 115: 673–680.

52. Vohr BR, Wright LL, Dusick AM, Mele L, Verter J, Steichen JJ, *et al.* (2000) Neurodevelopmental and functional outcomes of extremely low birth weight infants in the National Institute of Child Health and Human Development Neonatal Research Network, 1993–1994. *Pediatrics* 105: 1216–1226.

53. Kuban K, Allred E, O'Shea TM, Paneth N, Pagano M, Dammann O, *et al.* (2008) Cranial ultrasound lesions in the NICU predict cerebral palsy at age 2 years in children who were born at extremely low gestational age. *J Child Neurol* 24: 63–72.

54. O'Shea TM, Kuban KCK, Allred EN, Paneth N, Pagano M, Dammann O, *et al.* (2008) Neonatal cranial ultrasound lesions and developmental delays at 2 years of age among extremely low gestational age children. *Pediatrics* 122: E662–E669.

55. Van Meurs KP, Wright LL, Ehrenkranz RA, Lemons JA, Ball MB, Poole WK, *et al.* (2005) Inhaled nitric oxide for premature infants with severe respiratory failure. *N Engl J Med* 353: 13–22.

56. Kenyon SL, Taylor DJ, Tarnow-Mordi W. (2001) Broad-spectrum antibiotics for preterm, prelabour rupture of fetal membranes: the ORACLE I randomised trial. *Lancet* 357: 979–988.

57. Kenyon SL, Taylor DJ, Tarnow-Mordi W. (2001) Broad-spectrum antibiotics for spontaneous preterm labour: the ORACLE II randomised trial. *Lancet* 357: 989–994.

58. Rouse DJ, Hirtz DG, Thom E, *et al.* (2008) A randomized, controlled trial of magnesium sulfate for the prevention of cerebral palsy. *N Engl J Med* 359: 895–905.

59. Kuban KCK, Leviton A, Krishnamoorthy KS, Brown ER, Teele RL, Baglivo JA, *et al.* (1986) Neonatal intracranial hemorrhage and phenobarbital. *Pediatrics* 77: 443–450.

60. Ment LR, Oh W, Ehrenkranz RA, Philip AG, Vohr B, Allan W, *et al.* (1994) Low-dose indomethacin and prevention of intraventricular hemorrhage: a multicenter randomized trial. *Pediatrics* 93: 543–550.

61. Bandstra ES, Montalvo BM, Goldberg RN, Pacheco I, Ferrer PL, Flynn J, *et al.* (1988) Prophylactic indomethacin for prevention of intraventricular hemorrhage in premature-infants. *Pediatrics* 82: 533–542.

62. Shankaran S, Papile LA, Wright LL, Ehrenkranz RA, Mele L, Lemons JA, *et al.* (1997) The effect of antenatal phenobarbital therapy on neonatal intracranial hemorrhage in preterm infants. *N Engl J Med* 337: 466–471.

63. Paneth N, Rudelli R, Kazam E, Monte W. (1994) Prognosis. In: Paneth N, Rudelli R, Kazam E, Monte W, eds. *Brain Damage in the Preterm Infant.* London: Cambridge University Press; 171–185.

64. Limperopoulos C, Benson CB, Bassan H, DiSalvo DN, Kinnamon DD, Moore M, *et al.* (2005) Cerebellar hemorrhage in the preterm infant: ultra-sonographic findings and risk factors. *Pediatrics* 116: 717–724.

65. Luna JA, Goldstein RB. (2000) Sonographic visualization of neodatal posterior fossa abnormalities through the posterolateral fontanelle. *Am J Roentgenol* 174: 561–567.

66. DiSalvo DN. (2001) A new view of the neonatal brain: clinical utility of supplemental neurological imaging ultrasound windows. *Radiographics* 21: 943–955.

67. Buckley KM, Taylor GA, Estroff JA, Barnewolt CE, Share JC, Paltiel HJ. (1997) Use of the mastoid fontanelle for improved sonographic visualization of the neonatal midbrain and posterior fossa. *Am J Roentgenol* 168: 1021–1025.

68. Correa F, Enriquez G, Rossello J, Lucaya J, Piqueras J, Aso C, *et al.* (2004) Posterior fontanelle sonography: an acoustic window into the neonatal brain. *Am J Neuroradiol* 25: 1274–1282.

69. Krishnamoorthy KS, Shannon DC, Delong GR, Todres ID, Davis KR. (1979) Neurologic sequelae in the survivors of neonatal intra-ventricular hemorrhage. *Pediatrics* 64: 233–237.

70. Thorburn RJ, Stewart AL, Hope PL, Lipscomb AP, Reynolds EOR, Pape KE. (1981) Prediction of death and major handicap in very preterm infants by brain ultrasound. *Lancet* 1: 1119–1121.

71. Shankaran S, Slovis TL, Bedard MP, Poland RL. (1982) Sonographic classification of intra-cranical hemorrhage — a prognostic indicator of mortality, morbidity, and short-term neurologic outcome. *J Pediatr* 100: 469–475.

72. Levene MI, Starte DR. (1981) A longitudinal-study of post-haemorrhagic ventricular dilatation in the newborn. *Arch Dis Childhood* 56: 905–910.

73. Papile LA, Burstein J, Burstein R, Koffler H, Koops BL, Johnson JD. (1980) Post-hemorrhagic hydrocephalus in low-birth-weight infants — treatment by serial lumbar punctures. *J Pediatr* 97: 273–237.

74. Graziani LJ, Pasto M, Stanley C, Steben J, Desai H, Desai S, *et al.* (1985) Cranial ultrasound and clinical studies in preterm infants. *J Pediatr* 106: 269–276.

75. Stewart AL, Reynolds EO, Hope PL, Hamilton PA, Baudin J, Costello AM, *et al.* (1987) Probability of neurodevelopmental disorders estimated from ultrasound appearance of brains of very preterm infants. *Dev Med Child Neurol* 29: 3–11.

76. Costello AMD, Hamilton PA, Baudin J, Townsend J, Bradford BC, Stewart AL, *et al.* (1988) Prediction of neurodevelopmental impairment at 4 years from brain ultrasound appearance of very preterm infants. *Dev Med Child Neurol* 30: 711–722.

77. Roth SC, Baudin J, Mccormick DC, Edwards AD, Townsend J, Stewart AL, *et al.* (1993) Relation between ultrasound appearance of the brain of very preterm infants and neurodevelopmental impairment at 8 years. *Dev Med Child Neurol* 35: 755–768.

78. Levene MI. (1981) Measurement of the growth of the lateral ventricles in preterm infants with real-time ultrasound. *Arch Dis Child* 56: 900–904.

79. Kuban K, Teele RL. (1984) Rationale for grading intracranial hemorrhage in premature-infants. *Pediatrics* 74: 358–363.

80. Leviton A, Kuban K, Paneth N. (2007) Intraventricular haemorrhage grading scheme: time to abandon? *Acta Paediatr* 96: 1254–1256.

81. Paneth N, Rudelli R, Monte W, Rodriguez E, Pinto J, Kairam R, *et al.* (1990) White matter necrosis in very-low-birth-weight infants — neuropathologic

and ultrasonographic findings in infants surviving 6 days or longer. *J Pediatr* 116: 975–984.

82. Paneth N, Rudelli R, Kazam E, Monte W. (1994) Germinal matrix and intraventricular bleeding: location, extent, ultrasound imaging. In: Paneth N, Rudelli R, Kazam E, Monte W, eds. *Brain Damage in the Preterm Infant.* London: Cambridge University Press; 71–98.

83. Paneth N, Rudelli R, Kazam E, Monte W. (1994) The varieties of leukomalacia. In: Paneth N, Rudelli R, Kazam E, Monte W, eds. *Brain Damage in the Preterm Infant.* London: Cambridge University Press; 119–137.

84. Paneth N, Rudelli R, Kazam E, Monte W. (1994) Asssociated pathologic lesions: cerebellar hemorrhage, pontosubicular necrosis, basal ganglia necrosis. In: Paneth N, Rudelli R, Kazam E, Monte W, eds. *Brain Damage in the Preterm Infant.* London: Cambridge University Press; 163–170.

85. Limperopoulos C, Bassan H, Gauvreau K, Robertson RL, Sullivan NR, Benson CB, *et al.* (2007) Does cerebellar injury in premature infants contribute to the high prevalence of long-term cognitive, learning, and behavioral disability in survivors? *Pediatrics* 120: 584–593.

86. Paneth N, Rudelli R, Monte W, Rodriguez E, Pinto J, Kairam R, *et al.* (1990) White matter necrosis in very low birth weight infants: Neuropathologic and ultrasonographic findings in infants surviving six days or longer. *J Pediatr* 116: 975–984.

87. Pinto J, Paneth N, Kazam E, Kairam R, Wallenstein S, Rose W, *et al.* (1988) Interobserver variability in neonatal cranial ultrasonography. *Paediatr Perinat Epidemiol* 2: 43–58.

88. Pinto-Martin JA, Whitaker AH, Feldman JF, Van Rossem R, Paneth N. (1999) Relation of cranial ultrasound abnormalities in low-birthweight infants to motor or cognitive performance at ages 2, 6, and 9 years. *Dev Med Child Neurol* 41: 826–833.

89. Whitaker AH, Feldman JF, VanRossem R, Schonfeld IS, PintoMartin JA, Torre C, *et al.* (1996) Neonatal cranial ultrasound abnormalities in low birth weight infants: relation to cognitive outcomes at six years of age. *Pediatrics* 98: 719–729.

90. Whitaker AH, Van Rossem R, Feldman JF, Schonfeld IS, Pinto-Martin JA, Tore C, *et al.* (1997) Psychiatric outcomes in low-birth-weight children at age 6 years: relation to neonatal cranial ultrasound abnormalities. *Arch Gen Psychiatry* 54: 847–856.

91. Pape KE, Bennettbritton S, Szymonowicz W, Martin DJ, Fitz CR, Becker L. (1983) Diagnostic-accuracy of neonatal brain imaging — a postmortem correlation of computed-tomography and ultrasound scans. *J Pediatr* 102: 275–280.

92. Babcock DS, Bove KE, Han BK. (1982) Intracranial hemorrhage in premature infants: sonographic-pathologic correlation. *AJNR Am J Neuroradiol* 3: 309–317.

93. Szymonowicz W, Schafler K, Cussen LJ, Yu VY. (1984) Ultrasound and necropsy study of periventricular haemorrhage in preterm infants. *Arch Dis Child* 59: 637–642.

94. Thorburn RJ, Lipscomb AP, Reynolds EO, Blackwell RJ, Cusick G, Shaw DG, *et al.* (1982) Accuracy of imaging of the brains of newborn infants by linear-array real-time ultrasound. *Early Hum Dev* 6: 31–46.

95. Trounce JQ, Fagan D, Levene MI. (1986) Intraventricular haemorrhage and periventricular leucomalacia: ultrasound and autopsy correlation. *Arch Dis Child* 61: 1203–1207.

96. Corbett SS, Rosenfeld CR, Laptook AR, Risser R, Maravilla AM, Dowling S, *et al.* (1991) Intraobserver and interobserver reliability in assessment of neonatal cranial ultrasounds. *Early Hum Dev* 27: 9–17.

97. O'Shea TM, Volberg F, Dillard RG. (1993) Reliability of interpretations of cranial ultrasound examinations of very low birthweight neonates. *Dev Med Child Neurol* 35: 97–101.

98. Kuban K, Adler I, Allred E, Batton D, Bezinque S, Betz BW, *et al.* (2007) Observer variability assessing US scans of the preterm brain: the ELGAn study. *Pediatr Radiol* 37: 1201–1208.

99. Hintz SR, Slovis T, Bulas D, Van Meurs KP, Perritt R, Stevenson DK, *et al.* (2007) Interobserver reliability and accuracy of cranial ultrasound scanning interpretation in premature infants. *J Pediatr* 150: 592–596.

100. Harris DL, Bloomfield FH, Teele R, Harding JE. (2006) Variable interpretation of ultrasonograms may contribute to variation in the reported incidence of white matter damage between newborn intensive care units in New Zealand. *Arch Dis Childhood-Fetal* 91: F11–F16.

101. Kuban K, Adler I, Allred E, Batton D, Bezinque S, Betz BW, *et al.* (2007) Observer variability assessing US scans of the preterm brain: the ELGAN study. *Pediatr Radiol* 37: 1201–1208.

102. Wall SN, Partridge JC. (1997) Death in the intensive care nursery: physician practice of withdrawing and withholding life support. *Pediatrics* 99: 64–70.

103. Stevenson DK, Goldworth A. (2002) Ethical considerations in neuroimaging and its impact on decision-making for neonates. *Brain Cognition* 50: 449–454.

104. Levene MI, Wigglesworth JS, Dubowitz V. (1981) Cerebral structure and intraventricular hemorrhage in the neonate — a real-time ultrasound study. *Arch Dis Childhood* 56: 416–424.

105. Rademaker KJ, Groenendaal F, Jansen GH, Eken P, deVries LS. (1994) Unilateral hemorrhagic parenchymal lesions in the preterm infant — shape, site and prognosis. *Acta Paediatr* 83: 602–608.

106. Gould SJ, Howard S, Hope PL, Reynolds EOR. (1987) Periventricular intraparenchymal cerebral-hemorrhage in preterm infants — the role of venous infarction. *J Pathol* 151: 197–202.

107. Roze E, Kerstjens JM, Maathuis CGB, ter Horst HJ, Bos AF. (2008) Risk factors for adverse outcome in preterm infants with periventricular hemorrhagic infarction. *Pediatrics* 122: E46–E52.

108. Bassan H, Limperopoulos C, Visconti K, Feldman HA, Avery LM, Benson CB, *et al.* (2006) Ultrasonographic severity scoring of periventricular hemorrhagic infarction in relation to neurological outcome. *Ann Neurol* 60: S158–S159.

109. Bassan H, Limperopoulos C, Visconti K, Mayer DL, Feldman HA, Avery L, *et al.* (2007) Neurodevelopmental outcome in survivors of periventricular hemorrhagic infarction. *Pediatrics* 120: 785–792.

110. Amess PN, Baudin J, Townsend J, Meek J, Roth SC, Neville BGR, *et al.* (1998) Epilepsy in very preterm infants: neonatal cranial ultrasound reveals a high-risk subcategory. *Dev Med Child Neurol* 40: 724–730.

111. Whitelaw A. (1990) Randomized trial of early tapping in neonatal posthaemorrhagic ventricular dilatation. *Arch Dis Childhood* 65: 3–10.

112. Kennedy C, Campbell M, Elbourne D, Hope P, Johnson A, Darroch A, *et al.* (1998) International randomised controlled trial of acetazolamide and furosemide in posthaemorrhagic ventricular dilatation in infancy. *Lancet* 352: 433–440.

113. Whitelaw A, Thoresen M, Pople I. (2002) Posthaemorrhagic ventricular dilatation. *Arch Dis Childhood* 86: 72–74.

114. Sola-Visner M, Saxonhouse MA, Brown RE. (2008) Neonatal thrombocytopenia: what we do and don't know. *Early Hum Dev* 84: 499–506.

115. Whitelaw A, Pople I, Cherian S, Evans D, Thoresen M. (2003) Phase 1 trial of prevention of hydrocephalus after intraventricular hemorrhage in newborn infants by drainage, irrigation, and fibrinolytic therapy. *Pediatrics* 111: 759–765.

116. Whitelaw A, Evans D, Carter M, Thoresen M, Wroblewska J, Mandera M, *et al.* (2007) Randomized clinical trial of prevention of hydrocephalus after intraventricular hemorrhage in preterm infants: brain-washing versus tapping fluid. *Pediatrics* 119: E1071–E1078.

117. Horbar JD, Leahy K, Lucey JF. (1982) Real-time ultrasonography — its use in diagnosis and management of neonatal hydrocephalus. *Am J Dis Child* 136: 693–696.

118. Allan WC, Holt PJ, Sawyer LR, Tito AM, Meade SK. (1982) Ventricular dilation after neonatal periventricular-intraventricular hemorrhage — natural-history and therapeutic implications. *Am J Dis Child* 136: 589–593.

119. Donn SM, Goldstein GW, Silver TM. (1981) Real-time ultrasonography — its use in the evaluation of neonatal intra-cranical hemorrhage and posthemorrhagic hydrocephalus. *Am J Dis Childr* 135: 319–321.

120. Volpe JJ, Pasternak JF, Allan WC. (1977) Ventricular dilation preceding rapid head growth following neonatal intracranial hemorrhage. *Am J Dis Childr* 131: 1212–1215.

121. Korobkin R. (1975) Relationship between head circumference and development of communicating hydrocephalus in infants following intraventricular hemorrhage. *Pediatrics* 56: 74–77.

122. Perlman JM, Lynch B, Volpe JJ. (1990) Late hydrocephalus after arrest and resolution of neonatal posthemorrhagic hydrocephalus. *Dev Med Child Neurol* 32: 725–729.

123. Johnson ML, Mack LA, Rumack CM, Frost M, Rashbaum C. (1979) B-mode echoencephalography in the normal and high-risk infant. *Am J Roentgenol* 133: 3753–3781.

124. Brann BS, Qualls C, Wells L, Papile L. (1991) Asymmetric growth of the lateral cerebral ventricle in infants with posthemorrhagic ventricular dilation. *J Pediatr* 118: 108–112.

125. Grasby DC, Esterman A, Marshall P. (2003) Ultrasound grading of cerebral ventricular dilatation in preterm neonates. *J Paediatr Child Health* 39: 186–190.

126. Morony S, Marshall P, Langlois S. (1984) Periventricular hemorrhage and ventricular dilatation detected by real-time ultrasound in infants-less-than-1500G Birth-Weight. *Aust Paediatr J* 20: 252.

127. London DA, Carroll BA, Enzmann DR. (1980) Sonography of ventricular size and germinal matrix hemorrhage in premature-infants. *Am J Neuroradiol* 1: 295–300.

128. Dykes FD, Dunbar B, Lazarra A, Ahmann PA. (1989) Posthemorrhagic hydrocephalus in high-risk preterm infants — natural-history, management, and long-term outcome. *J Pediatr* 114: 611–618.

129. Adams-Chapman I, Hansen NI, Stoll BJ, Higgins R. (2008) Neurodevelopmental outcome of extremely low birth weight infants with posthemorrhagic hydrocephalus requiring shunt insertion. *Pediatrics* 121: E1167–E1177.

130. Brouwer A, Groenendaal F, van Haastert IL, Rademaker K, Hanlo P, de Vries L. (2008) Neurodevelopmental outcome of preterm infants with severe intraventricular hemorrhage and therapy for post-hemorrhagic ventricular dilatation. *J Pediatr* 152: 648–654.

131. de Vries LS, Liem KD, van Dijk K, Smit BJ, Sie L, Rademaker KJ, *et al.* (2002) Early versus late treatment of posthaemorrhagic ventricular dilatation: results of a retrospective study from five neonatal intensive care units in the Netherlands. *Acta Paediatr* 91: 212–217.

132. Paneth N, Rudelli R, Kazam E, Monte W. (1994) Ultrasonographic Methods. In: Paneth N, Rudelli R, Kazam E, Monte W, eds. *Brain Damage in the Preterm Infant.* London: Cambridge University Press; 171–185.

133. Vasileiadis GT. (2004) Grading intraventricular hemorrhage with no grades. *Pediatrics* 113: 930–931.

134. Morales WJ. (1987) Effect of intraventricular hemorrhage on the one-year mental and neurologic handicaps of the very-low-birth-weight infant. *Obstetr Gynecol* 70: 111–114.

135. Vasileiadis GT, Gelman N, Han VKM, Williams LA, Mann R, Bureau Y, *et al.* (2004) Uncomplicated intraventricular hemorrhage is followed by reduced cortical volume at near-term age. *Pediatrics* 114: E367–E372.

136. Nwaesei CG, Allen AC, Vincer M, Brown St. J, Stinson DA Evans JR, Byrne JM. (1988) Effect of timing of cerebral ultrasonography on the prediction of later neurodevelopmental outcome in high-risk preterm infants. *J Pediatr* 112: 970–975.

137. Kuban K, Allred EN, Dammann O, Pagano M, Leviton A, Share J, *et al.* (2001) Topography of cerebral white matter disease of prematurity studied prospectively in 1607 very-low-birthweight infants. *J Child Neurol* 16: 401–408.

138. Holling EE, Leviton A. (1999) Characteristics of cranial ultrasound white-matter echolucencies that predict disability: a review. *Dev Med Child Neurol* 41: 136–139.

139. Sherlock RL, Anderson PJ, Doyle LW. (2005) Neurodevelopmental seque-lae of intraventricular haemorrhage at 8 years of age in a regional cohort of ELBW/very preterm infants. *Early Hum Dev* 81: 909–916.

140. Vollmer B, Roth S, Riley K, O'Brien F, Baudin J, De Haan M, *et al.* (2006) Long-term neurodevelopmental outcome of preterm children with unilateral cerebral lesions diagnosed by neonatal ultrasound. *Early Hum Dev* 82: 655–661.

141. Hack M, Taylor HG, Klein N, Eiben R, Schatschneider C, Mercuriminich N. (1994) School-age outcomes in children with birth weights under 750 G. *N Engl J Med* 331: 753–759.

142. Mikkola K, Ritari N, Tommiska V, Salokorpi T, Lehtonen L, Tammela O, *et al.* (2005) Neurodevelopmental outcome at 5 years of age of a national cohort of extremely low birth weight infants who were born in 1996–1997. *Pediatrics* 116: 1391–1400.

143. Msall ME, Buck GM, Rogers BT, Merke DP, Wan CC, Catanzaro NL, *et al.* (1994) Multivariate risks among extremely low birth weight premature infants. *J Perinatol* 14: 41–47.

144. Whitaker AH, Feldman JF, Lorenz JM, Shen S, McNicholas F, Nieto M, *et al.* (2006) Motor and cognitive outcomes in nondisabled low-birth-weight adolescents — early determinants. *Arch Pediatr Adolescent Med* 160: 1040–1046.

145. D'Angio CT, Sinkin RA, Stevens TP, Landfish NK, Merzbach JL, Ryan RM, *et al.* (2002) Longitudinal, 15-year follow-up of children born at less than 29 weeks' gestation after introduction of surfactant therapy into a region: Neurologic, cognitive, and educational outcomes. *Pediatrics* 110: 1094–1102.

146. Perlman JM, Rollins N. (2000) Surveillance protocol for the detection of intracranial abnormalities in premature neonates. *Arch Pediatr Adolesc Med* 154: 822–826.

147. Nwafor-Anene VN, DeCristofaro JD, Baumgart S. (2003) Serial head ultrasound studies in preterm infants: how many normal studies does one infant need to exclude significant abnormalities? *J Perinatol* 23: 104–110.
148. Harris NJ, Palacio D, Ginzel A, Richardson CJ, Swischuk L. (2007) Are routine cranial ultrasounds necessary in premature infants greater than 30 weeks gestation? *Am J Perinatol* 24: 17–21.
149. O'Shea TM, Klinepeter KL, Dillard RG. (1998) Prenatal events and the risk of cerebral palsy in very low birth weight infants. *Am J Epidemiol* 147: 362–369.
150. van de BM, den Ouden L, Guit GL. (1992) Value of cranial ultrasound and magnetic resonance imaging in predicting neurodevelopmental outcome in preterm infants. *Pediatrics* 90: 196–199.
151. Woodward LJ, Anderson PJ, Austin NC, Howard K, Inder TE. (2006) Neonatal MRI to predict neurodevelopmental outcomes in preterm infants. *N Engl J Med* 355: 685–694.
152. Horsch S, Hallberg B, Leifsdottir K, Skiold B, Nagy Z, Mosskin M, *et al.* (2007) Brain abnormalities in extremely low gestational age infants: a Swedish population based Mill study. *Acta Paediatr* 96: 979–984.
153. Mirmiran M, Barnes PD, Keller K, Constantinou JC, Fleisher BE, Hintz SR, *et al.* (2004) Neonatal brain magnetic resonance imaging before discharge is better than serial cranial ultrasound in predicting cerebral palsy in very low birth weight preterm infants. *Pediatrics* 114: 992–998.
154. Valkama AM, Paakko EL, Vainionpaa LK, Lanning FP, Ilkko EA, Koivisto ME. (2000) Magnetic resonance imaging at term and neuromotor outcome in preterm infants. *Acta Paediatr* 89: 348–355.
155. Nanba Y, Matsui K, Aida N, Sato Y, Toyoshima K, Kawataki M, *et al.* (2007) Magnetic resonance imaging regional T1 abnormalities at term accurately predict motor outcome in preterm infants. *Pediatrics* 120: E10–E19.
156. Spittle AJ, Brown NC, Doyle LW, Boyd RN, Hunt RW, Bear M, *et al.* (2008) Quality of general movements is related to white matter pathology in very preterm infants. Pediatrics 121: E1184–E1189.
157. Krishnan ML, Dyet LE, Boardman JP, Kapellou O, Allsop JM, Cowan F, *et al.* (2007) Relationship between white matter apparent diffusion coefficients in preterm infants at term-equivalent age and developmental outcome at 2 years. *Pediatrics* 120: E604–E609.

158. Edgin JO, Inder TE, Anderson PJ, Hood KM, Clark CAC, Woodward LJ. (2008) Executive functioning in preschool children born very preterm: Relationship with early white matter pathology. *J Int Neuropsychol Soc* 14: 90–101.

159. Beauchamp MH, Thompson DK, Howard K, Doyle LW, Egan GF, Inder TE, *et al.* (2008) Preterm infant hippocampal volumes correlate with later working memory deficits. *Brain* 131: 2986–2994.

160. Shah DK, Guinane C, August P, Austin NC, Woodward LJ, Thompson DK, *et al.* (2006) Reduced occipital regional volumes at term predict impaired visual function in early childhood in very low birth weight infants. *Invest Ophth Vis Sci* 47: 3366–3373.

161. vanderKnaap MS, vanWezelMeijler G, Barth PG, Barkhof F, Ader HJ, Valk J. (1996) Normal gyration and sulcation in preterm and term neonates: appearance on MR images. *Radiology* 200: 389–396.

162. Roelants-van Rijn AM, Nikkels PGJ, Groenendaal F, Van der Grond J, Barth PG, Snoeck I, *et al.* (2001) Neonatal diffusion-weighted MR imaging: relation with histopathology or follow-up MR examination. *Neuropediatrics* 32: 286–294.

163. Counsell SJ, Maalouf EF, Fletcher AM, Duggan P, Battin M, Lewis HJ, *et al.* (2002) MR imaging assessment of myelination in the very preterm brain. *Am J Neuroradiol* 23: 872–881.

164. Counsell SJ, Rutherford MA, Cowan FM, Edwards AD. (2003) Magnetic resonance imaging of preterm brain injury. *Arch Dis Childhood* 88: 269–274.

165. Rutherford M, Malamateniou C, Zeka J, Counsell S. (2004) MR imaging of the neonatal brain at 3 Tesla. *Eur J Paediatr Neurol* 8: 281–289.

166. Rutherford M, Ward P, Allsop J, Malamatentiou C, Counsell S. (2005) Magnetic resonance imaging in neonatal encephalopathy. *Early Hum Dev* 81: 13–25.

167. Rutherford MA, Ward P, Malamatentiou C. (2005) Advanced MR techniques in the term-born neonate with perinatal brain injury. *Semin Fetal Neonat Med* 10: 445–460.

168. Cowan FM, Rutherford M. (2005) Recent advances in imaging the fetus and newborn. *Semin Fetal Neonat Med* 10: 401–402.

169. Arthur R. (2006) Magnetic resonance imaging in preterm infants. *Pediatr Radiol* 36: 593–607.

170. Leijser LM, Liauw L, Veen S, de Boer IP, Walther FJ, Wezel-Meijler G. (2008) Comparing brain white matter on sequential cranial ultrasound and MRI in very preterm infants. *Neuroradiology* 50: 799–811.

171. Wezel-Meijler G, Leijser LM, de Bruine FT, Steggerda SJ, Van der Grond J, Walther FJ. (2009) Magnetic resonance imaging of the brain in newborn infants: practical aspects. *Early Hum Dev* 85: 85–92.

172. Levene MI, Whitelaw A, Dubowitz V, Bydder GM, Steiner RE, Randell CP, *et al.* (1982) Nuclear magnetic-resonance imaging of the brain in children. *Brit Med J* 285: 774–776.

173. van de Bor M, Guit GL, Schreuder AM, Wondergem J, Vielvoye GJ. (1989) Early detection of delayed myelination in preterm infants. *Pediatrics* 84: 407–411.

174. Hart AR, Whitby EW, Griffiths PD, Smith MF. (2008) Magnetic resonance imaging and developmental outcome following preterm birth: review of current evidence. *Dev Med Child Neurol* 50: 655–663.

175. Bluml S, Friedlich P, Erberich S, Wood JC, Seri I, Nelson MD. (2004) MR imaging of newborns by using an MR-compatible incubator with integrated radiofrequency coils: Initial experience. *Radiology* 231: 594–601.

176. Whitby EH, Griffiths PD, Lonneker-Lammers T, Srinivasan R, Connolly DJA, Capener D, *et al.* (2004) Ultrafast magnetic resonance imaging of the neonate in a magnetic resonance-compatible incubator with a built-in coil. *Pediatrics* 113: 150–152.

177. Jones RA, Palasis S, Grattan-Smith JD. (2004) MRI of the neonatal brain: optimization of spin-echo parameters. *Am J Roentgenol* 182: 367–372.

178. Huppi PS, Inder TE. (2001) Magnetic resonance techniques in the evaluation of the perinatal brain: recent advances and future directions. *Semin Neonatol* 6: 195–210.

179. Schneider JF, Confort-Gouny S, Le Fur Y, Viout P, Bennathan M, Chapon F, *et al.* (2007) Diffusion-weighted imaging in normal fetal brain maturation. *Eur Radiol* 17: 2422–2429.

180. McArdle CB, Richardson CJ, Nicholas DA, Mirfakhraee M, Hayden CK, Amparo EG. (1987) Developmental features of the neonatal brain — MR imaging 2. Ventricular size and extracerebral space. *Radiology* 162: 230–234.

181. McArdle CB, Richardson CJ, Hayden CK, Nicholas DA, Crofford MJ, Amparo EG. (1987) Abnormalities of the neonatal brain — MR imaging 1. Intracranial hemorrhage. *Radiology* 163: 387–394.

182. McArdle CB, Richardson CJ, Nicholas DA, Mirfakhraee M, Hayden CK, Amparo EG. (1987) Developmental features of the neonatal brain — MR imaging 1. Gray-white matter differentiation and myelination. *Radiology* 162: 223–229.

183. Huppi PS, Warfield S, Kikinis R, Barnes PD, Zientara GP, Jolesz FA, *et al.* (1998) Quantitative magnetic resonance imaging of brain development in premature and mature newborns. *Ann Neurol* 43: 224–235.

184. Childs AM, Cornette L, Ramenghi LA, Tanner SF, Arthur RJ, Martinez D, *et al.* (2001) Magnetic resonance and cranial ultrasound characteristics of periventricular white matter abnormalities in newborn infants. *Clin Radiol* 56: 647–655.

185. Dyet LE, Kennea N, Counsell SJ, Maalouf EF, Ajayi-Obe M, Duggan PJ, *et al.* (2006) Natural history of brain lesions in extremely preterm infants studied with serial magnetic resonance imaging from birth and neurodevelopmental assessment. *Pediatrics* 118: 458–536.

186. Maalouf EF, Duggan PJ, Counsell SJ, Rutherford MA, Cowan F, Azzopardi D, *et al.* (2001) Comparison of findings on cranial ultrasound and magnetic resonance imaging in preterm infants. *Pediatrics* 107: 719–727.

187. Van Wezel-Meijler. (2007) *Neonatal Cranial Ultrasonography*. Heidelberg: Springer Verlag.

188. Leijser LM, de Bruine FT, Steggerda SJ, Van der Grond J, Walther FJ, Wezel-Meijler G. (2009) Brain imaging findings in very preterm infants throughout the neonatal period: Part I. Incidences and evolution of lesions, comparison between ultrasound and MRI. *Early Hum Dev* 85: 101–109.

189. Roelants-van Rijn AM, Groenendaal F, Beek FJ, Eken P, van Haastert IC, de Vries LS. (2001) Parenchymal brain injury in the preterm infant: comparison of cranial ultrasound, MRI and neurodevelopmental outcome. *Neuropediatrics* 32: 80–89.

190. de Vries L, Roelants-van Rijn AM, Rademaker KJ, Van Haastert IC, Beek FJ, Groenedaal F. (2001) Unilateral parenchymal haemorrhagic infarction in the preterm infant. Eur *J Paediatr Neurol* 5: 139–149.

191. Miller SP, Cozzio CC, Goldstein RB, Ferriero DM, Partridge JC, Vigneron DB, *et al.* (2003) Comparing the diagnosis of white matter injury in premature newborns with serial MR imaging and transfontanel ultrasonography findings. *Am J Neuroradiol* 24: 1661–1669.

192. Rademaker KJ, Uiterwaal CSPM, Beek FJA, van Haastert IC, Lieftink AF, Groenendaal F, *et al.* (2005) Neonatal cranial ultrasound versus MRI and neurodevelopmental outcome at school age in children born preterm. *Arch Dis Childhood-Fetal N* 90: F489–F493.

193. Leijser LM, de Vries LS, Rutherford MA, Manzur AY, Groenendaal F, de Koning TJ, *et al.* (2007) Cranial ultrasound in metabolic disorders presenting in the neonatal period: characteristic features and comparison with MR imaging. *Am J Neuroradiol* 28: 1223–1231.

194. de Vries LS, Verboon-Maciolek MA, Cowan FM, Groenendaal F. (2006) The role of cranial ultrasound and magnetic resonance imaging in the diagnosis of infections of the central nervous system. *Early Hum Dev* 82: 8198–8125.

195. Barkovich AJ, Kjos BO, Jackson DE, Norman D. (1988) Normal maturation of the neonatal and infant brain — Mr imaging at 1.5 T. *Radiology* 166: 173–180.

196. Barkovich AJ, Maroldo TV. (1993) Magnetic resonance imaging of normal and abnormal brain development. *Top Magn Reson Imaging* 5: 96–122.

197. Rutherford MA. (2001) *MRI of Neonatal Brain*. Edinburgh: Saunders.

198. Srinivasan L, Rutherford MA. (2008) MRI of the newborn brain. *Paediatr Child Health* 18: 183–195.

199. Kostovic I, Judas M. (2002) Correlation between the sequential ingrowth of afferents and transient patterns of cortical lamination in preterm infants. *Anat Record* 267: 1–6.

200. Kostovic I, Judas M, Rados M, Hrabac P. (2002) Laminar organization of the human fetal cerebrum revealed by histochemical markers and magnetic resonance imaging. *Cerebral Cortex* 12: 536–544.

201. Judas M, Rados M, Jovanov-Milosevic N, Hrabac P, Stern-Padovan R, Kostovic I. (2005) Structural, immunocytochemical, and MR imaging properties of periventricular crossroads of growing cortical pathways in preterm infants. *Am J Neuroradiol* 26: 2671–2684.

202. Chi JG, Dooling EC, Gilles FH. (1977) Gyral development of human-brain. *Ann Neurol* 1: 86–93.

203. *Development of the Human Foetal Brain: an Anatomical Atlas.* (1987) Paris, France: Inserm-CNRS: Masson.

204. Hansen PE, Ballesteros MC, Soila K, Garcia L, Howard JM. (1993) MR imaging of the developing human brain. 1. Prenatal development. *Radiographics* 13: 21–36.

205. Gilmore JH, Lin W, Prastawa MW, Looney CB, Vetsa YSK, Knickmeyer RC, *et al.* (2007) Regional gray matter growth, sexual dimorphism, and cerebral asymmetry in the neonatal brain. *J Neurosci* 27: 1255–1260.

206. Dubois J, Benders M, Cachia A, Lazeyras F, Leuchter RHV, Sizonenko SV, *et al.* (2008) Mapping the early cortical folding process in the preterm newborn brain. *Cerebral Cortex* 18: 1444–1454.

207. Battin MR, Maalouf EF, Counsell SJ, Herlihy AH, Rutherford MA, Azzopardi D, *et al.* (1998) Magnetic resonance imaging of the brain in very preterm infants: visualization of the germinal matrix, early myelination, and cortical folding. *Pediatrics* 101: 957–962.

208. Kagan J, Herschkowitz N. (2008) *A Young Mind in a Growing Brain.* Mahwah, New Jersey: Erlbaum; 2005.

209. Lawrence RK, Inder TE. Anatomic changes and imaging in assessing brain injury in the term infant. *Clin Perinatol* 35: 679–693.

210. de Vries LS, Groenendaal F, van Haastert IC, Eken P, Rademaker KJ, Meiners LC. (1999) Asymmetrical myelination of the posterior limb of the internal capsule in infants with periventricular haemorrhagic infarction: an early predictor of hemiplegia. *Neuropediatrics* 30: 314–319.

211 Sie LTL, van der Knaap MS, Wezel-Meijler G, van Amerongen AHMT, Lafeber HN, Valk J. (2000) Early MR features of hypoxic-ischemic brain injury in neonates with periventricular densities on sonograms. *Am J Neuroradiol* 21: 852–861.

212. Sie LTL, Hart AAM, van Hof J, de Groot L, Lems W, Lafeber HN, *et al.* (2005) Predictive value of neonatal MRI with respect to late MRI findings and clinical outcome. A study in infants with periventricular densities on neonatal ultrasound. *Neuropediatrics* 36: 78–89.

213. Miller SP, Ferriero DM, Leonard C, Piecuch R, Glidden DV, Partridge JC, *et al.* (2005) Early brain injury in premature newborns detected with magnetic resonance imaging is associated with adverse early neurodevelopmental outcome. *J Pediatr* 147: 609–616.

214. Huang BY, Castillo M. (2008) Hypoxic-ischemic brain injury: imaging findings from birth to adulthood. *Radiographics* 28: 417–439.

215. Barkovich AJ, Sargent SK. (1995) Profound asphyxia in the premature-infant — imaging findings. *Am J Neuroradiol* 16: 1837–1846.

216. Barkovich AJ, Westmark K, Partridge C, Sola A, Ferriero DM. (1995) Perinatal asphyxia — MR findings in the first 10 days. *Am J Neuroradiol* 16: 427–438.

217. Barkovich AJ. (2005) Brain and spine injuries in infancy and childhood. In: Barkovich AJ, ed. *Pediatric Neuroimaging*. Philadelphia, PA: Lippincott, Williams, and Wilkins; 190–290.

218. McQuillen PS, Ferriero DM. (2004) Selective vulnerability in the developing central nervous system. *Pediatr Neurol* 30: 227–235.

219. Back SA, Luo NL, Borenstein NS, Levine JM, Volpe JJ, Kinney HC. (2001) Late oligodendrocyte progenitors coincide with the developmental window of vulnerability for human perinatal white matter injury. *J Neurosci* 21: 1302–1312.

220. Back SA, Han BH, Luo NL, Chricton CA, Xanthoudakis S, Tam J, *et al.* (2002) Selective vulnerability of late oligodendrocyte progenitors to hypoxia-ischemia. *J Neurosci* 22: 455–463.

221. Flodmark O, Roland EH, Hill A, Whitfield MF. (1987) Periventricular leukomalacia — radiologic-diagnosis. *Radiology* 162: 119–124.

222. Flodmark O, Lupton B, Li D, Stimac GK, Roland EH, Hill A, *et al.* (1989) MR imaging of periventricular leukomalacia in childhood. *Am J Roentgenol* 152: 583–590.

223. Dubowitz LMS, Bydder GM, Mushin J. (1985) Developmental sequence of periventricular leukomalacia — correlation of ultrasound, clinical, and nuclear magnetic-resonance functions. *Arch Dis Childhood* 60: 349–355.

224. Inder TE, Wells SJ, Mogridge NB, Spencer C, Volpe JJ. (2003) Defining the nature of the cerebral abnormalities in the premature infant: a qualitative magnetic resonance imaging study. *J Pediatr* 143: 171–179.

225. Robertson RL, Ben Sira L, Barnes PD, Mulkern RV, Robson CD, Maier SE, *et al.* (1999) MR line-scan diffusion-weighted imaging of term neonates with perinatal brain ischemia. *Am J Neuroradiol* 20: 1658–1670.

226. Barkovich AJ. (1992) MR and CT Evaluation of profound neonatal and infantile asphyxia. *Am J Neuroradiol* 13: 959–972.

227. Grant PE, Yu D. (2006) Acute injury to the immature brain with hypoxia with or without hypoperfusion. *Radiol Clin North America* 44: 63–67.

228. Wijdicks EFM, Campeau NG, Miller GM. (2001) MR imaging in comatose survivors of cardiac resuscitation. *Am J Neuroradiol* 22: 1561–1565.

229. Forbes KPN, Pipe JG, Bird R. (2000) Neonatal hypoxic-ischemic encephalopathy: detection with diffusion-weighted MR imaging. *Am J Neuroradiol* 21: 1490–1496.

230. Heinz ER, Provenzale JM. (2009) Imaging findings in neonatal hypoxia: a practical review. *Am J Roentgenol* 192: 41–47.

231. Ashwal S, Majcher JS, Vain N, Longo LD. (1980) Patterns of fetal lamb regional cerebral blood-flow during and after prolonged hypoxia. *Pediatr Res* 14: 1104–1110.

232. Nelson KB. (2007) Perinatal ischemic stroke. *Stroke* 38: 742–745.

233. Raju TNK, Nelson KB, Ferriero D, Lynch JK. (2007) Ischemic perinatal stroke: summary of a workshop sponsored by the national institute of child health and human development and the national institute of neurological disorders and stroke. *Pediatrics* 120: 609-616.

234. Obenaus A, Ashwal S. (2008) Magnetic resonance imaging in cerebral ischemia: focus on neonates. *Neuropharmacology* 55: 271–280.

235. Volpe JJ. (2000) *Neurology of the Newborn*. Philadelphia: WB Saunders.

236. Simbrunner J, Riccabona M. (2006) Imaging of the neonatal CNS. *Eur J Radiol* 60: 133–151.

237 Triulzi F, Baldoli C, Parazzini C. (2001) Neonatal MRI imaging. *Magn Reson Imaging Clin N Am* 9: 57–82.

238. Connelly A, Chong WK, Johnson CL, Ganesan V, Gadian DG, Kirkham FJ. (1997) Diffusion weighted magnetic resonance imaging of compromised tissue in stroke. *Arch Dis Childhood* 77: 38–41.

239. Dudink J, Mercuri E, Al Nakib L, Govaert P, Counsell SJ, Rutherford MA, *et al.* (2009) Evolution of unilateral perinatal arterial ischemic stroke on conventional and diffusion — weighted MR imaging. *Am J Neuroradiol* 30: 998–1004.

240. Tortori-Donati P (ed.) (2005) *Pediatric Neuroradiology*. Berlin: Springer.

241. Aicardi J, Chevrie JJ, Baraton J. (1987) Agenesis of the corpus callosum. In: Vinken PJ, Bruyn GW, Klawans HL, ed. *Handbook of Clinical Neurology*, Revised Series, Vol. 6. New York: Elsevier Science. 149–173.

242. Vergani P, Ghidini A, Strobelt N, Locatelli A, Mariani S, Bertalero C, *et al.* (1994) Prognostic indicators in the prenatal-diagnosis of agenesis of corpus-callosum. *Am J Obstet Gynecol* 170: 753–758.

243. Barkovich AJ, Norman D. (1988) Anomalies of the corpus-callosum — correlation with further anomalies of the brain. *Am J Roentgenol* 151: 171–179.

244. Glenn OA, Barkovich AJ. (2006) Magnetic resonance imaging of the fetal brain and spine: an increasingly important tool in prenatal diagnosis, Part 1. *Am J Neuroradiol* 27: 1604–1611.

245. Boddaert N, Klein O, Ferguson N, Sonigo P, Parisot D, Hertz-Pannier L, *et al.* (2003) Intellectual prognosis of the Dandy-Walker malformation in children: the importance of vermian lobulation. *Neuroradiology* 45: 320–324.

246. Klein O, Pierre-Kahn A, Boddaert N, Parisot D, Brunelle F. (2003) Dandy-Walker malformation: prenatal diagnosis and prognosis. *Childs Nervous System* 19: 484–489.

247. Golden JA, Rorke LB, Bruce DA. (1987) Dandy-Walker Syndrome and associated anomalies. *Pediatr Neurosci* 13: 38–44.

248. Maria BL, Zinreich SJ, Carson BC, Rosenbaum AE, Freeman JM. (1987) Dandy-Walker Syndrome Revisited. *Pediatr Neurosci* 13: 45–51.

249. Bindal AK, Storrs BB, Mclone DG. (1991) Management of the Dandy-Walker Syndrome. *Pediatr Neurosurg* 16: 163–169.

250. Sonigo PC, Rypens FF, Carteret M, Delezoide AL, Brunelle FO. (1998) MR imaging of fetal cerebral anomalies. *Pediatr Radiol* 28: 212–222.

251. Beitzke D, Simbrunner J, Riccabona M. (2008) MRI in paediatric hypoxic-ischemic disease, metabolic disorders and malformations — a review. *Eur J Radiol* 68: 199–213.

Chapter 6

Monitoring and Intervention Therapies in Neonatal Intensive Care Units

Anjali Parish*

6.1 Introduction

As the field of neonatology has evolved, most rapidly over the last 50 years, invasive and noninvasive monitoring has become the cornerstone in the management of the critically ill neonates. Several trends in monitoring have declared themselves. For example, physicians have realized that clinical determination of "color" for the management of jaundice is no longer appropriate and measurement of bilirubin levels is clearly superior. On the other hand, need for frequent blood sampling to monitor oxygen levels has given way to the use of pulse oximetry for the management of respiratory support. In fact, oxygen saturation is considered a vital sign in neonatal intensive care units (NICUs) where continuous cardio-respiratory monitoring is routine. Another interesting phenomenon is that as inpatient newborn stays have shortened over time, the need for outpatient monitoring and intervention in order to prevent disease has become more involved. This chapter will review in detail some of these shifts in trends for monitoring and subsequent changes in interventions in the NICU setting.

*Assistant Professor of Pediatrics, Medical College of Georgia.

6.2 Monitoring and Managing Oxygen Support

Up until the 1960s, the primary option for respiratory support was administration of supplemental oxygen.[1] Clinical observation of color and "cyanosis" was the determinant for need to intervene with oxygen supplementation and improvement in color was the indicator that treatment was adequate. Furthermore, clinicians had to know the difference between peripheral and central cyanosis and depended on arterial blood specimens to determine percentage arterial oxygen saturation to help distinguish between the two.[2] However, it was recognized decades ago that too much oxygen can be detrimental, especially for the development of retrolental fibroplasia in the premature infant.

Recognizing the need for a way to monitor oxygen levels more continuously and less invasively than obtaining blood specimens for gas analysis, researchers developed transcutaneous monitoring. Huch and colleagues published the first report on the clinical use of transcutaneous PO_2 monitoring to evaluate asphyxiated newborns and avoid blood sampling.[3] Probes had to be calibrated and then used to warm the infant's skin to 44°. After about 10 minutes the tcPO$_2$ values were equivalent to the PaO$_2$ values and reflective of changes in the infant's circulatory system. Unfortunately sites had to be changed every few hours in order to prevent damage to the patient's skin. Frequency of skin damage was greater in the more immature infants. Several factors influenced these measurements. These included sensor temperature, probe placement, peripheral perfusion, skin thickness and response time. Some of these factors are especially important in preterm infants. Furthermore, over the next decade investigators would fail to demonstrate consistently a decrease in need for arterial blood gas sampling, overall cost reduction by use of these monitors, and improvement in morbidity and mortality rates in the neonatal population.[4] However, it was a safe and effective technique to noninvasively monitor the effects of medical treatment on PO_2 values.

In the 1970s, while transcutaneous monitoring became valued as a clinical tool, pulse oximetry was developed; yet, it was not introduced into clinical practice for 10 more years.[5] Pulse oximetry measures the proportion of hemoglobin molecules which are loaded with oxygen.

Deoxygenated hemoglobin absorbs more light in the red band (600–750 nm), whereas oxygenated hemoglobin absorbs more light in the infrared band (850–1000 nm). The ratio of the absorbance of red and infrared light sent through a tissue correlates with the proportion of oxygenated to deoxygenated hemoglobin. Conventional oximeters identify the peaks and troughs in absorbance over time to obtain pulse added absorbances which are then associated algorithmically with empirically determined arterial oxygen saturation values. One major draw back to pulse oximetry was that it was very susceptible to motion artifacts. Newer models have overcome this issue to a great extent utilizing vastly improved techniques and algorithms. For example, new generation Massimo pulse oximeters use Signal Extraction Technology and "noise reference" algorithms to identify and read through periods with low signal-noise ratio in order to reduce this vulnerability. Pulse oximetry was shown to be both an accurate and reliable measure of arterial oxygen saturation even during times that might restrict an infant's blood flow to the skin.[6] However, outside of a narrow SpO_2 range, partial pressures of arterial oxygen can vary greatly, thus requiring arterial blood sampling when accurate PaO_2 levels need to be known.[7] Recently it was shown that transcutaneous monitoring resulted in less time spent with low and high oxygen tensions when compared to management based on pulse oximetry.[8] It has been suggested that transcutaneous monitoring and pulse oximetry should ideally be used together but determination of arterial blood gases will remain the gold standard in critically ill patients.[9] The pros and cons of these two technologies are compared in Table 6.1.

Unlike transcutaneous monitoring, pulse oximetry has been used to decrease morbidity in the premature infant population, especially in regards to retinopathy of prematurity (ROP). Several studies have already shown that limiting oxygen saturation levels to 85–93% can reduce the incidence of both ROP and chronic lung disease.[10] However, limiting oxygenation has raised concerns about long-term neurodevelopmental consequences. Preliminary data suggests that practices to avoid hyperoxia do not have detrimental effects on long-term neurodevelopmental outcomes nor increased rates of cerebral palsy.[11,12] Studies are ongoing to determine the optimal range of oxygen saturations.

Table 6.1.   Pros and cons of noninvasive methods to monitor oxygenation

	Transcutaneous Monitoring	Pulse Oximetry
Pros	Does not require blood sample	Does not require blood sample
	Potential to provide tcPO$_2$ level equivalent to PaO$_2$	Does not require calibration
		Easy to use
	Provides moment to moment feedback on how medical care is affecting oxygenation	Minimal potential for injury
		Proven to help decrease common morbidities in preterm infants
	Potential to decrease frequency of arterial sampling	
Cons	Requires calibration during which time monitoring is interrupted	Very susceptible to motion and noise artifact
	Potential for skin injury	Large range of PaO$_2$ can produce same oximeter value so requires arterial sampling when PaO$_2$ value needed to manage care
	Can be cumbersome to use	

6.3 Management of Hemolytic Disease in the Fetus and the Newborn

Management of neonates with hemolytic disease has dramatically changed over the years. Rh hemolytic disease constituted the greatest risk to neonates. Antenatal use of anti-D immune globulin to Rh negative women has decreased the need for exchange transfusions in Rh hemolytic disease (see Chapter 11). Before the introduction of Rh(D) immune globulin, physicians caring for infants frequently saw babies born with severe anemia and hydrops. Often these infants died quickly in respiratory failure, while others with Rh hemolytic disease progressed to hyperbilirubinemia and kernicterus. Until the first publication of what is now referred to as the exchange transfusion technique, doctors had little options but to watch many kids progress to severe neurological dysfunction and sometimes death. It was further speculated that Rh sensitization placed children at a higher risk for long-term mental delay. In 1946, Dr. Harry Wallerstein published the technique of "simultaneous removal and replacement of the blood of the newborn infant" with severe erythroblastosis which had been performed in three infants with immediate improvement in their clinical symptoms and recovery without further therapy.[13] The principle behind exchange transfusion is that a significant portion of the antibody and sensitized cells from the infant's circulation is removed during a typical double volume exchange. Other physicians confirmed short-term improvement with use of exchange transfusions, both single and multiple transfusions, for treatment of erythroblastosis fetalis.[14] In 1952, researchers from Great Britain published results from a randomized controlled trial which showed exchange transfusion to be superior to simple transfusion for treatment of hemolytic disease of the newborn.[15] Although it is a relatively safe procedure, it is associated with multiple complications with reported mortality of approximately 0.1–0.5%.

Even after the introduction of exchange transfusion, mortality of preterm infants with hydrops due to Rh hemolytic disease remained high. The concept of correcting the anemia *in utero* by transfusion and prolonging gestation was introduced by Liley[16] in the 1960s. In the early days, the packed red blood cells were transfused into the fetal peritoneal cavity utilizing radiographs and fluoroscopy. With the advent of ultrasonography the technique of intravascular transfusion of red cells into the fetus emerged.[17] The volume of blood transfused depends on multiple factors such as initial fetal hematocrit, size of the fetus, hematocrit of the transfused RBCs, and the target hematocrit. Following transfusion, fetal hematocrit declines by approximately 1% per day. There are significant risks associated with intrauterine transfusion. These include fetal infection, preterm labor, excessive bleeding, amniotic fluid leakage and even fetal death. Today, fetuses with severe hemolytic disease who are unlikely to survive postnatally are being treated with intrauterine transfusions. Fetuses above 18 weeks are potential candidates. Overall survival is about 85%. However, the presence of hydrops fetalis reduces survival significantly.

There was concern that improved survival with use of exchange transfusions may lead to an increase in long-term neurological sequelae, having saved children whose high bilirubin levels had already caused irreversible brain damage. A little over five years after introduction of exchange transfusion, researchers published a trend towards improved mental test performance in infants who had received exchange transfusions for treatment of erythroblastosis fetalis though the improvement did not reach statistical significance.[18] With time other researchers would confirm survival without apparent increase in long-term neurological deficits, suggesting multiple exchange transfusions are effective for prevention of long-term neurological morbidities due to hyperbilirubinemia.[19]

Exchange transfusions require exposure to donor blood products and invasive removal of the patient's blood volume and it is also costly. Accordingly physicians sought a way to treat hemolytic disease of the newborn while minimizing the use of exchange transfusions. Sato *et al.* reported the potential benefits of IVIG in three infants with hemolytic disease in 1991.[20] In the following year, the first randomized controlled trial comparing the use of a single high dose intravenous immune globulin (IVIG) plus phototherapy to conventional management of phototherapy only with exchange transfusion used in both groups according to set guidelines.[21] Results showed use of exchange transfusion in only 12.5% of patients in the IVIG group versus 69% in the conventional group.[21] In 1995, Dagoglu *et al.*[22] showed the effectiveness of IVIG given soon after birth in decreasing the need for exchange transfusions in a randomized trial. Alpey *et al.*[23] showed high dose of IVIG reduces the need for exchange transfusion in the group of neonates receiving phototherapy due to hemolytic diseases. A group from Turkey in 2001 showed that use of three doses of IVIG given 24 hours apart reduced the need for exchange transfusion to zero.[24] It appears from these studies that the success of IVIG treatment depends on early initiation of therapy. Long-term outcome studies for IVIG therapy are not available.

6.4 Phototherapy and Management of Neonatal Jaundice

The concept of phototherapy developed in Great Britain in the 1950s and arose from the observation that jaundiced babies temporarily reduced their yellow color when nurses placed them in sunlight.[25] However it did not gain wide acceptance until "rediscovered" in the US almost 10 years later when a randomized controlled trial showed that phototherapy was effective in modifying hyperbilirubinemia of prematurity.[26]

Over the next three decades numerous studies confirmed the efficacy and safety of phototherapy for newborn infants of all birth weights and although the original authors felt phototherapy would not replace exchange transfusion for treatment of hemolytic jaundice, coupled with newer pharmacologic techniques, phototherapy has managed to drastically reduce the need for exchange transfusion after all.[27]

More than one mechanism has been implicated in the reduction of serum bilirubin during phototherapy. The most important mechanism is photoisomerization. The isomers are rapidly taken up in the liver and transported into the bile and account for more than 80% of increased elimination during phototherapy. Conversion into lumirubin, a structural isomer, is another mechanism by which phototherapy works. Again, lumirubin is excreted through the bile into the intestine. The third pathway involves bilirubin oxidation. Many of these byproducts which are colorless and odorless are excreted by the kidney and liver without the need for conjugation.

The efficacy of phototherapy depends on the wavelength of the light and energy output. A blue light in the wavelength of 420–500 nm is better than white lights. Minimally effective energy level is approximately 5 microW/cm^2/nm. Effective phototherapy must provide irradiance levels above this. Standard phototherapy units should be positioned between 15–20 cm of the patient. Third important variable in its effectiveness is surface area of the neonate exposed to phototherapy.

As always, one must be cognizant of any potential side effects. With regard to phototherapy temperature instability, and increased insensible water loss through the skin are factors that require attention. Neonates exposed to phototherapy should have their eyes covered to protect against retinal damage. Another recognized side effect is bronze baby syndrome. Skin in these infants develops a bronze discoloration after placing under phototherapy. Conjugated hyperbilirubinemia is common in these infants.

With treatment for hyperbilirubinemia well established, attention turned to how to accurately assess the degree of jaundice in infants. Visual inspection of the infant to determine jaundice levels has been proven as inaccurate and unreliable when deciding upon the treatment for jaundiced babies.[28] Blood sampling to determine total serum bilirubin (TSB) levels is the standard of care when managing hyperbilirubinemia. However, noninvasive modalities to determine bilirubin levels have been developed. Transcutaneous bilirubin (TcB) monitoring was first introduced by Japanese researchers in 1980[29]and since that time newer TcB monitors have been shown as reliable indicators of bilirubin levels.[30,31] However, it is recommended that TcB levels >13 mg/dl be corroborated with TSB measurement in the predischarge well-baby population.[32]

Historically, exchange transfusion was initiated for total serum bilirubin levels >20 mg/dL in newborns with hemolytic disease who were unquestionably at an increased risk for kernicterus. Without different data by which to judge, many physicians applied the same 20 mg/dl threshold to non-hemolytic jaundice as well. After reviewing the currently available literature, Dr. Newman and Dr. Maisels[33] recommended a "kindler, gentler approach" for managing the jaundiced infant in the early 1990s. In their approach different guidelines for hemolytic and non-hemolytic jaundice were offered, increasing the threshold for exchange transfusion in the non-hemolytic group. In 2001, the International Congress on Neonatal Jaundice was convened in Hong Kong and recommendations on the evaluation and treatment of jaundiced infants were further refined.

Despite this close attention to the management of the jaundiced infant, concern for rising rates of kernicterus began to surface in the early 1990s as well.[34] There was much concern in regards to changing hospital practices which led to discharge of mothers with their newborn infants within 48 hours of delivery during an era in which more mothers were breastfeeding for the first time. Since TSB levels peak in healthy term infants at 3–5 days, many infants were being discharged before maximum jaundiced levels were achieved and of course before adequate breastfeeding may have been established. Furthermore, a rise in late preterm infant deliveries was adding to the risk level for hyperbilirubinemia in these patients who were traditionally treated as "near-term" with management similar to that of term infants. These combined factors led to the American Academy of Pediatrics issuing revised guidelines in 2004[35] including recommendations for newborn follow-up within 48 hours after discharge. Whether or not these changes in recommendations improve overall outcomes in patient care remains to be seen. See Table 6.2.

6.5 Conclusion

The care of newborn infants is filled with historical similarities of treatments and interventions being introduced without strong evidence based medicine.

Table 6.2. Timeline on evolution of treatment for hyperbilirubinemia

1946	Dr. Wallerstein introduces concept of exchange transfusion
1956	Discovery of phototherapy
1980	Transcutaneous bilirubinometry invented
1992	Use of IVIG to treat hemolytic jaundice published
1992	Distinction in treatment of hemolytic versus non-hemolytic jaundice published
2001	International Congress on Neonatal Jaundice convened
2004	Amidst growing concerns for rise in rates of kernicterus, AAP revises guidelines for treatment of hyperbilirubinemia in infants > 35 weeks gestational age

Many of these modalities have become ingrained in daily practice despite such lack of evidence which current medicine so strongly covets. Although much of the time an intervention "just makes sense", in today's medical environment something like exchange transfusion would not become common practice without large randomized controlled trials preferably with blinding and long-term follow-up. Furthermore hospital administrators require proof that new, expensive technology can truly impact patient care in a positive, and many times cost-saving manner before large sums of money will be spent to purchase such equipment. As medicine evolves according to society's demands, neonatology continues to offer exciting new ways to discover innovative techniques to monitor and advance patient care.

References

1. Philip AGS. (1970) The evolution of neonatology. *Ped Res* 58: 799–815, 2005.
2. Lees MH. Cyanosis of the newborn infant. *J Pediatr* 77: 484–498.
3. Huch R, Huch A, Lubbers DW. (1973) Transcutaneous measurement of blood PO_2 ($tcPO_2$) — method and application in perinatal medicine. *J Perinat Med* 1: 183–191.
4. Guilfoile TD. (1986) Bedside monitoring of the acutely ill neonate: the impact of transcutaneous monitoring on neonatal intensive care. *Respir Care* 31: 507–513.
5. Poets CF, Southall DP. (1994) Noninvasive monitoring of oxygenation in infants and children: practical considerations and areas of concern. *Pediatrics* 93: 737–746.

6. Hay Jr. WW, Brockway JM, Eyzaguirre M. (1989) Neonatal pulse oximetry: accuracy and reliability. *Pediatrics* 83: 717–722.

7. Brockway J, Hay Jr. WW. (1998) Prediction of arterial partial pressure of oxygen with pulse oxygen saturation measurements. *J Pediatr* 133: 63–66.

8. Quine D, Stenson BJ. (2008) Does the monitoring method influence stability of oxygenation in preterm infants? A randomized crossover study of saturation versus transcutaneous monitoring. *Arch Dis Child: Fetal Neonatal Ed* 93: F347–F350.

9. Poets CF, Southall DP. (1994) Noninvasive monitoring of oxygenation in infants and children: practical considerations and areas of concern. *Pediatrics* 93: 737–746.

10. Saugstad OD. (2007) Optimal oxygenation at birth and in the neonatal period. *Neonatology* 91: 319–322.

11. Deulofeut R, Critz A, Adams-Chapman I, Sola A. (2006) Avoiding hyperoxia in infants ≤1250 g is associated with improved short- and long-term outcomes. *J Perinatol* 26: 700–705.

12. Tin W, Milligan DWA, Pennefather P, Hey E. (2001) Pulse oximetry, severe retinopathy, and outcome at one year in babies of less than 28 weeks gestation. *Arch Dis Child Fetal Neonatal Ed* 84: F106–F110.

13. Wallerstein H. (1946) Treatment of severe erythorblastosis by simultaneous removal and replacement of the blood of the newborn infant. *Science* 103: 583–584.

14. Allen FH, Diamond LK, Vaughan III VC. (1950) Erythroblastosis fetalis VI: prevention of kernicterus. *Am J Dis Child* 80: 779–791.

15. Mollison PL, Walker W. (1952) Controlled trials of the treatment of haemolytic disease of the newborn. *Lancet* 262: 429–433.

16. Liley, AW. (1963) Intrauterine transfusion of foetus in haemolytic disease. *BMJ* 2: 1107.

17. Rodeck CH, Kemp JR, Holman CA, *et al.* (1981) Direct intravascular fetal blood transfusion by fetoscopy in severe Rhesus isoimmunisation. *Lancet* 1: 625.

18. Day R, Haines MS. (1954) Intelligence quotients of children recovered from erythroblastosis fetalis since the introduction of exchange transfusion. *Pediatrics* 13: 333–338.

19. Johnston WH, Angara V, Baumal R, Hawke WA, Johnson RH, Keet S, Wood M. (1967) Erythroblastosis fetalis and hyperbilirubinemia: a five-year follow-up

with neurological, psychological, and audiological evaluation. *Pediatrics* 39: 88–92.

20. Sato K, Hara T, Kondo T, *et al.* (1991) High-dose intravenous gammaglobulin therapy for neonatal immune haemolytic jaundice due to blood group incompatibility. *Acta Paediatr Scand* 80: 163.

21. Rübo J, Albrecht K, Lasch P, *et al.* (1992) High-dose intravenous immune globulin therapy for hyperbilirubinemia caused by Rh hemolytic disease. *J Pediatr* 121: 93–97.

22. Dagoglu T, Ovali F, Samanci N, Bengisu E. (1995) High-dose intravenous immunoglobulin therapy for rhesus haemolytic disease. *J Int Med Res* 23: 264–271.

23. Alpay F, Sarici SU, Okutan V, *et al.* (1999) High-dose intravenous immunoglobulin therapy in neonatal immune haemolytic jaundice. *Acta Paediatr* 88: 216–219.

24. Tanyer G, Siklar Z, Dallar Y, *et al.* (2001) Multiple dose IVIG treatment in neonatal immune hemolytic jaundice. *J Tropl Pediatr* 47: 50–53.

25. Dobbs RH, Cremer RJ. (1975) Phototherapy. *Arch Dis Child* 50: 833–836.

26. Lucey J, Ferreiro M, Hewitt J. (1968) Prevention of hyperbilirubinemia of prematurity by phototherapy. *Pediatrics* 41: 1047–1054.

27. Maisels MJ. (2001) Phototherapy-traditional and nontraditional. *J Perinatol* 21: S93–S97.

28. Moyer VA, Ahn C, Sneed S. (2000) Accuracy of clinical judgment in neonatal jaundice. *Arch Pediatr Adolesc Med* 154: 391–394.

29. Yamanouchi I, Yamauchi Y, Ikuko I. (1980) Transcutaneous bilirubinometry: preliminary studies of noninvasive transcutaneous bilirubin meter in the Okayama national hospital. *Pediatrics* 65: 195–202.

30. Bhutani VK, Gourley GR, Kreamer BL, *et al.* (2000) Nonivasive measurement of total serum bilirubin using a multi-wavelength spectrophotometry in multiracial newborn population. *Pediatrics* 106: 17e–26e.

31. Rubaltelli FF, Gourley GR, Loskamp N, *et al.* (2001) Transcutaneous bilirubin measurement: a multicenter evaluation of a new device. *Pediatrics* 107: 1264–1271.

32. Bhutani VK, Johnson LH. (2001) Jaundice technologies: prediction of hyperbilirubinemia in term and near-term newborns. *J Perinatol* 21: S76–S82.

33. Newman TB, Maisels MJ. (1992) Evaluation and treatment of jaundice in the term newborn: a kinder, gentler approach. *Pediatrics* 89: 809–818.

34. Bhutani VK, Johnson L. (2009) Kernicterus in the 21st century: frequently asked questions. *J Perinatol* 29: S20–S24.

35. Subcommittee on Hyperbilirubinemia. (2004) Management of hyperbilirubinemia in the newborn infant 35 or more weeks of gestation. *Pediatrics* 114: 297–316.

Chapter 7

Regulation of Neonatal Environment 2010

Stephen Baumgart* and Suzanne Touch[†]

7.1 Basic Physics of Heat Transfer[1]

There are four avenues for infant physiologic heat exchange (loss) within the NICU, i.e., *conduction, convection, evaporation* and *radiation*. Conduction is the transfer of heat from a warm solid object to cooler solid object through surface-to-surface contact, conduction is minimized for infants with insulating foam and cotton bedding. Convection (loss of heat to cool air) occurs through two mechanisms, natural and forced, and is the largest loss in a non-incubated nursery. Evaporation is the loss of a tremendous amount of latent heat (i.e., when liquid water changes state to become invisible vapor) through transcutaneous evaporation. Radiant heat exchange (direct heat transfer through electromagnetic waves) is largely ignored. However, premature neonates radiate up to 60% of their metabolic thermal energy to cooler walls and windows (thermostatically controlled to adult comfort temperatures). Analyzing each of these mechanisms is necessary to understand each infant's unique thermal equilibrium. Probably infants achieve different quantitative equilibriums despite the fact that they may be

*Professor of Pediatrics, GWU School of Medicine and Health Sciences, Children's National Medical Center.
[†]Associate Professor of Pediatrics, Drexel University School of Medicine, St. Christopher's Hospital for Children.

213

nurtured in similar incubator devices and under similar physical conditions. No one incubation technique fits all sizes of babies.

7.1.1 *Conduction*

Conductive heat loss to cooler surfaces in contact with an infant's skin depends on the conductivity of the surface material and its temperature. Usually, babies are nursed on insulating mattresses and blankets that minimize conductive heat loss to nearly zero. Intuitively, care must be exercised to maintain dry layers of insulation in contact with a baby's skin to maintain external insulation, since preterm infants have little native insulating fat.

7.1.2 *Convection*

Convective heat transfer in general comprises movement of heat through a *fluid medium*, either a liquid (e.g. blood or water flow), or a gas (e.g. environmental and ventilator air). There are two mechanisms determining convective heat transfer from infants into their environmental air.

7.1.2.1 *Natural convection*

Natural convection results simply from the gradient of temperature between the infant's skin surface and the surrounding still air.[2,3] In general, this temperature gradient is approximately 10°C, (25°C air in the NICU to 35°C or 37°C skin). Natural convection forms *convection cells* similar to weather cells over the curved surfaces of the baby lying supine within an incubator or on an open cot. Convection cells form as warm air rises, conveying heat and body moisture away from the baby. As warm air rises, it subsequently cools and falls back towards the baby forming a convection heat exchange cell. Baby surface area, posture and body geometry play an important role in the rate of convective heat loss away from the skin. An infant flexed in the fetal position leaves less surface area exposed to the environment experiencing less convective heat loss.[4] An infant extended flaccidly is able to dissipate more heat. Hence, an infant's posture may be the first clinical clue to the thermal comfort or discomfort of an infant.

7.1.2.2 *Forced convection*

Forced convection is the result of forced air movement. Applied mechanical energy moves an air mass past the infant's skin at a longitudinal rate. The rate of forced convective heat loss is exponentially proportional to the rate of air movement.[3] The effect of forced convection in disrupting the warm, humid air layered near an infant's skin is not usually appreciated in the nursery, where drafts may be imperceptible to personnel. Within convection-warmed incubators, air is forced into the incubator by a fan capable of promoting evaporation, as well as convective heat transfer. Care should be exercised not to disrupt air flow inside incubators with padding, or equipment introducing or disrupting controlled air flow.[5]

7.1.3 *Radiation*

Radiant heat transfer is probably the least intuitive aspect of heat loss or heat gain in newborn infant incubation. When standing near a double-sealed window on a winter's day we say, "we feel a draft here". An anemometer, however, would not indicate the presence of forced convection. We *feel* cold because the window glass surface is cold. Radiant heat transfer occurs as the result of infrared electromagnetic energy transmission from one's own warm body to another (the window's) cooler one. Bodies of different temperatures determine the direction and amount of heat transfer. Heat goes from where it is to where it isn't, with the warm body irradiating to the cooler. The physical expression for describing radiant heat transfer may be summarized by:

$$Q_{radiant} = \sigma\, \varepsilon_{skin}\, \varepsilon_{environment}\, (T^{-4}_{mean\ skin} - T^{-4}_{radiant}) \times A \times F \times W^{-1}.$$

The radiant heat transfer constant (σ, Stefan-Boltzman constant), and the physical emissive properties of the infant's skin and his/her surrounding walls (ε_{skin}, ε_{walls}), the infant's exposed body surface area (A_{BSArea}), and posture ($F_{fraction\ exposed}$), per unit body weight (W^{-1}) and the temperature gradient $(T^{-4}_{\text{mean skin}}-T^{-4}_{\text{radiant}})$ (°Kelvin) determine the rate of infrared radiant heat loss or gain.[1] Characteristically, in a single-walled incubator, heat transfers from the infant's skin which is warmer, to the surrounding cooler walls of the plastic incubator's interior. The incubator plastic then re-radiates heat to the nursery walls and windows. The plastic incubator walls are opaque to the transmission of infrared heat, thus absorbing all irradiated heat from the infant ($\varepsilon_{\text{skin}}$, $\varepsilon_{\text{walls}} = 1$). The incubator's mean wall temperature is somewhere between the incubator's internally warmed air and the external air and walls of the surrounding nursery which is generally about 10°C cooler than the incubator. An infant's posture may also affect radiant heat loss. Hey and Katz estimated that non-evaporative heat loss (*incubator operant temperature*) is approximately 60% dependant on wall temperature and 40% on air temperature.[6]

$$T_{\text{operant}} = 0.6(T_{\text{mean wall}}) + 0.4(T_{\text{mean skin}})(°C).(1,6).$$

To quote the caption to their famous figure from their paper, "Approximately 1°C should be added to these operative (incubator air) temperatures in order to derive the appropriate neutral air temperature for a single-walled incubator when nursery room temperature is less than 27°C (80°F), and rather more if room temperature is very much less than this."[6] Our nursery's environmental temperature averaged over three days in October 2006 was median T_{ambient} (23.1°C, range 20.9–25.4°C).

7.1.4 *Evaporation*

Premature newborn infants lose large amounts of water through evaporation from the surface of the skin.[2,4,7–14] Evaporative heat loss occurs first in the delivery room, born wet with amniotic fluid and exposed to the cold, dry air of the delivery suite (usually quite cool for the laboring mother and staff). They experience excessive evaporative heat loss having only a thin epidermal layer and no keratin epithelium serving as a vapor barrier that is normally present in older infants and adults. They also have less subcutaneous fat providing insulation than for babies at term.

Premature neonates lose excessive water and heat due to increased body surface area-to-body mass ratio (Table 7.1).[15] A 70 kg adult having

Table 7.1. Geometric increase in body surface area in proportion to diminishing body mass in low birth weight premature infants. Reproduced with permission, Springer-Verlag (calculated after Haycock *et al.*)[15].

Weight kg	Calculated Surface Area cm^2	Ratio cm^2/kg
2.0	1600	800
1.5	3000	870
1.0	1000	1000
0.5	650	1300

1.73 m^2 body surface area has 250 cm^2/kg exposed, compared with the 1.5 kg premature infant by almost three-fold increase in surface area-to-body mass ratio, and the extremely low birth weight premature infant ($\leq$ 500 grams) has a ratio more than six times the adult. Therefore, insensible water loss evaporating from the skin of the extremely low birth weight premature infant will convey heat away from the body at a rate at least six times that of an adult! The extremely low birth weight infant's body comprises 80–90% water *exposed* to the external environment through a thin no-keratin epidermal barrier.[16]

Hammerlund *et al.*, summarized in a series of elegant studies the rate of transepidermal water (and evaporative heat) loss in premature newborn infants nurtured in incubators throughout the first month of life, at different gestational ages.[10] At $\leq$ 26 week gestation, the infant in the first 48 hours may lose as much as 60 grams of water/m^2/hour, in excess of 180 mL/kg/day. Approximately 0.6 Kcal/mL is lost through evaporation (latent heat converting water into vapor), in excess of 100 Kcal/kg/day through evaporation alone![1]

7.2 Physiology of Response to Heat Loss

7.2.1 *Transition from the uterine environment: physiology of cold stress*

These mechanisms are mitigated by the sympathetic nervous system and brown fat and are discussed in detail below.[17–19] Immediately upon birth, the fetal-maternal heat reservoir and placental blood flow stops abruptly. The infant is born wet into a cold and hostile environment. I have calculated this experience in an adult would be as if we stepped from a warm shower wet into a cool and cloudy autumn day (about 45°F).

Environmental surface cooling ensues, with body temperatures dropping up to 1.0°C/min in the term newborn, much faster in premature neonates. Shivering (sometimes occurring in non-mammalian species at birth) is not active in human newborns. Increased infant activity, vasoconstriction, and *non-shivering thermogenesis* comprise the human neonate's primary defense when acutely exposed to a cold environment.[17] Term infants are able to maintain an increased metabolic rate of heat production under such conditions for minutes only through these mechanisms. Thereafter, energy stores become depleted and lethal hypothermia ensues rapidly characterized by cardiovascular collapse.

An adrenaline surge occurs at parturition from both the sympathetic nervous system, and the neurohumoral axis emanating from the para-aortic sympathetic nodes (organs of Zuckerkandl) and the fetal adrenal gland. Peripheral vasoconstriction and pulmonary vasoconstriction occur with subsequent deterioration of oxygenation and circulation during critical transition. Tissue hypoxia accumulates lactic acidosis contributing to death in a cold neonate.[20] Hypoxia also blunts thermal response to accelerating acute hypothermia.

7.2.2 *Afferent limb*

Homeothermic response to a cold environment begins with temperature sensation. There are two sensitive sites, i.e. the hypothalamus and the skin. Sensation of cold by neonatal skin triggers an immediate cold-adaptive response. Core sensors in the hypothalamus (which are blunted) come into play. Some physiologists conjecture that neonatal cold reception resides primarily in the skin, whereas warm reception resides in the hypothalamus receiving warm bloodflow from para-aortic brown fat deposits (see below). Both sensors are integrated, because cold sensory response is inhibited by core sensor hyperthermia, and core hypothermia facilitates cutaneous sensory drive. Peripheral skin cold sensation as a first responder is important, because early detection of heat loss from the skin aids the infant's heat surge for maintaining core temperature.

7.2.3 *Central regulation*

Multiple skin temperature inputs are likely integrated in the hypothalamus. No single control temperature exists. Skin temperature varies from 8–10°C and temperature of the hypothalamus varies daily by ±0.5°C. There exist nocturnal and daytime temperature fluctuations, variations with sympathetic tone, and maladaptive regulation with asphyxia, hypoxemia, and central nervous system malformations. Premature infants regulate to maintain core temperature near 37.5°C (99.5°F), whereas term infants tend to regulate at a lower core temperature of 36.5°C (97.7°F). Because thermal regulation triggers at Δ0.5°C (about 1°F), deviation at any temperature sensory site (central or peripheral) is important.

7.2.4 *Efferents*

The effector limb of the neonatal thermal response is the sympathetic nervous system. More recently, studies have demonstrated that infant behavior may also be involved. Flexion versus extended posture to retain or dissipate heat respectively, and irritability versus depression of activity. The earliest maturing response is sympathetically innervated vasoconstriction in deep dermal arterioles, resulting in reduced blood flow of warmth from the infant's core into the exposed periphery of the skin. In mature neonates, reduction of skin blood flow also improves fat insulation (subcutaneous white fat). Therefore, diminished fat content in low birth weight babies limits insulation. Nonetheless, vasoconstriction is active in the premature newborn's defense, and this response is present even in the most immature infants that survive.[1]

Brown fat is a second sympathetic organ providing non-shivering thermalgenesis.[17] Brown fat is located under the axilla, subscapular, in the mediastinum, and para-aortic paraspinal, and perinephric regions of the newborn at term. Adipocyte membranes are copiously innervated with adrenergic receptors for norepinephrine and epinephrine, both sympathetic nervous and humorally sensitive. When cold stressed, these receptors result in formation of cyclic AMP, inducing lipoprotein lipase activity. Thyroid hormone is required for this effect, and a thyroid surge occurs as the result of cold stimulation from birth.[21–23] Moreover, brown fat adipocytes demonstrate an abundance of mitochondria to hydrolyze and re-esterify triglycerides and to oxidize free fatty acids.[24] In the term infant, these reactions are exothermic and may increase metabolic two- to three-fold. The appearance of this thermogenic organ (brown color) is the result of a penetrating web of blood vessels that conduct heat produced into the central venous circulation maintaining temperature and function of the myocardium and providing negative feedback to the thalamus in the central nervous system. Preterm babies have little brown fat and may not be capable of any increase in metabolic rate despite the most severe cold stress, rendering these infants functional poikilotherms.[25]

Finally, recent evidence suggests that control of voluntary muscle tone, posture, and increased motor activity with agitation may serve to augment heat production in skeletal muscle via mobilized muscle glycogen and glucose oxidation. These substrates are mostly deposited over the last trimester of gestation. Therefore, the premature infant remains particularly vulnerable to cold stress. Clinical observations of infant posture, behavior, and skin perfusion are useful signs for assessing infant comfort during incubation, and have been practiced by nurses over the past century.

7.2.5 *Intervention in early cold stress is intuitive*

Drying infants in the delivery room interrupts evaporative heat loss,[1] swaddling infants prevents exposure to cool air and provides insulation to retain metabolic heat generated,[2] and placing the newborn infant into the mother's arms to nurse, in particular, into her axillary fold as the warmest part of her body, promotes conductive heat transfer to the infant,[3] relieving cold stress. Alternatively, a convectively warmed incubator enclosure with air temperatures ranging 35–37°C, or a radiant warmer bed may be provided, and a variety of plastic or silver swaddling heat shields have been proposed to prevent excessive cold exposure in premature infants.[2,26–28]

Once outside the delivery room, infants are placed either into an incubator, or into a bassinette, and temperature is closely monitored and maintained through the first two to three hours of transitional care, either by warming the air within the incubator, or careful monitoring of the bundled, cot-nursed infant (generally one layer of clothing and two layers cotton blankets). Despite these measures, near term premature infants (32–37 weeks gestation) or small for gestation infants may suffer the consequences of a persistently cool environment where core temperature is maintained at the expense of metabolic heat generation, with subsequent failure to thrive.[29] Malnourishment and infection attend these conditions, increasing neonatal mortality.

7.3 Human Incubation

7.3.1 *General metabolic heat balance equation*

The general metabolic heat balance equation is given below:

$$Q_{metabolic} + Q_{stored} = Q_{conduction} + Q_{convection} + Q_{radiation} + Q_{evaporation}.$$

Q is the rate of heat change (Kcal/kg/hour, kilojoules/kg/day, or Watts/m^2) is positive for heat gain in the left expression of the equation, and by convention is also positive for heat losses expressed to the right of this equation (conduction, convection, radiation, and evaporation), either heat storage results in a rise in body temperature and metabolic heat produced through metabolism are balanced by the sum of the rates of heat losses.[30] At equilibrium (homeothermy), Q_{stored} = 0 (i.e. no change in body temperature). If an infant's environment is perturbed, physiologic response is stimulated, resulting in an increase in metabolic rate $Q_{metabolic}$ characteristic of homeotherms. Correction of body temperature occurs at the expense of energy. As with all mammals, even the smallest premature infant surviving displays this tendency.

Glass, Silverman and Sinclair investigated the effect of environmental temperature in premature infants maintained in dry, ambient air environments of either 35°C or 36.5°C in the first few days of life.[31] Significantly more weight gain was demonstrated for the warmer infants achieving better growth and regaining birth weight. Surprisingly, rectal temperatures in both groups of infants remained normal. They concluded that thermogenic activation in the slightly cooler environment resulted in the consumption of calories which might have been utilized for growth. They also suggested that graded temperature regulation within incubators (to maintain rectal temperature without thermogenic stimulation constituting a thermal neutral environment) was vital, not only to the survival of preterm infants, but also to reduce morbidity and to achieve optimal growth.

7.3.2 *The thermal neutral concept*[6,11,32-37]

To determine optimal environmental temperature (in most cases air temperature, see below), temperature is generally plotted on an X-axis against the infant's metabolic rate of heat produced on the Y-axis (indicated by oxygen consumption, determined by indirect calorimetry). Although newborn infants (particularly premature babies) cannot shiver, they nevertheless respond to environmental cooling by increasing metabolic rate (homeothermic response). The *thermal neutral temperature zone* is a narrow range of environmental temperatures (between low and high *critical temperatures*), within which the infant controls core body temperature using non-metabolic mechanisms (vasoconstriction, posture, and behavior). Below the critical temperature of the thermal neutral zone, metabolic rate increases to summit metabolism two to three times resting (minimal observed) metabolic rate.

Since core temperature is maintained at the expense of metabolic energy expenditure, simply monitoring core body temperature (rectal or axilla) will not detect whether an infant resides within the thermal neutral zone of environmental temperature. Once summit metabolism is exhausted, body cooling occurs, resulting in deep hypothermia myocardial suppression, and death (especially below 33°C, see Section 7.9).

An inappropriately high environmental temperature results in uncontrolled body heating. Beyond the infant's ability to dissipate body heat, the van't Hoff effect occurs with unstoppable body warming. When this occurs, body temperature rises to where infants sustain seizures (≥ 41.7°C, 107°F) and die. Therefore, thermal regulation for neonates requires maintenance of both physical and physiologic parameters to maintain homeothermy without excessive metabolic expenditure.

7.4 Convection Warmed Incubators

7.4.1 *Air versus skin temperature control*

Characteristically, the modern incubator has a transparent, plastic hood placed over the infant, who lies on an insulating foam mattress, and is provided with a variety of access options for handling and care. Like in an isolation glove-box for handling microbiologic, radioactive or toxic substances, hand ports provide access with the least interruption of warming. Additionally, however, a larger side-panel may be opened permitting access to the infant within for handling, physical or radiological examinations, and blood sampling or performance of minor surgical procedures. Underneath the bed surface upon which the infant lays is an electric warming element. Air is forced over the warming element by a fan. Warmed air is thus circulated within the hood, usually in a controlled fashion to maintain still and quiet air, undisturbed at the center of the box, near the infant's skin. Temperature may be regulated electronically at the incubator's control panel either to thermostatically determine the air temperature within the hood (i.e. to provide the optimal thermal neutral environment viz. Hey and Katz's nomograms), or alternatively, the infant's skin temperature may be servo-controlled to maintain a constant skin temperature, usually measured by an electronic thermistor attached to the skin on the infant's abdomen.[6,38]

7.4.2 *Air temperature control*

Hey and Katz's air temperature nomograms for incubation of premature, low birth weight infants within a single-wall device (London, UK, 1975), compares babies weighing 1.0 kg at birth to babies weighing 2.0 kg at birth, and defining thermal neutral incubator operating temperatures recommended (in degrees Fahrenheit or Centigrade).[6,36,38] These nomograms plot the horizontal axis representing the infant's postnatal age in days to approximately one month after birth. The principle of graded incubation is demonstrated in these nomograms. The authors, however, hastened to add in a figure caption, that nursery air temperatures below 27°C or relative humidity < 50% renders their nomogram inaccurate unless significant upwards correction of the incubator's *operant temperature* (a weighted mean of measured wall and air temperatures, see above) is made.

7.4.3 *Skin surface control*

As a result of the difficulties in determining the exact thermal neutral environment by defining all of the infant and environmental parameters described earlier (including air temperature, air velocity, relative humidity, mean inner wall temperature, and the infant's skin temperature, surface area, and posture), Silverman, Sinclair and Agate suggested that any set of environmental conditions that guaranteed a *normothermic* skin surface temperature would be sufficient to attenuate thermal regulatory response mediated in humans predominantly by skin sensation.[39] These authors defined a skin temperature set-point between 36.2–36.5°C over the anterior abdominal wall for thermostatic control of incubator air temperature warming to guarantee a minimal observed metabolic rate of oxygen consumption, and therefore, a thermal neutral environment. Servo-controlled skin temperature has now become the standard of care for regulating incubator heating.

7.4.4 *Evaporation and humidification in incubators*

Convection warmed incubators are complex environments, however. One example of this complexity is represented by Okken *et al.* reporting partitional calorimetry.[40] Two specially constructed incubators were compared. The first partition described a natural (still air) convection warmed incubator, with air rising passively from powerful heating elements located underneath the infant's mattress uniformly warming the interior of the incubator. The second partition described a fan-forced convection incubator as first described. Non-evaporative heat loss (the sum of convection, radiation and conduction) was 60%, compared to 47% in the forced convection incubator. Evaporative heat loss (E) was 13% higher in the forced convective environment. These authors attributed the increased evaporative heat loss in a forced convection warmed incubator to disturbance of the layer of moist air over the infant's skin (microenvironment). A relationship between convection and evaporation is demonstrated in this experiment.

Artificial humidification of air warmed to a higher capacity for water content (relative humidity) within an incubator has been used commonly to reduce excessive evaporative heat loss and to prevent dehydration, especially in very low birth weight premature infants. Humidification inside incubator hoods is usually accomplished by passive evaporation of water from a reservoir pan near the heating element and in the air pathway underneath the incubator mattress.[41] Other attempts at humidification of incubators in the past employed mist in an effort to saturate the infant's convective environment.[42,43] This strategy resulted in a proliferation of reports of *Pseudomonas* infections during 1950–1970 in the US and humidification of incubators was rejected in a series of case studies.[42–45]

Running incubator hoods dry, however, results in relative humidity levels ≤15%, when nursery air is warmed and re-circulated within the chamber, promoting excessive insensible water (and heat) loss.[46] The incubator compensates for this excessive heat loss by further increasing air temperature within the hood to maintain the infant's body temperature. Excessive evaporation results in increased incubator operating temperature, which in turn results in excessive evaporation. In response to these concerns, the American Academy of Pediatrics published in their incubator recommendations that an intermediate humidification level of 40–50% be employed using water in the vapor form (rather than nebulized particulate water "mist" which may foster bacterial growth).[47]

One investigation of incubator humidification was conducted by Harpin and Rutter in the UK.[41] In retrospect, 33 infants were nurtured in humidified incubators saturated between 80–90% relative humidity. Subjects receiving humidification were < 30 weeks gestation and were less than two weeks old. Two infants acquired *Pseudomonas* sepsis, one died. Twenty nine comparable subjects of similar gestation and postnatal age were nurtured in dry incubators, but one suffered an episode of *Pseudomonas* sepsis and died. Interestingly, none of these infants succumbed to infection during the course of the study in the first two weeks of life. The authors recommended that humidification be used routinely in VLBW infants only in the first two to four weeks of life, and only with intermittent periods of dry incubator operation for at least 12 hours to prevent colonization of the incubator. Until recently (see hybrid incubators below) this practice has not found favor in the US. Early humidification may be prudent for incubation of extremely low birth weight infants (<27 weeks gestation and <1000 grams at birth) where heat and water losses are excessive and pathologic (producing dehydration).[8,16] More modern hybrid incubators now incorporate both temperature and humidity servo-control devices to provide relative humidity levels between 60–80% without particulate water rain-out and diminish the risk of infection with this practice.

7.4.5 *Double-walled incubators*

An example of the importance of radiant heat transfer inside incubators was demonstrated by Bell *et al.*, comparing two different incubator designs.[5] Partitional calorimetry was demonstrated for a standard, single-walled incubator and a double-walled incubator. The double-walled incubator used (Air Shields, C100 Isolette^{TM}) constituted a plastic chamber from the single-walled incubator with an additional inner wall suspended several centimeters separate from the outer wall of the incubator. Warm air circulated between these two walls, warming both the outer and inner surfaces of the inner wall, as well as the inner surface of the outer wall of the incubator. The result is higher inner wall temperature ~10°C warmer than within the single wall device. The infant's skin radiates to the inner wall instead of to the cold outer wall of the incubator.

Thus, radiant heat loss to the doubled walls of the incubator (directly exposed to the infant's skin) is reduced. Convective heat loss is higher in the double-walled incubator since a less warm air temperature is required to warm the infant when radiant heat loss is conserved. As vapor pressure was constant in these studies (without artificial humidification) regardless of incubator air temperature, evaporative heat loss was almost the same in both incubator devices, although somewhat lower with the double-wall and lower air temperature. The benefit derived from the double-walled incubator was a more homogenous partition comparing evaporation (E), convection (C), and radiation (R) in the double-walled device to the single wall incubator. The complexity of controlling environmental variables with simple interventions is important for determining the net heat balance for babies in incubators.

7.4.6 *Incubator homeothermy*

All incubator studies demonstrating a *thermal neutral environment* under a variety of controlled conditions, and governing incubator air temperature, incubator air humidity, wall temperature, and nursery environmental temperature were performed at steady state conditions. Measurements of infant metabolic rates were similarly performed when the infant was at rest, post-prandial, and in general, naked and supine. Such steady state conditions may not be a reality for critically ill premature neonates nurtured within an incubator hood regulated by a servo-control system, and subjected to the many variations in the modern neonatal intensive care environment. Hand ports and doors may be open and closed several times a day in order to perform nursing procedures, minor surgical procedures, and X-ray, ultrasound and echocardiographic examinations. Incubator ports may be opened more than once in an hour in some nursery situations.

Bell and Rios demonstrated in 1983 the characteristics of two commercially available incubators and their servo-controllers for air temperature held at constant level near thermal neutral temperature for premature newborns when the major access panel is opened and then closed.[48] Some of these devices are able to respond in such a way as to maintain or slightly overshoot the thermal neutral temperature. Of course, any enclosure when opened for a significant amount of time cannot interrupt the entry of cold nursery air.

When subsequently closed, internal incubator air temperature rebounds. The servo-control system tends to overshoot and subsequently undershoot incubator air temperature for as long as one hour after the door has been closed. Such fluctuations become part of the infant's thermal experience during intensive care. Their study suggests that incubators should be interrupted as little as possible. This is impractical for managing our smallest critically ill neonates.

7.4.7 *Prematurity and conventional incubation*

In a classic study of partitional calorimetry, Wheldon and Rutter described the complete thermal balance of a series of infants nurtured in a partially humidified, single-walled, forced convection warmed incubator.[3] A group

of babies with a mean weight of 1.58 kg demonstrated nearly similar radiant (R), convective (C) and evaporative (E) heat losses, that when
summed (Σ) balanced the infant's metabolic rate (M). However, when the
same incubator device controlled body temperature for a 1.08 kg infant,
the incubator behaved quite differently. Radiant heat loss was quite low,
and convective heat loss became negative as the air warmed hotter than
the infant's skin. Convection heat gain is therefore necessary to maintain
an extremely low birth weight infant's body temperature.

As a result of super-heated warming, evaporative heat loss was very
high in this extremely low birth weight baby. Evaporative heat loss alone
was greater than the sum of non-evaporative heat losses, and was also
greater than the infant's metabolism. This unusual balance is the result
of the small size of the baby and large evaporative and radiant heat
losses. Most incubators incorporate temperature safety features that do not
permit air temperature above body temperature for longer than 30 minutes
to avoid cooking larger infants. Thus, many conventional incubator
designs may not adequately warm the extremely low birth weight infant
under 1.0 kg birth weight, particularly at birth when evaporative losses
are extremely high.[8,12] This tendency may be intervened by either
humidifying the incubator or defeating the temperature safety feature. The
liabilities with either infection or uncontrolled hyperthermia exist when
using conventional convection-warmed incubators in this population.

7.5 The Open Radiant Warmer Bed

The radiant warmer bed is an open bed platform exposed to the nursery's
cooler ambient air environment, and wall temperatures. Underneath the
platform accommodates X-ray plates, and the bed surface is topped with
a foam mattress, and usually covered with cotton blankets upon which the
critically ill newborn infant lies without a plastic enclosure. Suspended
from a pylon approximately 80–90 cm above this platform is a radiant
heat source comprised of an electrically heated metal alloy coiled within
a quartz tube. A thermostatic skin servo-control mechanism regulates
electrical power input to the wire, generating radiant heat in the middle
portion of the infrared spectrum (wavelengths between 1–3 μm).
The quartz envelope absorbs this relatively short-wave infrared energy

and re-emits electromagnetic radiation in longer, safer wavelengths ($> 3 \mu$m). At full power input (~600 watts), the sum of infrared irradiance output is < 100 mW/cm^2 of surface area irradiated on the bed platform below. The heat delivered in the near infrared spectrum ($< 1 \mu$m) is < 10 mW/cm^2 of surface area irradiated. These levels of radiant exposure in the infrared spectrum are felt to be biologically safe for the developing skin and eyes in the premature newborn infant.[49]

Polished aluminum baffles or a parabolic reflector distributes energy emitted by the radiant heating element evenly over the entire surface of the bed platform.[4] Within the operating range for premature newborn infants 1.0–1.5 kg, the radiant power density delivered is from 14.8–17.4 mW/cm^2, well below the 50–60 mW/cm^2 felt to be potentially dangerous for thermal injury.[49] The head, foot and sides of the radiant warmer bed platform receive less radiant power than the center of the bed platform. Optimally, infants are positioned in the center of this area. Overhead radiant warmers may feel uncomfortably warm for infant care providers working under the heat lamp.

The infant's posture and position under the radiant warmer may alter the effective radiant surface area exposed. Moreover, the infant's curved body surface varies direct versus skew radiant exposure. Laterally, the infant may actually irradiate heat away from the body to the much cooler walls of the surrounding nursery. Radiant delivery comprises both radiant heat delivery which is absorbed by the baby, as well as radiant heat losses to the sides.[50] We have modeled heat doses delivered to the rectangular or circular shadows cast by a series of cylinders representing the infant's torso, arms and legs, with a spherical head.[50]

7.5.1 *Partitional calorimetry under radiant warmers*

Figure 7.1 demonstrates complete partitional calorimetry performed under radiant warmers in a series of premature infants reported by Baumgart.[50] Calculated from our model and thermopile measurements, net radiant heat loss and gain (negative loss) are demonstrated graphically. The calculated effects of evaporation (measured insensible loss by weight, corrected for RQ), convection (calculated from mean skin and air temperatures and an anemometer), and conduction (insulated mattress temperature); and of

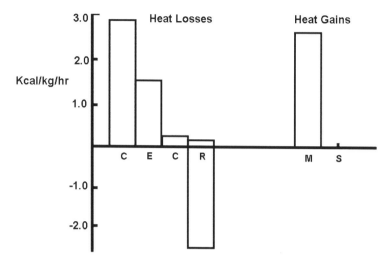

Fig. 7.1. Partitional calorimetry for premature infants nurtured naked and supine on a radiant warmer bed servo-controlled to maintain abdominal skin temperature between 36.5–37.2°C. Dynamic equilibrium is achieved when radiant heat delivered from the warmer balances large convective, evaporative and radiant heat losses. Metabolic rate of heat production is relatively small compared to the magnitude of physical heat exchange with the surrounding environment (adapted from Baumgart).[50]

infant metabolic heat production (calculated from measured oxygen consumption, carbon dioxide production, and RQ) are also depicted. Heat loss comprises 64% convection to the surrounding cool air of the nursery's environment (air temperature ~25°C). The majority of convective heat loss occurs through natural convection, while a minor component comprises forced convective air movement from doors opening and closing within the nursery, nursery personnel moving around the bedside, and cycling of heating and cooling vents supplying the nursery (sampled over about two years seasonal variation in Philadelphia, USA).

Turbulent convective air movements also contribute to evaporative heat loss that comprises 30% of total heat loss in Fig. 7.1. This is similar to the observation of Okken *et al.*,[40] where convection of forced air contributed to disruption of a thin microenvironment of humidified, warm air layered near the infant's skin, potentiating evaporative loss. Under a radiant warmer, due to indirect heating of the bed's surface, conductive heat loss in this diagram is <4%, and radiant heat losses from the infant's sides toward the nursery's walls comprises <2% of total heat loss.

Thermal equilibrium is maintained by a precarious balance of heat losses [through convection (C), evaporation (E), conduction (C) and (R) radiation], replaced by radiant heat gain (R) directly from the warming element. Fifty eight percent of heat replacement is derived from the servo-controlled radiant warmer. Metabolic heat production (M) comprises only 42% of the thermal balance, and is overpowered by convection + evaporation heat losses, and the radiant warmer's replenishment.

Thus, convective heat loss comprises the single largest component of heat loss for infants under radiant warmers, followed by evaporation. Heat loss is replaced in non-homogenously from above by radiant warming. Radiant temperature may be lower at the sides of the infant, as uneven heating and cooling affects the balance between convective turbulence and evaporation, and overhead radiant warming may be "felt" through sensation on the infant's skin, like a sunny day at the beach in October.

7.5.2 *Radiant warmers versus incubators*

7.5.2.1 *Insensible water loss under radiant warmers*

When open radiant warmer beds were first introduced in the early 1970s, several authors published studies suggesting an increased insensible water loss dehydrating critically ill premature babies.[9,15,51] However, these studies failed to control for ambient vapor pressure (a function of air temperature and relative humidity) for infants nurtured within closed incubator environments versus under open radiant warmers. There are two more recent studies on insensible water loss incurred within incubators and under radiant warmers.[20,52] Insensible water loss for a range of infants between 1.0 kg and 2.0 kg was reported by Wu and Hodgeman.[14] Insensible water loss for infants < 1.0 kg was extrapolated linearly. Infants in this study were nurtured within incubators accompanied by moderate humidification. In an analogous study, infants nurtured under radiant warmers were measured to determine their insensible water loss ranging in weights from 0.67–2.2 kg.[8] Notably, a geometric rise in insensible water loss occurred with infants < 1.0 kg in birth weight. Above 1.0 kg, insensible water loss between incubator and radiant warmer nurtured babies were nearly identical. Similar rates of water loss have been reported by Sedin *et al.*, measuring transcutaneous evaporation using another technique (transcutaneous evapoimetry).[12] Together, these studies suggest that insensible water loss is less a function of the heat source used, and rather reflects infant geometry, skin maturity, and ambient vapor pressure. For example, use of water saturated environments within incubators may all but eliminate insensible water loss and, therefore, evaporative heat loss.

One more recent report[52] suggests low birth weight infants may be imperiled shortly after birth insisting solely on conventional convection incubation preferred over radiant warming, as their population recovered normothermia more slowly following cold stress in the nursery.[52,53] These authors recommended stabilization under radiant warmers and fluid replenishment to avoid rigors of cold distress with slow recovery in incubators.

7.5.2.2 *Higher oxygen consumption under radiant warmers*

Due to the relatively large fluctuations in convective, evaporative and radiant heat transfer for infants nursed under radiant warmers, several authors have recently criticized these devices as ineffective in producing a thermal neutral environment. In particular, Le Blanc *et al.* in 1982 summarized several studies in a meta-analysis comparing radiant warmers to convection incubators for infants nurtured alternatively in each of these environments.[54] The thermal neutral environment was defined for each warming device as the minimal observed metabolic rate (MOMR) of oxygen consumption (mL/kg/min), over 30 minutes stable monitoring, when skin temperature was servo-controlled between 36.0°C and 36.5°C, and thermal equilibrium had been achieved at steady state conditions for several hours (an unreal world as stated above). Eleven of 16 infants demonstrated slightly higher rates of oxygen consumption when nursed at similar temperatures under radiant warmers. Mean results demonstrated oxygen consumption of 6.84 ± 0.37 SEM versus 7.45 ± 0.44 mL/kg/min, an increase of 8.8% in metabolic rate under radiant warmers.

7.5.2.3 *Thermal neutral temperature under radiant warmers*

We demonstrated the metabolic rate of oxygen consumption in mL/kg/min over three 90 minute study periods for a 1.2 kg mechanically ventilated infant in our Philadelphia NICU at three different radiant warmer servo-control skin temperatures: 35.5°C, 36.5°C and 37.5°C.[55] At the cooler temperature of 35.5°C, MOMR is equal to approximately 6 mL/kg/min, over the 90-minute study period, peaks and valleys in oxygen consumption occurred that paralleled periods of activity and quiet sleep. At 36.5°C, MOMR equaled about 4.3 mL/kg/min, which is significantly lower. At 37.5°C, metabolic rate was significantly lower, at about 4 mL/kg/min. From these studies over longer durations of real NICU time, it seems clear that infant behavior may constitute a significant part of the metabolic rate determination, and that behavioral comfort may significantly affect the thermal neutral zone. This result was corroborated by Bruck and Parmelee in the early 1960s for larger infants nurtured inside convection warmed incubators, where infant behavior indicated thermal comfort, describing irritability with cold stress, and placidity with appropriate warming.[32,33]

We extended our studies to 18 premature babies nurtured under radiant warmers and demonstrated a thermal neutral environmental temperature (approximately 36.2–36.5°C servo-controlled anterior abdominal wall skin temperature), wherein all infant behavior under real-world NICU conditions was incorporated.[55] Overall metabolic rate approximated 7.2 mL/kg/min at the warmer's 36.5°C skin temperature set point. Increasing anterior abdominal skin temperature above this point by 1°C resulted in no significant further reduction in metabolic rate, and occasional hyperthermia ≥ 37.5°C occurred (that is detrimental to infants recovering from hypoxia). Moreover, the gradient between peripheral skin temperature (measured on the heel), core temperature (deep rectal), and mean skin temperature (sampled at the heel, abdomen and cheek), widened with diminishing anterior abdominal wall skin servo-control temperature.[55] In particular, when servo-controlled to 37.5°C, these infants rapidly approached mean skin temperatures nearly equal to servo-controlled skin temperature. The gradient for heat loss (through convection) narrowed sufficiently for a number of these infants to develop hyperpyrexia (38.2–38.5°C). We therefore recommend avoiding skin control temperatures above 36.7–37.0°C for infants in the weight range we studied (between 0.87–1.60 kg).

In conclusion, a moderate skin temperature between 36.5–37.2°C corresponds to the thermal neutral zone for premature infants under a radiant warmer. The thermal neutral environment under a radiant warmer does not constitute a homeothermic steady state, however. Nevertheless, the radiant warmer environment seems necessary to deliver heat continuously to the critically ill infant requiring intensive care. The uninterrupted steady state studies performed in premature growing infants do not apply to a critically ill population. Care for such infants within incubators results in frequent interruption of the incubator's function and similar variability in thermal control. Some clinical adaptations evaluated for use with radiant warmers to improve the baby's microenvironment will be discussed in a following section.

7.6 Hybrid Incubator-Radiant Warmer Design

A more promising new development in commercial convection-warmed incubator and radiant warming technology is a hybrid design, combining these two separate warming modes into one device. Manufacturers in the US and Germany (Air-Shields, Hill-Rom, Drager and the General Electric, Ohmeda Corporations) each have launched such products. In the incubator mode, movable plastic walls enclose the tiny premature infant providing servo-controlled air warming, and the overhead radiant warmer is incorporated into the roof of this design pod but remains off in incubator mode. In the radiant warmer mode, the plastic walls are retracted, and the radiant warmer rises on to an appropriate height on a motorized pylon and rapidly fires-up to seamlessly maintain servo-controlled skin temperature during the performance of infant care procedures. The infant is not moved during the transition, and no plastic barrier is interposed between the infant and the radiant heater when on. The servo-control algorithms, and the integrity of the plastic enclosure in incubator mode are critical to the performance of such devices, and the utility of these products (survival, quality of life) is yet to be proven. I will review what has been published, for two products below.

7.6.1 *Versalet Incuwarmer*^{TM}

In a preliminary trial Touch *et al.* tested nine premature lambs randomized at delivery, to receive incubation from a conventional radiant warming bed (Resuscitaire^{TM}) with subsequent transfer into an incubator C550 Isolette^{TM}, or from the hybrid Versalet 7700 Care System^{TM} (Hill-Rom, Air-Shields, Hatboro, PA) in both the warmer bed and the incubator modes as previously described.[56] Deep lamb central and surface temperatures, heart rate, blood pressure and oxygenation (blood gas determinations) were measured first during warming in the radiant warmer bed mode, Versalet^{TM}, or on the radiant warmer bed Resuscitaire^{TM} and then during transition to the incubator mode, Versalet^{TM}, or Isolette^{TM}, and then back to the warmer bed, and bed mode. All the animals remained clinically stable throughout the entire transfer protocol on both arms of the study. Despite careful planning, however, adverse encounters resulting in loss of temperature probe data acquisition (probes became disattached) occurred in the control group during transfers from one device to the other. There were no significant differences in the temperature or physiologic profiles (including pH and blood gasses) during any of the transitions in either group. Compared with the standard warming techniques now used in NICU's (separate warmer bed for resuscitation and stabilization with transfer ASAP into an incubator device), the Versalet provides similar thermal and cardiovascular stability without adverse physiologic events during transition to different modes of warming. The authors warn that the contribution of this device to ease of management and improved outcomes in humans needs to be evaluated in a clinical trial.[56–58] To our knowledge, no such clinical trial has yet been conducted, and the Versalet is out of production (Greenspan, privileged communication).

7.6.2 *Giraffe Omnibed*^{TM}

As a radiant warmer, the Giraffe OmniBed evenly heats the infant's mattress utilizing a curved reflector surface to distribute heat generated by the shielded element. Babies are warmed uniformly, regardless of their position on the bed platform surface which may be rotated in a 360° (degree) arc, accommodating IV and ventilator tubing and monitoring wires. The same platform provides tilt up to 12° in Trendelenburg or reverse Trendelenburg positions. Three-sided access from drop-down walls in the radiant warmer mode allows caregivers to perform necessary procedures such as diaper and bedding changes, sampling blood, starting IV's, performing tracheal intubation, or administering medications, performing X-rays, and ultrasound examinations without interrupting warming. A stable thermal environment in either the incubator or radiant warmer mode eliminates the stress of moving premature babies from one incubator device to another, for example when performing chest tube insertion or other minor surgical procedures outside the OR. In an industry sponsored study,[59] Leef *et al.* report that when controlled for acuity of illness, infants were handled significantly less with the Giraffe OmniBed, especially when converted to incubator mode (from 6.9 handling events per hour maximum on a standard radiant warmer bed device to 1.6 times per hour OmniBed-closed). Authors concluded that the OmniBed is conducive to providing developmentally appropriate care, i.e. medically fragile newborns are exposed to a variety of visual, auditory, and tactile stimuli that would not occur within the mother's womb. Consequences of such stimulation are unknown, although it seems reasonable to avoid excessive handling and inappropriate touches due to documented physiological effects of procedural handling.[60]

In another industry sponsored study,[61] there were no differences found in mean skin temperature among the four tested conditions in real-world premature neonates (R = radiant warmer configuration of Omnibed, transition R to C = convection-warmed closed Omnibed, and transition C to R). Mean heart rate, respiratory rate, blood pressure, and oxygen saturation were not statistically different among the four test conditions. The authors concluded that the Giraffe OmniBed provides thermal and physiological stability across bed states eliminating the risk of infant stress or mishap as a result of bed transfer.

When transforming the Giraffe OmniBed from incubator to warmer bed and back, the closed-convection heat partition (above) adapts to form a uniform open-radiant heating configuration with sequential alterations of air warming temperature, fan power, and radiant heat density delivered from the warming canopy while displaying all equipment and baby parameters in one centralized control panel. For example, when returning to the closed-convection mode, the radiant warmer pylon retracts and immediately stops electrical power to the warming element, automatically opening an air vent to cool the reflector hood before over-warming the infant upon descent. In closed-convection mode, bidirectional airflow through double wall construction (see above) of the Giraffe OmniBed provides a stable thermal environment. When either door hand-port is opened, an air curtain minimizes heat loss from the device.

Light and sound levels are carefully controlled within the OmniBed to promote a healthy infant development.[62] An alarm light located out of the baby's field of view is easily visible to caregivers. The WhisperQuiet™ mode limits sound levels to create the quietest, most soothing environment possible. Alarm speakers minimize any noise experienced by the baby. An in-bed scale also reduces handling stress to the baby.

Additionally, a novel servo-regulated humidifier can be set to humidify the closed-incubator condition to the desired *relative humidity* between 70–80%, optimal to avoid excessive insensible water loss and electrolyte disturbances in extremely low birth weight premature neonates in the first week of life when incubated conventionally, dry. One recent preliminary report of a clinical series compared the use of initial stabilization of ELBW babies (< 1000 grams at birth) under a radiant warmer followed by conventional incubation, dry versus use of humidity control in Omnibeds, demonstrated that humidification improves care by decreasing fluid intake, improving electrolyte balance, and growth velocity (Boston AAP, Kim, *et al.*, #7933.24, 2007). The authors did not address the risk-benefit issue of humidification and infection.

The Giraffe® Humidifier is an immersion heater in a reservoir of sterile, distilled water. Water temperature at equilibrium ranges 52–58°C, which is bactericidal to most organisms thriving at temperatures of 20–45°C (i.e. human pathogens). For an added safety measure against accidental reservoir contamination, a small amount of water is boiled off the immersion element just before the humidity is distributed into the air circulated inside the infant's compartment. Sterile humidity is created in a vapor state, with no airborne water droplets. In an industry sponsored study,[63] humidified Omnibeds (*in vitro*, air control mode at 35°C and servo-humidified to 65% relative humidity) were cultured (bacterial swabs were repeated at 24 hours, 48 hours, 72 hours, and 168 hours following reservoir contamination with four water-borne pathogens over a four-week period). No infant environmental culture revealed growth of any pathogen. The authors conclude that there is no concern for an increased risk of infection to an infant when the reservoir is filled daily with sterile distilled water and the bed is routinely cleaned, according to their protocol.

7.7 Other Warming Strategies

7.7.1 *Rigid plastic body hoods as heat shields*

Differing authors have proposed a 1–3 mm thickness of plastic used as a miniature incubator hood placed over infants on open radiant warmer beds (in lieu of a true hybrid device). Yeh *et al.* reported lower insensible water loss using such a device.[64] However, Bell *et al.* failed to replicate this effect.[65] The configuration of the plastic hoods used in each of these studies was different, neither simulated the specialized design of the manufactured double-walled incubators, nor represented a true hybrid device. Moreover, in our study, the interposition of heat opaque plastic between the infant and the radiant warmer interfered with heat delivery. In our study, the hood covering premature subjects on a radiant warmer bed absorbed nearly 85% of radiant warmer energy.[66] Typically the plastic heated to $\geq 42°C$. In response, the radiant warmer's servo-controlled heater output increased dramatically to maintain subjects' abdominal skin temperature.

Use of plastic hoods with a respiratory humidifier (called "swamping") encourages particulate condensation within the hood and onto the baby rendering them prone to bacterial colonization with water-born pathogens (*Pseudomonas, Stenotrophomonas, Clostridia, Citrobacter, Candida*, etc.). This practice is not recommended. Disruption of the servo-control mechanism by the interposition of an opaque, plastic heat sink between the infant and the warmer seems a poor strategy.

7.7.2 *Occlusive plastic blankets or bags*

In contrast to a body hood (and less expensive than the hybrid design), we have advocated the use of a flexible saran plastic blanket.[2,67] This device is thin and transparent to permit free radiant heat exchange between the infant and the radiant warmer.[66] The blanket conforms to the infant's body reducing the effect of convection disrupting the microenvironment of warm, humid air layered near the infant's skin, and does not require an external source of humidification, warmer power is not increased, and insensible water loss reduces 30–40%.[2] Indeed, the servo-controlled radiant heat required to maintain thermal equilibrium is reduced by as much as 30%.[67] Oxygen consumption is reduced from approximately 9.0 mL/kg/min to 8.0 mL/kg/min. This is enough to compensate for the 8.8% increase associated with the radiant warmer bed (see above) versus a convection warmed incubator in steady state. The net effect of saran blanket heat shielding under radiant warmers allows the baby's own small rate of metabolic heat production to determine their core temperature.

Recently, a polyethylene plastic bag was evaluated by Vohra *et al.* to promote temperature maintenance during resuscitation performed at delivery under radiant warmers, and during the transport of infants to the NICU in convection warmed (dry) transport incubators.[68] A significantly higher admission rectal temperature and subsequently improved survival was reported for infants < 28 weeks gestation. This result has recently been replicated.[69]

There may be adverse effects of such plastic wraps for the ELBW infant. The immature skin may stick to the plastic causing maceration. In rare cases where temperature probes have loosened, life-threatening hyperthermia has resulted with the warmer switching to full power. Nursing care requires vigilance and periodic infant temperature assessment independent of the servo-controller skin temperature. We recommend axilla temperature monitoring at least every two hours under radiant warmers. The use of a thin plastic blanket is presently the most effective technique for rendering infants under radiant warmers more consistently thermal neutral.

7.7.3 *Semi-occlusive artificial "skin"*

Another method for reducing insensible water loss in extremely low birth weight premature infants nurtured under radiant heaters (and in dry incubators) is covering the skin exposed to air with semi-occlusive polyurethane dressings (Tegederm™ or Opsite™).[70] In early studies using this technique covering the chest and abdomen of premature infants, we evaluated transcutaneous evaporation directly using an evaporimeter. Compared to skin sites that were not dressed with the artificial polyurethane skin, insensible water loss from days 1–4 of life was reduced by 30–50%. Care must be used when removing such dressings as the delicate epidermis may easily be damaged.

Porat and Brodsky reported results applying an adherent polyurethane layer over the entire torso and extremities of extremely low birth weight infants ≤ 800 grams.[71] They reported less hypernatremic dehydration and lower fluid maintenance volume required, a reduced incidence of PDA and IVH, as well as improved survival. We caution that further studies are required before routine application of adherent artificial polyurethane to premature neonates be performed.

7.7.4 *Petroleum emollients*

Another popular water impermeable dressing for skin of low birth weight preterm neonates is the application of Aquaphor™. Although early results were encouraging for preserving skin integrity and perhaps controlling excessive dehydration in incubators,[72] the findings of a multi-center randomized trial (Vermont Oxford Network, 2001),[73] and other reports suggest bacterial and fungal blood stream infections may be more common with use of this technique.[74] We do not advocate this practice.

7.8 Other Clinical Scenarios

7.8.1 *Kangaroo care*

Kangaroo care is warming newborns by skin-to-skin contact with the mother or father where premature infants are held naked in the axilla or between the breasts. Pioneered in Bogotá, Columbia for nurturing near-term premature neonates, this method was adopted in Scandinavian and other countries for earlier premature babies in the 1980s. Kangaroo care promotes a thermal neutral metabolic rate and temperature stability. Early studies suggested a significant reduction in mortality and morbidity, through enhanced maternal-infant attachment, increased infant alertness, more stable sleep patterns, better weight gain, and earlier hospital discharge. Moreover, during kangaroo care, infants with BPD have demonstrated better oxygenation, and other infants show less periodic breathing and apnea. Even in the NICU, kangaroo care may be performed. Infants should be covered with a cotton blanket for insulation, and sessions should initially be limited to 30 minutes. Thereafter, sessions can be increased gradually in our experience up to four hours. To my knowledge, no adverse effects have been reported.[75]

7.8.2 *Extremely low birth weight (ELBW) infants*

Temperature maintenance of an extremely premature infant (≤750 g) should be part of neonatal resuscitation. Despite radiant warming and convective incubation during transport, these babies frequently exhibit moderate to severe hypothermia <32°C, exhibiting bradycardia and hypotension.[76] Suboptimal radiant heating, early transfer into a dry incubator, and the pressure for performing procedures contribute to heat loss. Lower pH has been demonstrated for premature infants ≤28 weeks gestation.[53]

Quickly drying these babies, proper placement directly under the radiant heater (not maternal bonding), and covering their heads are important steps for temperature resuscitation. Other techniques might be considered, such as use of the plastic bag described by Vohra, or a saran or blanket or polyurethane drape during umbilical catheterization.[68] Finally, these subjects should be adequately warmed under a radiant warmer before transferring to a dry incubator that may prolong thermal recovery in these infants.[52] Probably, if available, the hybrid Giraffe Omnibed could best be employed at birth in the DR, and during transport to NICU. Procedures might be instigated with smooth transformation of the thermal and physiological environment between warmer and closed incubator modes, with the addition of humidity 60–80% relative, to avoid evaporative water and heat loss.

There are no data describing the best rate of re-warming for hypothermic babies, however recent experience from our therapeutic hypothermia program (see below) suggest slower is better regarding cardiac arrhythmias, glucose and electrolyte shifts, and strokes. A closely monitored rate of temperature rise of about +0.5°C/hour seems the best using a radiant warmer servo-controlled to skin temperature, but may not be achievable in incubators delivering air temperatures <37°C. Hybrid incubators can also be used as radiant warmer beds, and may be helpful in re-warming.

7.9 Therapeutic Hypothermia for Term and Near-Term Neonates — Cerebral Protection

More recently (2005–2010), therapeutic hypothermia has been established as the standard of care for a highly selected population of near-term/term neonates with hypoxic-ischemic events after birth. Two recent randomized studies suggest that cerebral cooling with either whole body cooling (to 33.5°C core esophageal temperature — moderate hypothermia), or selective head cooling (10°C along with mild whole-body cooling to 34°C) reduces the risk for death or moderate to severe neurological injury from more than or equal to 60% to less than 50%.[77,78] The National Institutes of Health's Institute of Child Health and Human Development (NICHD) Experts Panel Workshop held in May 2005, emphasized using standardized protocols adapted from these randomized trials for hypothermia treatment, and recommended continual follow-up until school age to develop, and to better refine new therapies for treating moderate-to-severe clinical neonatal encephalopathy in term or near-term neonates.[79]

We adopted the Neonatal Network's whole-body hypothermia protocol. Additionally, we provide continuous EEG neurological-monitoring as part of our hypothermia protocol. A full montage video-EEG (using a modified International 10–20 system for neonates) is recorded by computer for 120 hours after birth to include cooling and re-warming recovery. Amplitude-integrated EEG (aEEG) was also reviewed for characterization of background pattern and for detection of seizures. Automated seizure detection by aEEG was confirmed on raw EEG signals. To receive cooling therapy, infants must be more than or equal to 36 weeks completed gestation, must arrive for treatment within six hours of birth and have experienced a hypoxic-ischemic (HI) insult. Evidence of HI injury includes that the baby required resuscitation at delivery, an umbilical vessel blood gas pH of less than or equal to 7.00 or having a significant base deficit of at least −16. Also qualifying for therapy are blood gas disturbances within the first hour of life with pH 7.01–7.15 and a base deficit of −10 to −15.9, along with an ominous perinatal history (fetal heart rate decelerations, umbilical cord prolapse or rupture, uterine rupture, severe maternal trauma preceding birth, and abruption of the placenta, or the mother experienced a life-threatening event requiring CPR). Signs of moderate to severe neonatal encephalopathy must also be present (an infant who is lethargic, or completely stuporous, has diminished or completely absent activity and muscle tone, having weak or absent sucking and Moro reflexes, with pupils fixed and constricted or unresponsive and dilated, having fixed flexion or extension posturing of extremities, or a clinically observed seizure. Although definable, EEG/aEEG recordings are not part of our institutional criteria. Infants with such symptoms persisting for several days have about a 60% risk for death before hospital discharge, while a majority of survivors experience moderate to severe life-long neurodevelopmental disabilities (cerebral palsy, deafness, blindness, mental retardation, or recurrent seizures disorder, epilepsy).

Infants meeting criteria are placed at admission supine onto a water-filled cooling blanket, pre-cooled to 5°C (41°F). We use a Blanketrol II (Cincinnati Sub-Zero Inc., Ohio), a device used commonly in our ER to reduce high fevers and in our OR where it is used to promote hypothermia before and during cardiac surgery. After softening in warm water, an esophageal temperature probe is placed into the distal third of the esophagus, and the water mattress cooling unit's thermostatic controller is set to 33.5°C. A second larger pediatric-size blanket is also attached in parallel to the cooling system. Water circulates through both blankets with the larger blanket hung on an IV rack at bedside (termed a "sail") serving as thermal capacitance with room air temperature to diminish fluctuations in the esophageal temperature (to less than ±0.5°C). Although we use a warmer bed platform as a crib of convenience for ready access, the overhead warmer is not turned on during the cooling period. Abdominal wall skin temperature is also monitored with a surface probe, available with the warmer bed (in monitor mode). Temperatures of the esophagus, skin, and axilla are thus monitored and recorded every 15 minutes for the first four hours of cooling, every hour for the next eight hours, and every four hours during the remaining 72 hour period of hypothermia. Our electronic medical record provides hourly esophageal temperature recording. After 72 hours, the set point of the controller on the cooling system is increased by +0.5°C per hour to promote gradual (slow) re-warming. The Neonatal Network reported febrile rebound and seizures during re-warming. This has not been our experience. After six hours, the esophageal probe and cooling blankets are removed, and anterior abdominal wall skin temperature is then regulated using the radiant warmer's servomechanism set at 36.5°C (warmer on). The purpose for re-warming slowly is to avoid rapid shifts in critical electrolytes (calcium and potassium), cardiac arrhythmias, and in particular re-warming overshoot, since fever promotes further brain injury.[80] Infants otherwise receive routine care, with continuous monitoring of vital signs (mild bradycardia 80–90 and small decrease in mean arterial blood pressure ≤ 20 mmHg are commonly observed and easily treated with volume and pressor infusions). Frequent blood samples are monitored for (1) glucose regulation (infants are restricted to 4–6 mg/kg/min dextrose infusion, (2) coagulopathy in particular treating fibrinogen levels < 150 mg/dL, and platelet levels < 80,000 per mm,[3] and (3) for major organ failure (e.g. electrolytes, BUN, creatinine, liver enzymes and PT).

Our clinical experience over the past three years in over 90 babies meeting strict criteria for therapeutic hypothermia has been commensurate with that reported from the Neonatal Network. We achieved target esophageal temperature at 33.5 ± 1.0°C in 30–60 minutes without major circulatory mishap. Continuous EEG monitoring has been instructive for intervening seizure activity (observed on EEG in about one-quarter). We have generally observed improvements in background voltages and patterns on EEG recordings during and after hypothermia. Specifically, improvement of background activity, appearance of sleep-wake cycle and disappearance of seizures is observed at the time of re-warming.[81] Neonatal Network observed seizures emerging frequently during re-warming, hence our caution is to re-warm more slowly.[77] We presently are acquiring and reviewing infant neurological and developmental follow-up data.

We made the clinical observation that the water mattress felt warm to touch (i.e. warmer than our hand) during the majority of the cooling period.[82] Median ambient temperature in our NICU during October 2007

$T_{ambient}$ (23.1°C, range 20.9–25.4°C) was usually less than both the blanket water and baby temperatures. No infant had acidemia during cooling. Temperature gradients suggest that whole body cooling is achieved through surface cooling from skin exposed to the ambient environment, and not actually cooling from the water-blanket. Except in the first 30 minutes, the blanket more often provided warmth to maintain $T_{esophageal}$ at 33.5°C. Whole body cooling might also be provided by regulating an incubator air temperature, or a radiant heater's output to maintain esophageal temperature.

7.10 Summary

The complexity of neonatal environmental care has expanded rapidly in recent years to include many techniques and manipulations for our most fragile patients. For tiny and critically ill premature neonates, care must be taken to provide an uninterrupted source of warmth, adequate to maintain body temperature, and also to reduce thermal stress and the physiologic/metabolic demand associated with it. As we salvage smaller infants, we must be hyperalert to that the problem of geometrically increasing heat loss and cold stress. New technology is introduced about every 10 years as we rediscover historical studies in smaller patients. The converse is applicable with therapeutic cooling for birth asphyxia, i.e. we must avoid application of excessive warming. In the hectic intensive care nursery environment, all too frequently temperature regulation is either forgotten or delegated to machinery to respond to thermal fluctuations in a timely manner. Temperature assessments should be performed frequently, separate from the warming/cooling devices servo-control monitored temperature. Extremes of environments are best avoided. Hybrid incubators are probably best for the nurturance and growth of premature infants. Radiant warming may thus be provided seamlessly for the delivery of intensive care with uninterrupted heat delivery. As much as possible, shielding infants from the harsh extrauterine environment is desirable. Preservation of the delicate, microenvironment of warm, humid air that resides near to a premature infant's skin within 1–2 mm is important for maintaining homeothermy.

References

1. Sinclair JC. (1976) Metabolic rate and temperature control. In: Smith CA, Nelson NM, eds. *The Physiology of the Newborn Infant.* Thomas, Springfield, Illinois; 354–415.

2. Baumgart S, Engle WD, Fox WW, *et al.* (1981) Effect of heat shielding on convective and evaporative heat losses and on radiant heat transfer in the premature infant. *J Pediatr* 99: 948–956.

3. Wheldon AE, Rutter N. (1982) The heat balance of small babies nursed in incubators and under radiant warmers. *Early Hum Develop* 6: 131–143.

4. Baumgart S, Engle WD, Fox WW, Polin RA. (1981) Radiant warmer power and body size as determinants of insensible water loss in the critically ill neonate. *Pediatr Res* 15: 1495–1499.

5. Bell EF, Rios GR. (1983) A double-walled incubator alters the partition of body heat loss of premature infants. *Pediatr Res* 17: 135–140.

6. Hey EN, Katz G. (1970) The optimum thermal environment for naked babies. *Arch Dis Child* 45: 328–334.

7. Baumgart S, Engle WD, Fox WW, Polin RA. (1980) Radiant energy monitoring as a measurement of insensible water loss in critically ill neonates under radiant warmers. *Pediatr Res* 14: 590A.

8. Baumgart S, Langman CB, Sosulski R, *et al.* (1982) Fluid, electrolyte and glucose maintenance in the very low birth weight infant. *Clin Pediatr* 21: 199–206.

9. Bell EF, Neidich GA, Cashore WJ, *et al.* (1979) Combined effect of radiant warmer and phototherapy on insensible water loss in low-birth weight infants. *J Pediatr* 94: 810–813.

10. Hammarlund K, Sedin G. (1983) Transepidermal water loss in newborn infants. VIII. Relation to gestational age and post-natal age in appropriate and small for gestational age infants. *Acta Paediatr Scand* 72: 721–728.

11. Hey EN, Katz G. (1969) Evaporative water loss in the newborn baby. *J Physiol (Lond)* 200: 605–619.

12. Sedin G, Hammarlund K, Nilsson GE, *et al.* (1985) Measurements of transepidermal water loss in newborn infants. *Clin Perinatol* 12: 79–96.

13. Williams PR, OH W. (1974) Effects of radiant warmer on insensible water loss in newborn infants. *Am J Dis Child* 128: 511–514.

14. Wu PYK, Hodgman JE. (1974) Insensible water loss in preterm infants: changes with postnatal development and non-ionizing radiant energy. *Pediatrics* 54: 704–712.

15. Costarino AT, Baumgart S. (1991) Water metabolism in the neonate. In: Cowett RM, ed. *Principles of Perinatal-Neonatal Metabolism*. New York, Springer-Verlag; 623–649.

16. Costarino AT, Baumgart S. (1986) Modern fluid and electrolyte management of the critically ill premature infant. *Pediatr Clin North Am* 33: 153–178.

17. Alexander G, Williams D. (1968) Shivering and non-shivering thermalgenesis during summit metabolism in young lambs. *J Physiol (Lond)* 198: 251–276.

18. Hodgkin DD, *et al.* (1988) *In vivo* brown fat response to hypothermia and norepinephrine in the ovine fetus. *J Dev Physiol* 10: 383–391.

19. Schroder H, Huneke B, Klug A, *et al.* (1987) Fetal sheep temperatures *in utero* during cooling and application of triiodothyronine, norepinephrine, propranolol and suxamethonium. *Pflugers Arch* 410: 376–384.

20. Baumgart S. (1992) Incubation of the human newborn infant. In: Pommerance J, Richardson CJ, eds. *Issues in Clinical Neonatology*, Norwalk, CT, Appleton & Lange; 139–150.

21. Bray GA, Goodman HM. (1965) Studies on the early effects of thyroid hormones. *Endocrinology* 76: 323–328.

22. Klein AH, Reviczky A, Padbury JF. (1984) Thyroid hormones augment catecholamine-stimulated brown adipose tissue thermalgenesis in the ovine fetus. *Endocrinology* 114: 1065–1069.

23. Swanson HE. (1956) Interrelations between thyroxin and adrenalin in the regulation of oxygen consumption in the albino rat. *Endocrinology* 59: 217–225.

24. Silva JE, Larsen PR. (1983) Adrenergic activation of triiodothyronine production in brown adipose tissue. *Nature* 305: 712–713.

25. Hull D, Smales ORC. (1978) Heat production in the newborn. In: Sinclair JC, ed. *Temperature Regulation and Energy Metabolism in the Newborn*, New York, Grune and Stratton; 129–156.

26. Baum JD, Scopes JW. (1968) The silver swaddler. *Lancet* 1: 672–673.

27. Besch NJ, Perlstein PH, Edwards NK, *et al.* (1971) The transparent baby bag. *N Engl J Med* 284: 121–124.

28. Dahm LS, James LS. (1972) Newborn temperature: heat loss in the delivery room. *Pediatrics* 49: 504–513.

29. Silverman WA, Fertig JW, Berger AP. (1958) The influence of the thermal environment upon the survival of the newly born premature infant. *Pediatrics* 22: 876–886.

30. Hardy JD, Gagge AP, Rapp GM. (1969) Proposed standard system of symbols for thermal physiology. *J Appl Physiol* 27: 439–440.

31. Glass L, Silverman WA, Sinclair JC. (1968) Effect of the thermal environment on cold resistance and growth of small infants after the first week of life. *Pediatrics* 41: 1033–1046.

32. Bruck K, Parmelee AH, Bruck M. (1962) Neutral temperature range and range of "thermal comfort" in premature infants. *Biol Neonate* 4: 32–51.

33. Bruck K. (1978) Heat production and temperature regulation. In: Stave U, ed. *Perinatal Physiology*, New York, Plenum Publishing; 455–498.

34. Bruck K. (1961) Temperature regulation in the newborn infant. *Biol Neonate* 3: 65–119.

35. Cross KW, Dawes GS, Mott JC. (1959) Anoxia, oxygen consumption and cardiac output in newborn lambs and adult sheep. *J Physiol* 146: 316–343.

36. Hey EN. (1969) The relation between environmental temperature and oxygen consumption in the new-born baby. *J Physiol* 200: 589–603.

37. Hill JR, Rahimtulla KA. (1965) Heat balance and the metabolic rate of newborn babies in relation to environmental temperature, and the effect of age and of weight on basal metabolic rate. *J Physiol* 180: 239–265.

38. Hey EN. (1975) Thermal neutrality. *Br Med Bull* 31: 69–74.

39. Silverman WA, Sinclair JC, Agate FJ Jr. (1966) The oxygen cost of minor changes in heat balance of small newborn infants. *Acta Pediatr Scand* 55: 294–300.

40. Okken A, Blijham C, Franz W, *et al.* (1982) Effects of forced convection of heated air on insensible water loss and heat loss in preterm infants in incubators. *J Pediatr* 101: 108–112.

41. Harpin VA, Rutter N. (1985) Humidification of incubators. *Arch Dis Child* 60: 219–224.

42. Moffet HL, Allan D, Williams T. (1967) Survival and dissemination of bacteria in nebulizers and incubators. *AJDC* 114: 13–20.

43. Moffet HL, Allan D. (1967) Colonization of infants exposed to bacterially contaminated mists. *AJDC* 114: 21–25.

44. Brown DG, Baublis J. (1977) Reservoirs of pseudomonas in an intensive care unit for newborn infants: mechanism of control. *J Pediatr* 90: 453–457.

45. Hoffman MA, Finberg L. (1955) Pseudomonas infections in infants associated with high humidity environments. *J Pediatr* 46: 626–630.

46. Hill JR. (1959) The oxygen consumption of newborn and adult mammals: its dependence on the oxygen tension in the inspired air and on the environmental temperature. *J Physiol* 149: 346–373.

47. *Guidelines for Perinatal Care.* (1988) 2nd ed., AAP/ACOG; 278.

48. Bell EF, Rios GR. (1983) Performance characteristics of two double-walled infant incubators. *Crit Care Med* 11: 663–667.

49. Baumgart S, Knauth A, Casey FX, *et al.* (1993) Infrared eye injury not due to radiant warmer use in premature neonates. *Am J Dis Child* 147: 565–569.

50. Baumgart S. (1990) Radiant heat loss versus radiant heat gain in premature neonates under radiant heaters. *Biol Neonat* 57: 10–20.

51. Engle WD, Baumgart S, Schwartz JG, Fox WW, Polin RA. (1981) Insensible water loss in the critically III neonate. Combined effect of radiant-warmer power and phototherapy. *Am J Dis Child* 135: 516–520.

52. Meyer MP, Payton MJ, Salmon A, Hutchinson C, de Klerk A. (2001) A clinical comparison of radiant warmer and incubator care for preterm infants from birth to 1800 Grams. *Pediatrics* 108: 395–401.

53. Meyer M, Bold GT. (2007) Admission temperatures following radiant warmer or incubator transport for preterm infants, 28 weeks: a randomized study. *Arch Dis Child Fetal Neonatal Ed* 92: F295–F297.

54. LeBlanc MH. (1984) Relative efficacy of radiant and convective heat in incubators in producing thermalneutrality for the premature. *Pediatr Res* 18: 425–428.

55. Malin S, Baumgart S. (1987) Optimal thermal management for low birth weight infants nursed under high-power radiant warmers. *Pediatrics* 79: 47–54.

56. Touch SM, Greenspan JS, Cullen AB, Wolfson MR, Shaffer TH. (2001) *Biol Neonate* 80: 286–294.

57. Greenspan JS, Cullen AB, Touch SM, Wolfson MR, Shaffer TH. (2001) Thermal stability and transition studies with a hybrid warming device for neonates. *J Perinatol* 21(3): 167–173.

58. Sherman TI, Greenspan JS, St. Clair N, Touch SM, Shaffer TH. (2006) Optimizing the neonatal thermal environment. *Neonatal Network* 25: 251–260.

59. http://www.Medical.com/BedMasterEx/Physical%20and%20Developmental%20Touch%20Abstract

60. Gressens P, Rogido M, Paindaveine B, Sola A. (2002) The impact of neonatal intensive care practices on the developing brain. *Pediatrics* 140(6): 646–653.

61. http://www.excel-medical.com/BedMasterEx/Giraffe%20Thermal%20 Abstract%20Modified.doc

62. Lynam L. (2003) The impact of the microenvironment on newborn care a facility report: Christiana Care Health System. *Neonatal Intensive Care* Vol. 1 No. 1.

63. Lynam L, Biagotti L, BS. (2002) Testing for bacterial colonization in a Giraffe humidification system. *Neonatal Intensive Care* Vol. 15 No. 2.

64. Yeh TF, Amma P, Lillian LD, *et al.* (1979) Reduction of insensible water loss in premature infants under the radiant warmer. *J Pediatr* 94: 651–653.

65. Bell EF, Weinstein MR, Oh W. (1980) Heat balance in premature infants: comparative effects of convectively heat incubator and radiant warmer, with and without plastic heat shield. *J Pediatr* 96: 460–465.

66. Baumgart S, Fox WW, Polin RA. (1982) Physiologic implications of two different heat shields for infants under radiant warmers. *J Pediatr* 100(5): 787–790.

67. Baumgart S. (1984) Reduction of oxygen consumption, insensible water loss and radiant heat demand using a plastic blanket for low birth weight infants under radiant warmers. *Pediatrics* 74: 1022–1028.

68. Vohra S, Frent G, Campbell V, Abbott M, Whyte R. (1999) Effect of polyethylene occlusive skin wrapping on heat loss in very low birth weight infants at delivery: a randomized trial. *J Pediatr* 134: 547–551.

69. Mathew B, Lakshminrusimha S, Cominsky K, Schroder E, Carrion V. (2007) Vinyl bags prevent hypothermia at birth in pretermInfants. *Indian J Pediatr* 74(3): 249–253.

70. Knauth A, Gordin M, McNelis W, *et al.* (1989) A semipermeable polyurethane membrane as an artificial skin in premature neonates. *Pediatrics* 83: 945–950.

71. Porat R, Brodsky N. (1993) Effect of Tegederm use on outcome of extremely low birth weight (ELBW) infants. *Peds Res* 33: 231(A).

72 Nopper AJ, Horii KA, Sookdeo-Drost S, Wang TH, Mancini AJ, Lane AT. (1996) Topical ointment therapy benefits premature infants. *J Pediatr* 128: 660–669.

73. Edwards WH, Conner JM, Soll RF, for the Vermont Oxford Network. (2001) The effect of Aquaphor™ original emollient ointment on nosocomial sepsis

rates and skin integrity in infants of birth weight 501–1000 grams. *Pediatr Res* 49: 388A.

74. Oski K, Pappagallo M, Lerer T, Hussain N. (2001) Does use of Aquaphor™ (Aq) in extremely low birth weight infants (ELBW) increase the risk for nosocomial sepsis? *Pediatr Res* 49: 227A.

75. Anderson GC. (1991) Current knowledge about skin-to-skin (kangaroo care) for preterm infants. *J Perinatol* 11: 216–226.

76. McCall EM, Alderdice FA, Halliday HL, Jenkins JG, Vohra S. (2008) Interventions to prevent hypothermia at birth in preterm and/or low birth-weight infants. *Cochrane Database Systematic Review* 23(1): CD004210.

77. Shankaran S, Laptook AR, Ehrenkkranz RA, Tyson JE, McDonald SA, Donovan EF, Fanaroff AA, Poole WK, Wright LL, Higgins RD, Finer NN, Carlo WA, Duara S, Oh W, Cotton CM, Stevenson DK, Stoll BJ, Lemons JA, Guillet R, Jobe AH, for the NICHHD, Neonatal Research Network. (2005) Whole-body hypothermia for neonates with Hypoxic-ischemic encephalopathy. *N Engl J Med* 353: 1574–1584.

78. Gluckman PD, Wyatt JS, Azzopardi D, Ballard R, Edwards DA, Ferriero DM, Polin RA, Robertson CM, Thoreson M, Whtelaw A, Gunn AJ, CoolCap study group. (2005) Selective head-cooling with mild systemic hypothermia after neonatal encephalopathy: multi-center randomized trial. *Lancet* 365: 663–670.

79. Higgins RD, *et al.* (2006) Hypothermia and perinatal asphyxia: executive summary of the National Institute of Child Health and Human Development Workshop. *J Pediatr* 148: 170–175.

80. Yager JY, Armstrong EA, Jaharus C, Saucier DM, Wirrell EC. (2004) Preventing hyperthermia decreases brain damage following neonatal hypoxic-ischemic seizures. *Brain Res* 1011: 48–57.

81. El-Dib M, Massaro AN, Baumgart S, Tsuchida T, Short BL, Chang T. (2007) Amplitude integrated electroencephalogram (aEEG) background changes and seizures during therapeutic whole-body hypothermia. (Abstract) Pediatric Academic Societies' Annual meeting, Toronto, Canada.

82. Baumgart S, Massaro A, Chang T, Glass P, Tsuchida T, Short BL. (2007) Whole body cooling therapy: is it really a cooling mattress? (Abstract) Pediatric Academic Societies' Annual meeting, Toronto, Canada.

Chapter 8

Advances in Neonatal Nutritional Care

David H. Adamkin*

Over the past few decades, there has been a tremendous change in the way neonatal care is delivered. Advances in technology, introduction of surfactant, attention to growth and outcomes have all impacted positively on the care of the high risk neonate. This is particularly important given that in the US, rate of prematurity is increasing in the face of increasing survival of high risk neonates.

8.1 Historical Aspects

Two important aspects of nutritional support are nutritional content and mode of delivery. Chemical composition of milk was discovered in the 1890s and the concept of formula feeds was developed in the 1920s. Evaporated milk was the basic ingredient to which water and other substances such as Karo syrup was added. By 1940s, preterm infants were fed formulas with increased protein, saturated fats and minerals such as calcium and phosphorous. Metabolic acidosis and azotemia were not uncommon during this period. Introduction of whey predominant formula was introduced in the 1980s. We continue to tweak the content so that special formulas for various digestive and metabolic problems are available

*Professor of Pediatrics, University of Louisville.

and enhance the nutritional contents of both preterm and term formulas. Soft rubber catheters were used for feeding neonates as early as 1850s, while polyethylene tubes were introduced in the 1950s. Various types of tube feeding regimens such as intermittent bolus feeding and continuous gastric and transpyloric feeding remain the mainstay in delivering nutrition to preterm infants.

Immaturity of the gastrointestinal system of the premature infant is associated with poor motility and delayed transit. Difficulties in providing adequate enteral nutrition in many preterm infants as well as contraindication to enteral feedings in others, stimulated the development of intravenous feeding. Initially this consisted of intravenous glucose to which a protein hydrolysate was added. Metabolic acidosis, azotemia and hyperammonemia were common in the early days of intravenous feeding. These complications have been minimized with current generation of amino acid formulations. These parenteral nutrition solutions were administered into major veins. Peripherally inserted central venous catheters are used nowadays to provide longer term total parenteral nutrition and peripheral venous lines are often used for short term nutritional support.

8.2 Protein Strategies

The past 50 years have seen major advances in the clinical care and survival of extremely premature infants. Major strides and innovations have resulted in a survival of well over 90% of very low birth weight infants (VLBW). Nevertheless, the vast majority of these infants experience extrauterine growth restriction (EUGR). Their weights and frequently even head circumferences are less than that for the corresponding conceptional age by the time they are discharged from the neonatal intensive care unit. The outcome for these extremely low birth weight (ELBW < 1000 g) infants may be influenced by the intensity and duration of less than adequate nutrition. Since growth failure is associated with impaired neurocognitive development[1,2] later in life, its prevention is important. Thus, nutritional management of these infants remains the major challenge and hopefully an opportunity to improve outcomes.

Neonatologists and nutritionists have been developing new and innovative modalities for nutrient delivery. We have ongoing epidemiologic studies examining the impact of such new interventions and strategies on long term neurodevelopmental and even adult outcomes.

One of the major innovations has been the use of the factorial method developed by Ziegler *et al.*,[3] which estimated requirements of macronutrients. Traditionally, methods of estimating requirements have been as listed below.

(a) Analogy with the breast-fed infant. Although this has been the gold standard for term neonates, it is less applicable for the preterm infants who still need fortified human milk.

(b) Direct experimental evidence. This approach has been used in both term and preterm infants.

(c) Extrapolation from studies of human adults or adult animals. This approach has been taken in setting requirements for vitamins.

(d) Data on intakes by healthy subjects. Not applicable to the high risk neonate.

(e) Theoretically based calculations or the factorial method. This has been the basis for estimating requirements and then designing studies that resulted for example, in different generations of infant formulas.

The focus of this book and specifically this chapter is to examine therapies that have changed the way we deliver care to these patients. Protein is the principal growth nutrient for VLBW infants and has been the focus for new strategies that not only promote growth and neurodevelopment but also may contribute to the quality of adult health for these individuals.

8.2.1 *Requirements*

Nutrient requirements for VLBW infants may be defined as those intakes that promote postnatal growth that approximates *in utero* growth of a fetus of the same gestational age.[4] The most commonly used method for estimating the protein intake necessary to maintain the intrauterine rate of protein accretion is the factorial method, which includes an estimate of inevitable urinary nitrogen losses (i.e. the losses that occur in the absence of nitrogen intake) and an estimate of the amount deposited *in utero* corrected for efficiency of absorption and deposition. An alternative method is to determine the actual intakes that support intrauterine rates of growth and nitrogen accretion (empirical method).

The main advantages of the factorial method are that it provides estimates of energy requirements in addition to protein and may also be applied to very premature infants where there are no empirical estimates available. However, it does not determine nutrient needs for catch-up growth. The empirical approaches are more useful when one needs estimates for catch-up growth. The empirical methods do not estimate energy requirements. Table 8.1 shows enteral protein and energy requirements determined by the factorial approach. It also emphasizes that the requirements are more closely related to body weight than to gestational age. Table 8.2 shows protein recommended intake for an ELBW infant at 800 g versus a larger

Table 8.1.   Enteral protein and energy requirements of preterm infants*

Body Weight, g	Protein, g/kg/day	Energy, kcal/kg/day	P/E, g/100 kcal
500–700	4.0	105	3.8
700–900	4.0	108	3.7
900–1200	4.0	119	3.4
1200–1500	3.9	127	3.1
1500–1800	3.6	128	2.8
1800–2200	3.4	131	2.6

*Adapted from Ref. 5.
P/E = Ratio of protein to energy, expressed as grams of protein per 100 kcal.

Table 8.2.   Recommended protein intakes for premature infants*

	Weight 800 g		Weight 1600 g	
	g/kg/day	g/100 kcal	g/kg/day	g/100 kcal
Ziegler[5]	4.0	3.7	3.6	2.8
Kashyap and Heird[6]	—	—	3.0	2.5
Denne[7]	3.5–4.0	—	3.0	—
Klein[8]	3.4–4.3	2.5–3.6	3.4–4.3	2.5–3.6
Rigo[9]	3.8–4.2	3.3	3.4–3.6	2.8

*At energy intake of 120 kcal/kg/day. Modified from Ref. 4.

preterm infant at 1600 g. As shown, protein requirements decrease with increasing body size. Finally, Table 8.3 offers a composite of recommended enteral protein intakes from a number of expert organizations and the factorial method.

8.2.2 *Early postnatal intravenous amino acid administration*

Immaturity of the gastrointestinal tract in these ELBW infants precludes substantive nutritional support from enteral nutrition, thus nearly all of these infants are supported with parenteral nutrition (PN). From a nutritional point of view, the liberal use of PN has been a huge success particularly in the ELBW infant.

Until recently, the initiation of PN has been delayed by a number of days. Reasons for this delay have not been clear but, probably have been related to ELBW infants' ability to catabolize amino acids and, in general concerns about tolerance during the first days of life in critically ill infants.[13] This reluctance is often based on the report of azotemia, hyperammonemia, and metabolic acidosis seen in infants who received the early protein hydrolysate solutions.[14] Elevated blood urea nitrogen (BUN) concentrations are often cited as the predominant reason for limiting amino acid intake.

An understanding of fetal nutrition may be helpful in designing postnatal strategies in ELBW infants. Extending this data to clinical application, we know that at 70% of gestation there is little fetal lipid uptake. Fetal energy metabolism is not dependent on fat until early in the third trimester

Table 8.3. Recommended enteral protein intakes for VLBW infants*

Recommendation	g/kg/day
Ziegler *et al.*, 2007[5]	4.0
Life Science Research Office, 2002[10]	3.4–4.3
AAP Committee on Nutrition, 2004[11]	3.5–4.0
Canadian Paediatric Society, 1995[12]	
Birth Weight < 1000 g	3.5–4.0
Birth Weight ≥ 1000 g	3.0–3.6

*Adapted from Ref. 22.

and then it increases only gradually toward term. Glucose is delivered to the fetus from the mother at low fetal insulin concentrations, generally at a rate that matches fetal energy expenditure. The human placenta actively transports amino acids into the fetus and animal studies indicate that fetal amino acid uptake greatly exceeds protein accretion requirements. Approximately 50% of the amino acids taken up by the fetus are oxidized and serve as a significant energy source. Urea production is a byproduct of amino acid oxidation. Relatively high rates of fetal urea production are seen in human and animal fetuses as compared with the term neonate and adult, suggesting high protein turnover and oxidation rates in the fetus. Therefore, a rise in BUN which is often observed after the start of PN is not an adverse effect or sign of toxicity. Rather, an increase in urea nitrogen is a normal accompaniment of metabolizing amino acids.

Studies comparing high versus low intakes of amino acids in the first several days after birth have further diminished most of the safety concerns.[15,16] Evidence is building for the importance of this strategy to decrease catabolism, increase growth, head circumference and even neurodevelopment with higher amino acid intakes.[17]

A strong argument for the early aggressive use of amino acids is the prevention of metabolic shock. Concentrations of some key amino acids begin to decline in the VLBW infant at the time the cord is cut. This metabolic shock may trigger the starvation response, of which endogenous glucose production is a prominent feature. Irrepressibly, glucose production may be the cause of the so-called glucose intolerance that often limits the amount of energy that can be administered to the ELBW infant. It makes sense to ease the metabolic transition from fetal to extrauterine life. Withholding PN for days, or even for hours, sends the infant unnecessarily into a metabolic emergency. Thus, the need for PN may never be more acute than right after birth. It is noteworthy that Rivera *et al.*[18] made the surreptitious observation that glucose tolerance was substantially improved in the group receiving early amino acids. Early amino acids may stimulate insulin secretion. This is consistent with the notion that forestalling the starvation response improves glucose tolerance.

Finally, without initiation of early parenteral amino acids, plasma concentrations of certain amino acids (e.g. arginine and leucine) decrease. Secretion of insulin depends on the plasma concentrations of these amino acids as well as that of glucose. A shortage of amino acids limits glucose transport and energy metabolism via a reduction in insulin and insulin-like growth factors. This scenario leads to a downregulation of glucose transporters at the cellular membrane level, resulting in intracellular energy failure via a decrease in Na^+, K^+ ATPase activity. This directly contributes to leakage of intracellular potassium and is associated with nonoliguric hyperkalemia.[19] Early PN with amino acids minimizes the abrupt postnatal deprivation of amino acid supply and meets the following goals:

- prevention of protein catabolism,
- prevention of a decrease in growth-regulating factors such as insulin and downregulation of glucose transporters,
- prevention of hyperglycemia and hyperkalemia.

From a practical standpoint, this strategy should be associated with less extreme postnatal weight loss and an earlier return to birthweight. An earlier return to birthweight means the VLBW infant will be less likely to develop extrauterine growth restriction.

We recently published eight years of experience promoting and developing an early amino acid strategy paying particular attention to clinical and metabolic responses.[20] Table 8.4 shows the benefits of early amino acids which include a decrease in postnatal weight loss and age at return to birthweight especially with earlier initiation of amino acids by hour of age and higher dosage over the first five days of life at 3.0 g/kg/day.[20] The same relationship for decreasing the prevalence of EUGR by weight was seen with higher dose and earlier initiation.[20]

We also confirmed that there is no demonstrable relationship between the preceding days amino acid intake and BUN.[20] This is because BUN is not only related to amino acid intake but also renal function, hydration and acuity of illness as well as degree of prematurity.[20] Therefore, in most situations a modest rise in BUN (a major earlier concern) is consistent with the utilization of amino acids as a source of energy.[21]

Early intravenous amino acids improved energy intakes while at the same time allowing for more conservative fluid management, which may benefit ELBW infants in prevention of chronic lung disease.[20] Our data suggests that higher insulin activity accompanies increased amino acid

Table 8.4. Outcome data (mean ± s.d.)*

	Epoch 1 2000–2001	Epoch 2 2002–2004	Epoch 3 2006–2007	P
Age at TPNi	22.4 ± 22.3	9.5 ± 12.2	4.6 ± 6.3	< 0.001 (a)
Days of TPN	25.8 ± 12.4	31.5 ± 26.9	25.2 ± 21.3	NS
Age at weight nadir	4.9 ± 3.4	4.4 ± 6.2	2.9 ± 3.2	0.044 (b)
Return to BW	13.9 ± 6.3	10.7 ± 5.7	8.3 ± 5.0	≤ 0.001 (b,c)
Sepsis	27%	36%	10%	0.032 (d)
Cholestasis	11%	26%	5%	0.030 (c)
Max dBR	1.1 ± 1.6	2.7 ± 4.3	1.3 ± 3.2	0.002 (c)
Survival (%)	90%	90%	95%	NS
LOS	83.3 ± 24.9	105.2 ± 55.5	83.4 ± 28.8	0.003 (c)
GA at d/c	38.3 ± 2.7	40.9 ± 7.4	38.1 ± 3.4	0.008 (c)
Weight at d/c	2168 ± 436	2799 ± 966	2541 ± 573	< 0.001 (c)
HC at d/c	32.4 ± 2.2	33.9 ± 2.9	32.1 ± 3.5	< 0.015 (c,d)
EUGRw at d/c (e)	57.1%	34.7%	25.0%	0.005 (c)
EUGRhc at d/c (e)	10.0%	6.1%	10.0%	NS

*Adapted from Ref. 20.

Abbreviations: BW, birth weight; dBR, direct bilirubin; d/c, discharge; EUGR, extrauterine growth restriction (< 3rd percentile for GA); EUGRhc, HC < 3rd percentile for GA; EUGRw, weight < 3rd percentile for GA; GA, gestational age; LOS, length of stay; Max, maximum; NS, not significant; TPN, total parental nutrition; TPNi, TPN initiation.

(a) = All epochs, (b) = Epoch 1 versus 3, (c) = Epoch 1 versus 2, (d) = Epoch 2 versus 3, (e) = EUGR: weight or HC, < 3rd percentile for GA.

dosage. Thureen *et al.*[15] showed higher insulin concentrations in infants receiving amino acids at 3 g/kg/day compared to those receiving 1 g/kg/day. (Therefore this demonstrated improved glucose tolerance with higher amino acid intake.) The higher insulin concentrations are also associated with the avoidance of nonoliguric hyperkalemia, thus another good reason to start amino acids shortly after birth in ELBW infants.

8.2.3 *It is the Protein — Enteral*

The growth limiting nutrient for VLBW infants is almost always protein, whereas energy seldom limits growth as long as intakes of energy are at least 90 kcal/kg/day to 100 kcal/kg/day.[5] The ELBW nutritional challenge is the linkage between inadequate nutrition, postnatal growth failure and ultimately impaired neurocognitive development. Ziegler estimates inadequate protein intake being responsible for about 80% of the inadequate intakes.[22] Therefore despite caloric requirements being met enterally and all other nutrient needs are adequate, those of protein may still be inadequate.

Rigo and Sentere recently reviewed protein requirements and suggest the following:[23]

(1) Fetal lean body mass gain and the contribution of protein gain to lean body mass (LBM) gain appear a more suitable reference than does weight gain.
(2) An additional protein supply needs to be provided for early catch-up growth, compensating for the cumulative protein deficit developed during the first weeks of life.
(3) An increase in the protein-energy ratio is mandatory to improve LBM accretion and limit fat deposition (Fig. 8.1).
(4) Recommended dietary protein allowance needs to be adapted for postconceptional age instead of gestational age or birthweight to integrate the dynamic aspect of growth and protein metabolism.[23]

Tables 8.5 and 8.6 are adapted from Rigo and Sentere to illustrate these important protein recommendations. Many of the recommendations from Table 8.2 are based on healthy premature infants and designed to provide stable growing period equivalent to intrauterine growth. The cumulative nutritional period of deficit is not considered nor the need to obtain an early catch-up growth as they are with these revised recommendations.[23]

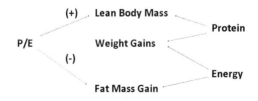

To increase LBM accretion and limit fat mass deposition, an
increase in P/E is mandatory.

Fig. 8.1.   Impact of protein/energy ratio (P/E) on body compostion.[23]

Table 8.5.   Revised recommended protein intake for premature infants*

	Without Need for Catch-up Growth	With Need for Catch-up Growth
26–30 weeks PCA: 16–18 g/kg/d LBM	3.8–4.2 g/kg/d	4.4 g/kg/d
30–36 weeks PCA: 14–15 g/kg/d LBM	3.4–3.6 g/kg/d	3.6–4.0 g/kg/d
36–40 weeks PCA: 13 g/kg/d LBM	2.8–3.2 g/kg/d	3.0–3.4 g/kg/d

*Adapted from Ref. 23.
PCA, postconceptual age; LBM, lean body mass; PER, protein/energy ratio — gram of protein/100 cal.

Table 8.6.   Revised recommended protein intake and protein-energy ratio for premature infants requiring catch-up growth*

PCA	Protein (g/k/day)	P/E (g/100 cal)
26–30	4.4	3.3
30–36	3.6–4.0	3.0
36–40	3.0–3.4	2.6–2.8

*Adapted from Ref. 23.

Analysis of studies of preterm infants fed human milk, human milk fortifiers and a variety of preterm formulas[9] allows evaluation of the determinants of weight gain, nitrogen retention and fat mass deposition. Figure 8.1 shows these important relationships with the sentinel goal being to increase LBM and limit fat mass deposition in premature infants by increasing protein-energy ratio.[9]

Protein intake and protein energy ratio are the main determinants of lean body mass gain, in contrast to fat mass gain, which is positively related to energy intake and negatively to the protein energy ratio.[24] The only way to increase the lean body mass accretion and limit fat mass deposition in premature infants is to increase the protein to energy ratio.

A comparison of protein requirements from three references[5,10,11] shows that when fed at 120 cal/kg/day, the various enteral options that we utilize to feed our VLBW infants are not adequate in proteins. Feeding typically provides less protein than is required, at least until the infant reaches a weight of 1500 g.

Protein levels in preterm human milk vary according to days of lactation.[24] The protein content of human milk decreases over time with duration of lactation. Even with standard fortification (100 ml human milk with four packets of human milk fortifier adding 0.94 g of protein), the protein intake decreases significantly over time. This may affect growth particularly in ELBW infants.

Formulas for preterm infants provide either 3.0 or 3.3 g/100 kcal. The higher protein preterm formula more closely meets the protein requirement and protein energy ratio for the ELBW infant.

Feeding strategies that provide 4.0 g/kg/day of protein are shown on Table 8.7. Some of these are unconventional like adding additional powder to human milk or mixing human milk with caloric dense formula. All have their disadvantages, e.g. mixing with caloric dense formula where the majority of the mixture is formula. This may decrease the benefit of human milk. There is also a fortifier made from human milk to make a 24 kcal/ounce milk (Prolacta + 4). The benefits are a purely human system and the avoidance of powders that are not sterile. The comparison of the preterm formulas suggests the provision of excessive energy with the standard preterm formula versus the high protein to reach 4.0 g/kg/day. The higher protein preterm formula has an increased protein-energy ratio, thus providing more protein but without additional energy.

Table 8.7.   Feeding strategies that can provide 4.0 grams of protein per kilogram per day

When using human milk:
- Use additional powder fortifier
- Use fortified donor milk
- Mix with 30 kcal/oz preterm formula

When using preterm formula:

High-Protein Preterm Formula 24 kcal	Preterm Formula 24 kcal
150 mL/kg/day	180 mL/kg/day
120 kcal/kg/day	144 kcal/kg/day
Protein/energy ratio = 3.3	Protein/energy ratio = 3.0

8.3 Future Implications of Feeding Strategies

Increased visceral adiposity in adults is recognized as a marker for metabolic syndrome.[25] A fascinating study in preterm infants using magnetic resonance to identify fat content showed a mean excess of intra-abdominal fat in those infants who had required the greatest level and intensity of neonatal care, i.e. stress.[26] It contradicts the speculation that there was increased propensity to metabolic syndrome in infants who grew faster.[27,28] Therefore, early stress and not under-nutrition or catch-up growth leads to deposition of a major indicator of early metabolic syndrome, i.e. increased abdominal visceral fat.[29] Therefore, strategies that promote the accretion of LBM and decreasing visceral fat deposition appear to be important to promote healthy adults.

The best description of today's growth in ELBW infants is that of extrauterine growth restriction with head sparing and abnormal visceral adiposity. Relative visceral adiposity occurs even in under-nutrition and growth restriction because of early growth deceleration, cumulative nutritional deficits and altered body fat distribution in ELBW infants. Therefore, early postnatal relative under-nutrition to avoid catch-up growth would most likely compromise neurodevelopment without the benefit of preventing the development of metabolic X syndrome later in life.

References

1. Morley R. (1999) Early growth and later development. In: Ziegler EE, Lucas A, Moro G, (eds.) *Nutrition of the Very Low Birthweight Infant.* Philadelphia: Lippincott; 19–32.
2. Latal-Hajnal B, von Siebenthal K, Kovari H, *et al.* (2003) Postnatal growth in VLBW infants: significant association with neurodevelopmental outcome. *J Pediatr* 143: 163–170.
3. Ziegler EE, O'Donnell AM, Nelson SE, Fomon SJ. (1976) Body composition of the reference fetus. *Growth* 40: 329–341.
4. American Academy of Pediatrics Committee on Nutrition. (1985) Nutritional needs of low-birth-weight infants. *Pediatrics* 76: 976–986.
5. Ziegler E. (2007) Protein requirements of very low birth weight infants. *J. Pediatric Gastroenterology and Nutrition* 45: S170–S174.

6. Kashyap S, Heird WC. (1994) Protein requirements of low birthweight, very low birthweight and small for gestational age infants. In: Räihä, NCCR, ed. *Protein Metabolism During Infancy*. New York: Raven Press; 133–151.

7. Denne SC. (2001) Protein and energy requirements in preterm infants. *Semin Neonatol* 6: 377–382.

8. Klein CJ. (2002) Nutrient requirements for preterm infant formulas. *J Nutr* 132(Suppl 1): 1395S–577S.

9. Rigo J. (2005) Protein, amino acids, and other nitrogen compounds. In: Tsang RC, Uauy R, Koletzko B, *et al.*, eds. *Nutrition of the Preterm Infant*. 2nd ed. Cincinnati: Digital Educational Publishing; 45–80.

10. Klein CJ. (2002) Nutrient requirements for preterm infant formulas. *J Nutr* 132(Suppl 1): 1395S–1577S.

11. Kleinman RE, ed. (2004) *Pediatric Nutrition Handbook*. Elk Grove Village, IL, American Academy of Pediatrics; 23–54.

12. Canadian Paediatric Society, Nutrition Committee. (1995) *Can Med Assoc J* 152: 1765–1785.

13. Kleigman RM, Fanaroff AA. (1981) Neonatal necrotizing enterocolitis: a nine-year experience. *Am J Dis Child* 135: 603–607.

14. Johnson JD, Albritton WL, Sunshine P. (1972) Hyperammonemia accompanying parenteral nutrition in newborn infants. *J Pediatr* 81: 154–161.

15. Thureen PJ, Melara D, Fennessey PV, Hay WWJ. (2003) Effect of low versus high intravenous amino acid intake on very low birth weight infants in the early neonatal period. *Pediatr Res* 53: 24–32.

16. Ibrahim HM, Jeroudi MA, Baier RJ, Dhanireddy R, Krouskop RW. (2004) Aggressive early total parental nutrition in low-birth-weight infants. *J Perinatol* 24: 483–486.

17. Poindexter BB, Langer JC, Dusick AM, Ehrenkranz RA. (2006) Early provision of parenteral amino acids in extremely low birth weight infants: relation to growth and neurodevelopmental outcome. *J Pediatr* 148: 300.

18. Rivera A Jr, Bell EF, Bier DM. (1993) Effect of intravenous amino acids on protein metabolism of preterm infants during the first three days of life. *Pediatr Res* 33: 106–111.

19. Stefano JL, Norman ME, Morales MC, Goplerud JM, Mishra OP, Delivoria-Papadopoulos M. (1993) DeNa-K+- ATPase activity associated with cellular potassium loss in extremely-low-birth-weight infants with nonoliguric hyperkalemia. *J Pediatr* 122: 276–284.

20. Radmacher PG, Lewis SL, Adamkin DH. (2009) Early amino acids and the metabolic response of ELBW infants (≤1000 g) in three time periods. *J Perinatol* 29: 433–437.

21. Neu J, ed. (2009) Is it time to stop starving premature infants? *J. Perinatology* 29: 399–400.

22. Ziegler E, Adamkin D, Ehrenkranz R. (2009) *Nutritional Strategies to Improve Outcomes in Premature Infants.* Abbott Webinar, New York City, NY.

23. Rigo J, Senterre J. (2006) Nutritional needs of the premature infants: current issues. *J Pediatr* 149(Suppl 5): S80–S87.

24. Schanler RJ, Atkinson SA. In: Tsang RC, *et al.* eds. (2005) *Nutrition of the Preterm Infant.* 2nd ed. Digital Educational Publishing.

25. Goodpaster BH, Krishnaswami S, Harris TB, Katsiaras A, Kritchevsky SB, Simonsick EM, *et al.* (2005) Obesity, regional body fat distribution, and the metabolic syndrome in older men and women. *Arch Intern Med* 165(7): 777–783.

26. Utaya S, Thomas EL, Hamilton G, Dore CJ, Bell J, Modi N. (2005) Altered adiposity after extremely premature birth. *Ped Res* 57(2): 211–215.

27. Singhal A, Fewtrell M, Cole TJ, Lucas A. (2003) Low nutrient intake and early growth for later insulin resistance in adolescents born preterm. *Lancet* 361(9363): 1089–1097.

28. Singhal A, Cole TJ, Fewtrell M, Deanfield J, Lucas A. (2004) Is slower early growth beneficial for long-term cardiovascular health? *Circulation* 109(9): 1108–1113.

29. Neu J, Hauser N, Douglas-Escobar M. (2007) Postnatal nutrition and adult health programming. *Sem Fetal Neonat Med* 12(1): 78–86.

Chapter 9

Advances in Ventilatory Care of the Neonate

Rangasamy Ramanathan*

Nearly 13 million infants are born prematurely each year with more than 85% of the premature births occurring in the developing countries of Africa and Asia. Even though significant progress in neonatal-perinatal care has been achieved over the past three decades, more than one million premature infants die each year in their first month. Despite the improvement in perinatal care, preterm birth rate in the US has risen more than 30% over the past two decades from 9.4% in 1981 to 12.3% in 2003.[1,2] The annual cost of caring for preterm babies and their associated health problems tops $26 billion in the US alone.

Respiratory distress syndrome (RDS) is the leading cause of respiratory failure and is a major cause of mortality and morbidity in very low birth weight (VLBW, < 1500 g) infants. Respiratory distress requiring support is also a major reason in late preterm infants admitted to the neonatal intensive care unit. Incidence of RDS is inversely proportional to gestational age at birth. Pathophysiology of RDS is characterized by insufficient production of a surface active agent, namely, surfactant. This results in high surface tension at the air-liquid interphase in the alveoli, leading to alveolar collapse. Until surfactant replacement therapy was approved in 1990, the only available therapy for RDS was supportive care in the form of supplemental oxygen, continuous positive pressure and mechanical ventilation.

---

*Professor of Pediatrics, Keck School of Medicine, University of Southern California.

9.1 Historical Perspective

Mechanical ventilation of the neonate has its root in the 18th century. Creation of the first practical medical respirator by Forrest Bird freed patients from the confines of iron lungs. The 1955 release of "Bird Universal Medical Respirator" was a land mark event in the evolution of mechanical ventilation. This unit was sold as the Bird Mark 7 Respirator, which was a pneumatic device and therefore required no electrical power source to operate. In the early 1960s, researchers and pioneer physicians began to intubate babies using a Cole rubber tube and a Bird Mark VIII ventilator with the infant J circuit system at the Toronto Hospital for Sick Children. Initially it was fraught with severe complications. The first newborn survived without air leak or cerebral abnormalities, albeit with chronic lung disease in 1963. Continuous respiratory support was being provided in the mid-1960s for infants with severe respiratory disease. A group of investigators in several different centers began to adapt mechanical ventilators to assist ventilation of infants with RDS. Bronchopulmonary dysplasia, a form of chronic lung disease in mechanically ventilated infants, was first described by Northway and coworkers[3] in 1967. The introduction in 1970 of the "Baby Bird" respirator saved the lives of innumerable neonates with respiratory distress syndromes, stimulating the development of a new era in neonatology. The first generation of ventilators designed specifically for neonatal use (Baby Bird I® and Bournes BP 200®) introduced time-cycled, pressure-limited, continuous flow with intermittent mandatory ventilation. Outcome of ventilated infants was less than desired as reflected in the commentary by Dr. Behrman[4] in 1970: "Evidence is still not strong enough and the indications for treatment are not sharply enough defined to establish the effectiveness of assisted ventilation for all premature infants with severe hyaline membrane disease." By mid-1970s, survival of these infants had increased to nearly 70%.[5,6]

9.2 Basics of Mechanical Ventilation

Application of continuous positive airway pressure (CPAP) helps to stabilize the lung with surfactant deficiency or dysfunction, especially at the end of expiration when the surface tension is at its highest. Ever since Gregory *et al.*[7] introduced the concept of providing CPAP to stabilize the lung and maintain functional residual capacity, numerous advances have been made in mechanical ventilation. The ultimate goal of mechanical ventilation is to provide effective gas exchange and support infants with apnea of prematurity with back up breaths, while causing minimal side effects, such as barotrauma or volutrauma and bronchopulmonary dysplasia (BPD). This requires that the ventilator perform a number of functions, i.e. move heated and humidified gas into the gas exchange units, hold it there for the desired amount of time before allowing it to escape, allow unimpeded gas egress to a preset positive end-expiratory pressure (PEEP), provide the desired concentration of inspired oxygen, and provide continuous monitoring of ventilator functions that affect the patient-ventilator interaction. The most important part of a ventilator is the exhalation valve. Currently, exhalation valves are of two types: variable pressure-flow valves and threshold resistors. Variable pressure-flow valves provide a constant resistance to flow. The level of pressure within the system is equal to the product of gas flow through the valve and the resistance of the valve (pressure = flow × resistance). This type of valve mechanism results in higher expiratory work of breathing when an infant attempts to exhale into a fixed-resistance expiratory valve. By controlling the resistance applied to this valve, one can set the peak inspiratory pressure (PIP) and PEEP. In contrast, threshold resistors provide a constant level of pressure within the system, independent of flow. This is accomplished by submerging the expiratory tube within a fluid column. The amount of pressure generated is simply determined by the depth of submersion. Since pressure is independent of flow, these systems are generally considered to be more stable, and are used to provide CPAP. In addition, oscillations produced by the exhaled gas bubbling through the fluid column appear to have a beneficial effect on ventilation.

Introduction of continuous gas flow respirators allowed for spontaneous breathing of newborn infants along with intermittent mandatory ventilation (IMV). During mechanical ventilation, triggering refers to how a mechanical breath is initiated, cycling refers to how a breath is terminated and limit refers to the variable that is limited or controlled by the operator. By setting the inspiratory time, time-cycled, pressure-limited IMV breath is provided, which is the most common mode used in newborn infants. Limiting variable can be pressure or volume. Pressure limited mode is more often used than volume limited ventilator mode in newborn infants, because of leaks around an uncuffed endotracheal tube. Furthermore, decelerating flow pattern generated during pressure limited ventilation results in less turbulence as compared to constant flow generated during volume limited ventilation. One of the issues with IMV mode is asynchrony between the ventilator and the patient breathing.[8] With the advent of microprocessor based technology, further refinements have been made in the provision of mechanical ventilatory support to neonates with respiratory failure. To minimize asynchrony between the ventilator and patient effort, modern ventilators offer patient triggered ventilation (PTV) or synchronized IMV (SIMV).[9] Continuous measurement of changes in flow or pressure at the patient interphase also made it feasible to synchronize patient efforts with the mechanically delivered breaths as well as providing pressure support (PS) to all spontaneous breath efforts. Addition of PS to spontaneous breaths decreases the work of breathing imposed by the high resistance of the endotracheal tube. There are several types of PTV available for clinical use: (1) SIMV, (2) assist-control (A/C) ventilation, (3) nasal or nasopharyngeal IMV/SIMV, (4) pressure support ventilation (PSV), (5) volume support (VS) ventilation, (6) volume targeted ventilation, (7) proportional assist ventilation (PAV), (8) mandatory minute ventilation (MMV), and (9) airway pressure release ventilation (APRV). Of these modes, SIMV, A/C and PSV modes have been studied more extensively than other modes in newborns.

During PTV, each inspiratory effort that exceeds the trigger threshold results in delivery of a mechanical breath, resulting in a more consistent delivery of tidal volume (Vt). During SIMV, each inspiratory effort that exceeds the trigger threshold during a "time window" results in a mechanical breath, resulting in larger Vt with mechanical breaths than with spontaneous breaths. SIMV provides a preset number of mechanical breaths as in IMV, but these are synchronized with the infant's spontaneous respiratory effort. However, spontaneous breaths in excess of the preset number are not supported, resulting in uneven tidal volumes. In A/C, every spontaneous breath effort that exceeds the trigger threshold is supported by the ventilator, providing more consistent tidal volume delivery. Consistent delivery of Vt, more rapid weaning from mechanical ventilation, and smaller fluctuations in blood pressure have been documented with A/C, as compared to SIMV. Pressure support ventilation is a patient-triggered, pressure-limited, flow-cycled mode of ventilation. Inspiratory "pressure support or boost" is provided to overcome the resistance of the endotracheal tube during spontaneous breath effort. Pressure support level above CPAP level is set by the clinician, and flow termination is set at 10% of peak flow. PS level is set at 30% to 50% of the delta pressure (PIP-PEEP). Typically, it is not necessary to wean the PS level, unless PS breath delivers Vt that is larger than the spontaneous tidal volume generated by the patient.

Studies evaluating PTV or SIMV have shown improvement in gas exchange, consistent delivery of Vt, decreased fluctuations in blood pressure and cerebral blood flow velocity, decrease in IVH, decreased need for sedation and paralysis, and fewer days on oxygen and mechanical ventilation.[10–17] None of these studies demonstrated a significant benefit in terms of reducing BPD. However, PTV is more "physiological", and therefore, should be used whenever feasible. Furthermore, by terminating the flow at certain value of the peak inspiratory flow, for example, flow cycling a breath at 10% of peak inspiratory flow delivered by the ventilator, both inspiratory and expiratory synchrony can be achieved. Incorporation of devices to measure flow and pressure at the endotracheal tube, such as hotwire anemometers and pneumotachometers made it possible to monitor breath to breath changes in lung mechanics in real-time at the bedside, thus, providing the clinician another dimension in the ventilatory care of neonates. Efficacy and feasibility of a newly developed mode of mechanical ventilation, namely, neurally adjusted ventilatory assist, commonly known as NAVA, is being evaluated in preterm infants.

During NAVA, the timing and magnitude of pressure delivered are controlled by the infants' diaphragmatic electrical activity (EAdi), a validated measurement of neural respiratory drive. Clinical trials in adults and term infants have shown that NAVA is more synchronous than conventional pressure support ventilation, and that NAVA delivers lower mean airway pressures to achieve the same ventilation and respiratory muscle unloading. NAVA has recently been approved for use in neonates by Health Canada and the FDA in the US. Principles of noninvasive nasal ventilation are similar to that of endotracheal tube ventilation, except for the use of nasal prongs to deliver the flow of inspired gases.

9.3 Tidal versus Non-tidal Ventilation via the Endotracheal Tube

Both tidal volume ventilation using conventional mechanical ventilators and non-tidal ventilation using high frequency ventilators (HFV) have been extensively evaluated in neonates requiring ventilatory support. High frequency ventilators deliver smaller tidal volumes at supraphysiogical respiratory frequencies. With the use of tidal volumes that are near to or less than dead space volumes, pressure excursions around mean pressure are kept minimal, and lung over distention can be avoided. HFV also allows maintenance of optimal lung volume in the desired range, while avoiding cyclical collapse and reexapnsion of terminal lung units. Three basic HFV modes that are available include high frequency oscillatory ventilation (HFOV), high frequency flow interruption (HIFI), and high frequency jet ventilation (HFJV). With both HFJV and HIFI, inspiration is active, and expiration is a passive process dependent on the recoil properties of the lung and chest wall. In contrast, during the expiratory phase of HFOV, a negative pressure is created at the airway, producing a pressure gradient that enhances gas egress. The time available for expiration is limited during HFV, thus gas trapping is a potential problem with HFJ and HIFI modes. The presence of active expiration phase with HFOV allows the safe use of higher frequencies with this technique. Non-tidal ventilation using HFOV, HIFI and HFJV have all been studied in the management of RDS before and after surfactant therapy became available and have been compared with IMV as well as SIMV modes (Table 9.1).[18] Among the six trials published during the pre-surfactant era, Clark *et al.*[19] reported a decrease in BPD with HFOV when compared to IMV. However, the incidence of severe intraventricular hemorrhage (IVH) or periventricular leukomalacia (PVL) was significantly higher in one of the HIFI trials published in 1989.[20] Three trials[21–23] were published after surfactants became available for treatment of RDS. Two of these studies[21,22] reported lower BPD incidence among infants randomized to HFV when compared to IMV, while the third study[23] had to be terminated because of an increase in IVH and or PVL among infants randomized to HFJV. Among the eight HFV trials[24–31] published between 1998 and 2003, when surfactant therapy and SIMV were commonly used, only two studies reported a decrease in BPD[24,25] with HFOV mode, and two studies[26,27]

Table 9.1. High frequency ventilation versus conventional ventilation studies from 1989 to 2003 in preterm infants and bronchopulmonary dysplasia[#]

	Number	Study population	Results
Pre-surfantant Era Trials (n = 6)			
HIFI, 1989	673	750–200 g	HFOV: no change in BPD; increase in IVH/PVL
Carlo, 1990	42	1000–2000 g	HFJV: no change in BPD
Keszler, 1991	144	≥ 750 g with PIE	HFJV: improved survival
Clark, 1992	83	≤ 1750 g	HFOV: decrease in BPD
HiFO, 1993	176	≥ 500 g	No change in BPD
Ogawa, 1993	92	750–2000 g	HFOV: no change in BPD
Surfactant Era Trials (n = 3)			
Gerstmann, 1996	125	≤ 35 weeks	HFOV: decrease in BPD and surfactant use
Wiswell, 1996	73	> 500 g; < 33 weeks	HFJV: no change in BPD; increase in severe IVH/PVL; trial stopped early
Keszler, 1997	130	700–1500 g; ≤ 35 weeks	HFJV: decrease in BPD
Surfactant and SIMV Era Trials (n = 8)			
Rettwitz-Volk, 1998	96	< 32 weeks	HFOV: no change in BPD
Plavka, 1999	43	500–1500 g	HFOV: decrease in BPD
Thome, 1999	284	24–30 weeks	HIFI: no change in BPD; increase in air leaks
Moriette, 2001	273	24–29 weeks	HFOV: no change in BPD
Courtney, 2002	498	601–1200 g	HFOV: decrease in BPD
Johnson, 2002	797	23–28 weeks	HFOV: no change in BPD
Craft, 2003	46	< 1000 g	HIFI: no change in BPD; increase in air leaks
Van Reempts, 2003	300	< 32 weeks	HFOV/HIFI: no change in BPD

[#] Adapted from Ref. 18; HIFI = high frequency flow interruption; HFOV = high frequency oscillatory ventilation; HFJV = high frequency jet ventilation; SIMV = synchronized intermittent mandatory ventilation; IVH = intraventricular hemorrhage; PVL = periventricular leukomalacia.

reported an increase in air leaks with HIFI mode. Three large trials compared elective use of HFV in the management of RDS. One study[25] reported a decrease in BPD, and a second study[28] reported a nonsignificant increase in IVH among infants treated with HFOV with no pulmonary benefit. Third trial showed no difference in pulmonary or central nervous system outcomes.[29] Differences in outcomes between HFV and IMV trials are primarily related to whether a lung protective ventilatory strategy was employed or not in both of these modes of ventilation. In the cumulative meta-analysis studies where optimal lung volume strategy was used were compared, there were no differences in pulmonary or non-pulmonary outcomes between HFV and IMV modes.[30]

9.4 Noninvasive Ventilation

9.4.1 *Nasal continuous positive airway pressure*

Since the duration of mechanical ventilation via the endotracheal tube has a direct correlation with BPD, clinicians are increasingly using noninvasive ventilation with nasal continuous positive airway pressure (NCPAP) or nasal intermittent positive pressure ventilation (NIPPV) to protect the preterm infant's lungs.[31] Noninvasive ventilation appears to be beneficial in the management of apnea of prematurity, for prevention of extubation failures, as well as in the initial management of RDS.[32–34] NCPAP has been used as a primary mode for RDS treatment, to prevent extubation failures, or extubation following surfactant administration. NCPAP can be delivered using conventional mechanical ventilators, bubble CPAP, or infant flow driver systems. Bubble CPAP is accomplished by submerging the expiratory limb of respiratory circuit within a fluid column. The amount of pressure maintained within the system is determined by the depth of submersion, and is generally independent of flow rate. Infant flow driver uses fluidic flip system which has been shown to assist spontaneous breathing and reduce work of breathing by reducing expiratory resistance and maintaining a stable airway pressure throughout the respiratory cycle.[35] NCPAP patient interfaces commonly used include single or binasal prongs and nasopharyngeal prongs. In some centers, nasal mask or high flow (> 2 LPM) nasal cannula are used to deliver CPAP. Binasal prongs are more effective than single prongs in preventing extubation failures. Extubation failures were significantly lower even among extremely low birth weight infants when binasal prongs were used (24% versus 88%).[36] It has been a routine practice in many centers to intubate extremely low birth weight (ELBW, < 1000 g) infants at birth.

Lindner *et al.*[37] in a retrospective, cohort study showed that adopting a policy of selective intubation in ELBW infants resulted in a significantly reduced need for intubation, lower incidence of BPD, IVH and reduced length of stay. Success rate with NCPAP use from the delivery room to avoid subsequent endotracheal intubation is still low in the USA. In a multicenter, randomized study, 80% of ELBW infants required intubation by seven days of age.[38] Observational studies using bubble NCPAP have shown a decrease in the BPD. In a prospective observational study, Meyer *et al.*[39] demonstrated that use of bubble CPAP in ELBW infants was associated with significantly improved survival without BPD. Sahni *et al.*[40] reported a very low incidence of BPD (7.4%) in infants < 1250 g who are at the highest risk for BPD, managed with bubble NCPAP. Lee *et al.*[41] reported 2–4 cm H_2O amplitude at a frequency of 15–30 Hz when bubble CPAP was used. The frequencies recorded by them are close to the resonant frequency of the lungs, where gas movement in and out of lungs is independent of lung compliance. This may account for improved ventilation despite smaller tidal volumes in infants on bubble CPAP compared to conventional NCPAP. However, Morley *et al.*[42] showed that bubbling rates during bubble CPAP had no effect on ventilation or oxygenation. In preterm lambs, lung volumes were higher with bubble CPAP as compared to conventional CPAP.[43] Furthermore, bubble CPAP use in preterm lambs was associated with a significant decrease in neutrophil recruitment into the lungs and the cells in alveolar wash had less H_2O_2.[43] Bubble CPAP system produces noisy pressure waveforms superimposed on pressure fluctuations, resulting in stochastic resonance. This results in improved lung recruitment in a poorly compliant lung and may also augment the efficiency of gas exchange.[44] Limited number of studies compared NCPAP delivered using conventional mechanical ventilators and infant flow drivers. Stefanescu *et al.*[45] found no difference in clinical outcomes when applying CPAP with the infant flow driver versus a conventional nasal CPAP device. Mechanical ventilation via the ET tube even for less than 48 hours is associated with a longer length of stay.[46] Success with CPAP depended on the experience of the staff and gestational age of infants, especially infants < 29 weeks.[46] Sandri *et al.*[47] A multicenter trial demonstrated no difference in BPD in infants between 28 and 31 weeks gestational age treated with prophylactic or rescue NCPAP. A major limitation of NCPAP is the need for intubation due to frequent apnea, bradycardia or desaturation in preterm infants. Approximately 30% to 40% of infants extubated from mechanical ventilation to NCPAP fail extubation, requiring reintubation. At present, there are no good tests to predict successful extubation in preterm infants. Kamlin *et al.*[48] used spontaneous breathing test (SBT) to predict successful extubation in preterm infants with a birth weight < 1250 g. A failed SBT was recorded if the infant had either bradycardia lasting for longer than 15 seconds and/or a drop in saturation below 85% despite a 15% increase in FiO_2 when infants were on CPAP via endotracheal tube (ET CPAP) prior to a planned extubation. No pressure support for spontaneous breaths was given during ET CPAP in this study. Sensitivity and specificity for SBT in predicting successful extubation were 97% and 73% respectively. Further studies are needed to evaluate if SBT may be used as a predictor of infant's readiness prior to extubation.

Nasal cannulae have been used to deliver oxygen at flow rates of 0.5 liters per minute (LPM) to as high as 6 LPM flow, usually with no intention of delivering CPAP. However, a significant amount of CPAP is generated, and is not measured continuously at the bedside. For example, use of flow rates of 2 LPM via a nasal cannula with an outer diameter of 3 mm results in a mean CPAP of 9.8 cm H_2O.[49] Complications reported with the use of high flow nasal cannula included increased incidence of air leaks, gas trapping, and volutrauma. One must exercise caution when delivering flow rates greater than 2 LPM via nasal cannula without knowing the amount of pressure delivered. Techniques to measure pressure delivered at the level of nasal interface is urgently needed, since nasal cannula to deliver CPAP intentionally or not has become very common in the US. Use of portable devices, such as Neopuff™ Infant Resuscitator (Fisher & Paykel Healthcare Corporation Limited, Irvine, CA) to deliver consistent positive end-expiratory pressure in the delivery room and during transport from the delivery room, is gaining popularity.[50]

9.4.2 *Nasal intermittent positive pressure ventilation*

NIPPV is an alternative option when infants are extubated from mechanical ventilation or for infants failing NCPAP. NIPPV is a form of noninvasive ventilation that combines NCPAP with IPPV breaths. NIPPV may augment NCPAP, prevent post-extubation failures, minimize SIMV duration, and potentially decrease BPD. NIPPV has been shown to decrease post-extubation failures significantly compared to NCPAP. Two randomized studies using synchronized NIPPV at the time of extubation showed significant reduction in extubation failures with NIPPV as compared to NCPAP.[33,51] In a retrospective study, Kulkarni *et al.*[52] showed that after introduction of NIPPV in their unit following a two-week education to their staff, there was a significant reduction in BPD. Recently, studies comparing NIPPV versus SIMV have shown promising results. Kugelman *et al.*[53] compared NCPAP with NIPPV as a primary mode of respiratory support in preterm infants < 35 weeks gestational age with RDS. NIPPV was more successful than NCPAP in decreasing the need for endotracheal intubation, and in the incidence of BPD. These authors did not report any adverse effects of NIPPV. This was the first study on using NIPPV as a primary mode for RDS treatment. However, study infants were larger and more mature. Only 40 of the 84 infants studied were VLBW (< 1500 g) infants. Ramanathan *et al.*[54] in a multicenter trial compared SIMV versus NIPPV in preterm infants requiring intubation and surfactant therapy at birth and showed that NIPPV mode was associated with a significant decrease in the need for mechanical ventilation at seven days of age and a reduction in BPD.

9.4.3 *Sustained inflation followed by CPAP*

Lung over distention even with one or two large inflations during resuscitation of ELBW infants immediately after birth initiates lung injury, eventually leading to BPD. Recently, te Pas *et al.*[55] reported results from a randomized, controlled trial of sustained inflation in the delivery room respiratory management of VLBW infants. These authors compared sustained inflation for 10 seconds at 20 cm H_2O applied via a nasopharyngeal tube followed by NCPAP versus manual inflations with a self-inflating bag and mask followed by NCPAP in 207 preterm infants. They showed that need for intubation, days on mechanical ventilation, days on NCPAP, air leaks, and moderate to severe BPD were significantly lower when a sustained inflation was used to recruit the lung instead of bag and mask ventilation.

Surfactant therapy and mechanical ventilation using conventional or high frequency ventilation have been the standard of care in the management neonates with RDS. Bronchopulmonary dysplasia continues to remain as a major morbidity in very low birth weight infants despite these treatments. BPD is associated with short- and long-term adverse pulmonary and non-pulmonary outcomes. Lung injury is directly related to the duration of invasive ventilation via the endotracheal tube. When an optimal lung volume strategy is employed, there does not appear to be any significant difference in pulmonary outcome between conventional and high frequency ventilation. Studies using noninvasive ventilation, such as nasal continuous positive airway pressure and nasal intermittent positive pressure ventilation have shown to decrease post-extubation failures, and a significant decrease in BPD. However, there are no guidelines for the use of noninvasive ventilation in preterm infants. More studies are needed before noninvasive ventilation becomes a routine lung protective strategy.

Short binasal prongs are more effective than single nasal prongs to deliver NCPAP. Use of caffeine has also been shown to be independently associated with a lower rate of BPD. Lung protective ventilatory strategy may involve noninvasive ventilation as a primary therapy or following surfactant administration in very preterm infants with respiratory distress syndrome. Initial steps in the management of preterm baby at risk for BPD may also include sustained inflation to establish functional residual capacity, followed by noninvasive ventilation and caffeine treatment to minimize lung injury and subsequent development of bronchopulmonary dysplasia.

References

1. Mathews TJ, Menacker F, MacDorman MF. (2004) Infant mortality statistics from the 2002 period: linked birth/infant death data set. *Natl Vital Stat Rep* 53: 1–29.

2. Davidoff MJ, Dias T, Damus K, Russell R, Bettegowda VR, Dolan S, *et al.* (2006) Changes in the gestational age distribution among US singleton

births: impact on rates of late preterm birth, 1992 to 2002. *Semin Perinatol* 30: 8–15.

3. Northway WH Jr, Rosan RC, Porter DY. (1967) Pulmonary disease following respiratory therapy of hyaline-membrane disease. Bronchopulmonary dysplasia. *N Engl J Med* 276: 357–368.

4. Behrman RE. (1970) Commentary: the use of assisted ventilation in the therapy of hyaline membrane disease. *J Pediatr* 76: 169–173.

5. Jones MD Jr, Murton LJ. (1977) Mechanical ventilation in newborn infants with hyaline membrane disease. *Pediatr Ann* 6: 253–261.

6. Schreiner RL, Kisling JA, Evans GM, Phillips S, Lemons JA, Gresham EL. (1980) Improved survival of ventilated neonates with modern intensive care. *Pediatrics* 66: 985–987.

7. Gregory GA, Kitterman JA, Phibbs RH, *et al.* (1971) Treatment of the idiopathic respiratory-distress syndrome with continuous positive airway pressure. *N Engl J Med* 284: 1333–1340.

8. Jarreau PH, Moriette C, Mussat P, *et al.* (1996) Patient-triggered ventilation decreases the work of breathing in neonates. *Am J Respir Crit Care Med* 153: 1176–1181.

9. Sinha SK, Donn SM. (2000) Advances in neonatal conventional ventilation. *Arch Dis Child Fetal Neonatal Ed* 75: F135–F140.

10. Hummler H, Gerhardt T, Gonzalez A, Claure N, Everett R, Bancalari E. (1996) Influence of different methods of synchronized mechanical ventilation on ventilation, gas exchange, patient effort, and blood pressure fluctuations in premature neonates. *Pediatr Pulmonol* 22: 305–313.

11. Chen JY, Ling UP, Chen JH. (1997) Comparison of synchronized and conventional intermittent mandatory ventilation in neonates. *Acta Paediatr Jpn* 39(5): 578–583.

12. Greenough A. (2001) Update on patient-triggered ventilation: clinics in perinatology. *Clin Perinatol* 28(3): 533–546.

13. Servant GM, Nicks JJ, Donn SM, Bandy KP, Lathrop C, Dechert RE. (1992) Feasibility of applying flow-synchronized ventilation to very low birth-weight infants. *Respir Care* 37: 249–253.

14. Donn SM, Nicks JJ, Becker MA. (1994) Flow-synchronized ventilation of preterm infants with respiratory distress syndrome. *J Perinatol* 14: 90–94.

15. Baumer JH. (2000) International randomized controlled trial of patient triggered ventilation in neonatal respiratory distress syndrome. *Arch Dis Child Fetal Neonatal Ed* 82: F5–F10.

16. Beresford MW, Shaw NJ, Manning D. (2000) Randomized controlled trial of patient triggered and fast rate ventilation in neonatal respiratory distress syndrome. *Arch Dis Child Fetal Neonatal Ed* 82: F14–F18.

17. Bernstein G, Mannino FL, Heldt GP, *et al.* (1996) Randomized multicenter trial comparing synchronized and conventional intermittent mandatory ventilation in neonates. *J Pediatr* 128: 453–463.

18. Keszler M. (2006) High-frequency ventilation: evidence-based practice and special clinical indications. *NeoReviews* 7: e234–249.

19. Clark RH, Gerstmann DR, Null DM, deLemos RA. (1992) Prospective randomized comparison of high frequency oscillatory and conventional ventilation in respiratory distress syndrome. *Pediatrics* 89: 5–12.

20. The HIFI Study Group. (1989) High-frequency oscillatory ventilation compared with conventional ventilation in the treatment of respiratory failure in preterm infants. *N Engl J Med* 320: 88–93.

21. Gerstmann DR, Minton SD, Stoddard RA, *et al.* (1996) The Provo multicenter early high frequency oscillatory ventilation trial: improved pulmonary and clinical outcome in respiratory distress syndrome. *Pediatrics* 98: 1044–1057.

22. Keszler M, Modanlou HD, Brudno DS, *et al.* (1997) Multicenter controlled clinical trial of high frequency jet ventilation in preterm infants with uncomplicated respiratory distress syndrome. *Pediatrics* 100: 593–599.

23. Wiswell TE, Graziani LJ, Kornhauser MS, *et al.* (1996) High-frequency jet ventilation in the early management of respiratory distress syndrome is associated with a greater risk for adverse outcomes. *Pediatrics* 98: 1035–1043.

24. Plavka R, Kopecky P, Sebron V, Svihovec P, Zlatohlavkova B, Janus V. (1999) A prospective randomized comparison of conventional mechanical ventilation and very early high frequency oscillatory ventilation in extremely premature newborns with respiratory distress syndrome. *Intensive Care Med* 25: 68–75.

25. Courtney SE, Durand DJ, Asselin JM, Hudak ML, Aschner JL, Shoemaker CT and The Neonatal Ventilation Study Group. (2002) High-frequency oscillatory ventilation versus conventional mechanical ventilation for very low birth weight infants. *N Engl J Med* 347: 643–652.

26. Thome U, Kossel H, Lipowsky G, *et al.* (1999) Randomized comparison of high-frequency ventilation with high-rate intermittent positive pressure ventilation in preterm infants with respiratory failure. *J Pediatr* 135: 39–46.

27. Craft AP, Bhandari V, Finer NN. (2003) The sy-fi study: a randomized prospective trial of synchronized intermittent mandatory ventilation versus a

high-frequency flow interrupter in infants less than 1000 g. *J Perinatol* 23: 14–19.

28. Moriette G, Paris-Llado J, Walti H, *et al.* (2001) Prospective randomized multicenter comparison of high-frequency oscillatory ventilation and conventional ventilation in preterm infants of less than 30 weeks with respiratory distress syndrome. *Pediatrics* 107: 363–372.

29. Johnson AH, Peacock JL, Greenough A, *et al.* (2002) High-frequency oscillatory ventilation for the prevention of chronic lung disease of prematurity. *N Engl J Med* 347: 633–642.

30. Bollen CW, Uiterwal CSPM, van Vught AJ. (2003) Cumulative metaanalysis of high-frequency versus conventional ventilation in premature neonates. *Am J Respir Crit Care Med* 168: 1150–1155.

31. De Paoli AG, Morley C, Davis PG. (2003) Nasal CPAP for neonates: what do we know in 2003? *Arch Dis Child Fetal Neonatal Ed* F168–F172.

32. Lin CH, Wang ST, Lin YJ, Yeh TF. (1998) Efficacy of nasal intermittent positive pressure ventilation in treating apnea of prematurity. *Pediatr Pulmonol* 26: 349–353.

33. Friedlich P, Lecart C, Posen R, Ramicone E, Chan L, Ramanathan R. (1999) A randomized trial of nasopharyngeal-synchronized intermittent mandatory ventilation versus nasopharyngeal continuous positive airway pressure in very low birth weight infants after extubation. *J Perinatol* 19: 413–418.

34. Santin R, Brodsky N, Bhandari V. (2004) A prospective observational pilot study of synchronized nasal intermittent positive pressure ventilation (SNIPPV) as a primary mode of ventilation in infants ≥ 28 weeks with respiratory distress syndrome (RDS). *J Perinatol* 24: 487–493.

35. Courtney SE, Aghai ZH, Saslow JG, Pyon KH, Habib RH. (2003) Changes in lung volume and work of breathing: a comparison of two variable-flow nasal continuous positive airway pressure devices in very low birth weight infants. *Pediatr Pulmonol* 36: 248–252.

36. Davis P, Davies M, Faber B. (2001) A randomized controlled trial of two methods of delivering nasal continuous positive airway pressure after extubation to infants weighing less than 1000 g: binasal (Hudson) versus single nasal prongs. *Arch Dis Child Fetal Neonatal Ed* 85: F82–F85.

37. Lindner W, Vobbeck S, Hummler H, Pohlandt F. (1999) Delivery room management of extremely low birth weight infants: Spontaneous breathing or intubation? *Pediatrics* 103: 961–967.

38. Finer NN, Carlo WA, Duara S, *et al.* (2004) Delivery room continuous positive airway pressure/positive end-expiratory pressure in extremely low birth weight infants: a feasibility trial. *Pediatrics* 114: 651–657.

39. Meyer M, Mildenhall M, Wong M. (2004) Outcome for infants weighing less than 1000 grams cared for with a nasal continuous positive airway pressure-based strategy. *J Paediatr Child Health* 40: 38–41.

40. Sahni R, Ammari A, Suri MS, *et al.* (2005) Is the new definition of bronchopulmonary dysplasia more useful? *J Perinatol* 25: 41–46.

41. Lee KS, Dunn MS, Fenwick M, Shennan AT. (1998) A comparison of underwater bubble continuous positive airway pressure with ventilator-derived continuous positive airway pressure in premature neonates ready for extubation. *Biol Neonate* 73: 69–75.

42. Morley CJ, Lau R, De Paoli A, Davis PG. (2005) Nasal continuous positive airway pressure: does bubbling improve gas exchange? *Arch Dis Child Fetal Neonatal Ed* 90: F343–F344.

43. Jobe AH, Kramer BW, Moss TJ, Newnham JP, Ikegami M. (2002) Decreased indicators of lung injury with continuous positive expiratory pressure in preterm lambs. *Pediatr Res* 52: 387–392.

44. Pillow JJ, Travadi JN. Bubble CPAP: Is the noise important? (2005) An in vitro study. *Pediatr Res* 57: 826–830.

45. Stefanescu BM, Murphy WP, Hansell BJ, Fuloria M, Morgan TM, Aschner JL. (2003) A randomized, controlled trial comparing two different continuous positive airway pressure systems for the successful extubation of extremely low birth weight infants. *Pediatrics* 112: 1031–1038.

46. Aly H, Massaro AN, Patel K, El-Mohandes AA. (2005) Is it safer to intubate premature infants in the delivery room. *Pediatrics* 115: 1660–1665.

47. Sandri F, Ancora G, Lanzoni A, Tagliabue P, Colnaghi M, Ventura ML. (2004) Prophylactic nasal continuous positive airways pressure in newborns of 28–31 weeks gestation: multicenter randomized controlled clinical trial. *Arch Dis Child Fetal Neonatal Ed* 89: F394–F398.

48. Kamlin COF, Davis PG, Morley CJ. (2006) Predicting successful extubation of very low birth weight infants. *Arch Dis Child Fetal Neonatal Ed* 91: F180–F183.

49. Locke RG, Wolfson MR, Shaffer TH, Rubenstein SD, Greenspan JS. (1993) Inadvertent administration of positive end-expiratory pressure during nasal cannula flow. *Pediatrics* 91: 135–138.

50. Finer NN, Rich W, Craft A, Henderson C. (2001) Comparison of methods of bag and mask ventilation for neonatal resuscitation. *Resuscitation* 49: 299–305.

51. Barrington KJ, Bull D, Finer NN. (2001) Randomized trial of nasal synchronized intermittent mandatory ventilation compared with continuous positive airway pressure after extubation of very low birth weight infants. *Pediatrics* 107: 638–641.

52. Kulkarni A, Ehrenkranz RA, Bhandari V. (2006) Effect of introduction of synchronized nasal intermittent positive-pressure ventilation in a neonatal intensive care unit on bronchopulmonary dysplasia and growth in preterm infants. *Am J Perinatol* 23: 1–8.

53. Kugelman A, Feferkorn I, Riskin A, Chistyakov I, Kaufman B, Bader D. (2007) Nasal intermittent mandatory ventilation versus nasal continuous positive airway pressure for respiratory distress syndrome: a randomized, controlled, prospective study. *J Pediatr* 150: 521–526.

54. Ramanathan R, Sekar K, Rasmussen R, Bhatia J, Soll R. (2009) Nasal Intermittent Positive Pressure Ventilation (NIPPV) versus Synchronized Intermittent Mandatory Ventilation (SIMV) After Surfactant Treatment for Respiratory Distress Syndrome (RDS) in Preterm Infants < 30 Weeks' Gestation: Multicenter, Randomized, Clinical Trial. Pediatric Academic Society Meetings, A3212.6.

55. te Pas AB, Walther FJ. (2007) A randomized, controlled trial of delivery-room respiratory management in very preterm infants. *Pediatrics* 120: 322–329.

Chapter 10

Respiratory Distress Syndrome: Impact of Surfactant Therapy and Antenatal Steroid

Oommen P. Mathew*

10.1 Introduction

Approximately 4.3 million babies were born in the USA in 2006. At the current rate of premature birth (almost 13%), this accounts for more than half a million premature infants. Prematurity is associated with significant morbidity and mortality. The vast majority of neonatal deaths occur in the first few days of life due to respiratory distress syndrome (RDS) secondary to surfactant deficiency of the immature lungs. Enhanced maturation of lungs by antenatal steroids and surfactant replacement therapy have revolutionized the care of preterm infants and reduced the mortality and morbidity substantially. Incidence of RDS increases with decreasing gestational age. Before surfactant replacement therapy and antenatal steroid, approximately 20% of infants born at 30–32 weeks of gestation and 60–80% at 26–28 weeks of gestation developed RDS and 5–10,000 infants died each year. In 1980, for example, 4989 infants died of RDS compared to 860 in 2005, the most recent year for which such data are available.[1] A remarkable achievement indeed!

---

*Professor of Pediatrics, Medical College of Georgia.

285

RDS, formerly known as hyaline membrane disease, primarily affects premature infants. Surfactant is critical for proper respiratory function. Surfactant, a contraction for surface active agent, reduces surface tension in the lung, prevents the collapse of the alveoli and distal airways, and facilitates gas exchange. It also reduces the work of breathing. Surfactant deficiency, therefore, leads to alveolar collapse and compromised pulmonary function. Clinically it is manifested as tachypnea, retractions, cyanosis and increased work of breathing. Surfactant deficient lungs are less compliant (more stiff) and consequently, infants are unable to expand them adequately even with increased respiratory efforts resulting in collapsed or atelectatic lungs. Before surfactant replacement therapy became available, supportive care, such as supplemental oxygen, continuous positive airway pressure and mechanical ventilation, was the only option. The lungs of infants who died of RDS were airless with a Swiss cheese pattern of atelectasis. The distended bronchioles contained hyaline membranes, a proteinaceous material derived from circulation but not seen in preterm infants who died soon after birth. In addition to primary surfactant deficiency which manifests soon after birth, surfactant deficiency can also occur due to surfactant inactivation or dysfunction. For example, aspiration of meconium or development of pulmonary edema or hemorrhage can lead to secondary surfactant deficiency.

10.2 Surfactant

10.2.1 *History*

The seminal observation by Avery and Mead in 1959 that lung extracts from infants who died from hyaline membrane disease failed to lower surface tension on a Wilhelmy surface tension balance lead to the emergence of the concept that surfactant deficiency is the underlying problem.[2] A number of important discoveries preceded and followed this observation and are well documented in several reviews.[3] Briefly, the relationship between pressure, surface tension and radius of curvature of surfaces was first described by Laplace in the early 19th century. Neergaard in 1929 described the extensive air-liquid interface within the lung and was able to measure the contribution of surface forces to elastic recoil of the lungs.

The observation of Pattle that stable bubbles are absent in lungs of immature animal was another important milestone. However, it was the experiment by Clements[4] showing that surface tension changes when surface area decreases that set the stage for the seminal discovery by Avery and Mead. These important discoveries were not enough to save Patrick Kennedy, the second son of President Kennedy. He was born prematurely in 1963 at 34 weeks gestation and died at the age of two days from RDS, commonly known as hyaline membrane disease at that time.

10.2.2 *Composition*

Surfactant is a type of biological soap, a complex mixture of phospholipids. It stabilizes alveoli and prevents them from collapsing in expiration by lowering surface tension. The composition of the alveolar lining layer was a focus of intense research in the 1960s. Nearly 90% of lipid fraction is phospholipids. Dipalmitoylphosphatidyl choline (DPPC) is its main surface tension-lowering component (Fig. 10.1). It also has four distinct surfactant-associated proteins designated as: SP-A, SP-B, SP-C, and SP-D (3). The role of these proteins in surfactant function has been clarified in various *in vivo* and *in vitro* studies. Their affinity for water is a key

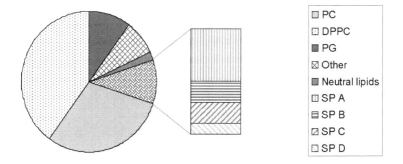

Fig. 10.1.   Surfactant composition.

PC = phosphatidyl choline, PG = phosphatidyl glycerol,

DPPC = Dipalmitoyl phosphatidyl choline,

SP A = surfactant protein A, SP B = surfactant protein B,

SP C = surfactant protein C, SP D = surfactant protein D.

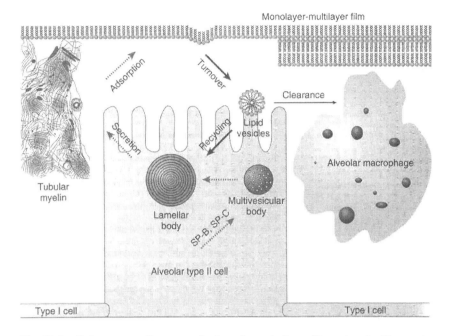

Fig. 10.2. Pulmonary surfactant synthesis and metabolism. (Reproduced with permission from Ref. 5.)

differentiating factor: SP-A and SP-D are hydrophilic, whereas SP-B and SP-C are hydrophobic. SP-B and SPC play an integral part in interacting with phospholipids in lowering surface tension. Surfactant is synthesized by the type II alveolar cell in a multi-step process and secreted as lamellar bodies, which are highly enriched phospholipids. This is schematically depicted in Fig. 10.2.[5] SP-B and SP-C are also enriched in lamellar bodies and co-secreted with phospholipids. Lamellar bodies are subsequently converted into a lattice structure known as tubular myelin[6] (Fig. 10.3). Spreading and adsorption characteristics of surfactants are critical to form a stable monolayer in the alveolus. Surfactant proteins, especially SP-B, play a critical role in this process. It is a small polypeptide comprising 79 amino acids. Human SP-B gene is composed of 10 exons located on chromosome 2. Mice lacking the SP-B protein, SP-B gene-knockout mice, die of respiratory failure soon after birth, whereas those mice lacking SP-C may develop various forms of interstitial lung disease much

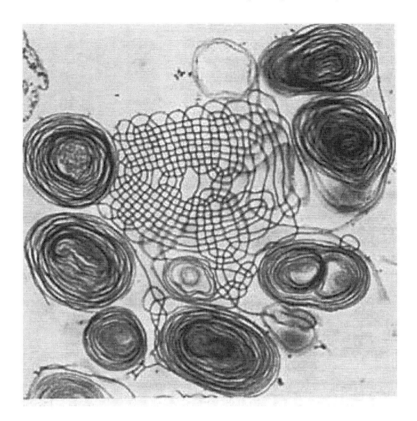

Fig. 10.3. Electron micrograph of lamellar bodies forming tubular myelin. (Reproduced with permission from Ref. 6.)

later in life. Human infants with mutations in SP-B gene often develop respiratory distress within hours of birth. They develop progressive respiratory failure and are unresponsive to surfactant replacement therapy. Hereditary SP-B deficiency was recognized in 1993 with the report of three siblings with fatal neonatal lung disease despite maximal supportive therapy.[7] The vast majority of infants with this disease die within the first three months. Lung transplantation is the only viable treatment option, besides compassionate care. Both partial and transient SP-B deficiencies have been recognized. Alveolar proteinosis is a frequent, but not path gnomonic, sign of SP-B deficiency. Congenital alveolar proteinosis should not be used synonymously with hereditary SP-B deficiency. More than 15 distinct mutations have been identified with the neonatal presentation of respiratory disease.

10.2.3 *Surfactant replacement therapy*

The era of surfactant replacement therapy was heralded by the successful treatment of human infants by Fujiwara and co-workers in 1980.[8] The goal of surfactant therapy is to replace and restore surfactant function. The road to surfactant replacement therapy for RDS was long and arduous. Initial treatment attempts with aerosols of DPPC in the 1960s were met with little success. However, Enhorning and colleagues subsequently provided experimental evidence in animals that RDS could be treated by exogenous administration of surfactant[9] and put the research for replacement therapy back on track. Fujiwara's work ignited a series of multi-center trials of various types of surfactants leading to the FDA approval of the first synthetic surfactant in 1990 and first natural surfactant in 1991. Extensive trials involving synthetic and natural surfactant mixtures derived from bovine and porcine lungs or human amniotic fluid followed. These trials unequivocally demonstrated a prompt and sustained response to surfactants with minimal side effects. Compared to control, surfactant replacement reduced the incidence of pneumothorax, pulmonary interstitial emphysema, and the combined outcome of death or bronchopulmonary dysplasia[10] (Table 10.1). However, surfactant replacement

Table 10.1.   Meta-analyses of prophylaxis and rescue treatment with animal-derived and synthetic surfactant[+]

	Prophylaxis, Relative Risk (95% CI)		Rescue, Relative Risk (95% CI)	
Outcome	Animal Derived	Synthetic	Animal Derived	Synthetic
Mortality	0.60 (0.44–0.83)	0.70 (0.58–0.85)	0.67 (0.58–0.76)	0.73 (0.61–0.88)
Pneumothorax	0.35 (0.26–0.49)	0.67 (0.50–0.90)	0.37 (0.25–0.50)	0.64 (0.55–0.76)
Pulmonary interstitial emphysema	0.46 (0.35–0.60)	0.68 (0.50–0.93)	Not available	0.62 (0.54–0.71)
Bronchopulmonary dysplasia or death	0.84 (0.75–0.93)	0.89 (0.77–1.03)	Not available	0.73 (0.65–0.83)

[+]Modified from Ref. 10.

therapy did not change the incidence of other morbidities such as bronchopulmonary dysplasia, intraventricular hemorrhage, necrotizing enterocolitis, nosocomial infections, retinopathy of prematurity and patent ductus arteriosus.[10] Effectiveness of surfactant replacement is not limited to the very low birth weight infants. Larger and more mature preterm infants with established respiratory distress syndrome also benefit from such therapy.

Initial trials focused on whether a single dose was adequate or multiple doses were required for the treatment of RDS as well as on the timing of the first dose of the drug. In prophylaxis studies preterm infants at high risk for developing RDS were given surfactant soon after birth, whereas in rescue treatment infants exhibited clinical and X-ray evidence of RDS before surfactant was administered. These studies clearly showed that prophylaxis is better than rescue treatment. Both a lower incidence and severity of RDS and fewer complications (Table 10.2) were observed among infants receiving prophylactic surfactant.[11] Early studies showed that multiple doses are superior to single dose regimen.[12,13] Although definitions of prophylaxis were not uniform among all studies, Committee on Fetus and Newborn recently defined prophylaxis "as surfactant administration before the onset of respiratory symptoms or efforts, before initial resuscitation efforts, or, most commonly, after initial resuscitation but within 10 to 30 minutes after birth." They also defined early rescue "as surfactant treatment within one to two hours of birth" and late rescue "as surfactant treatment two or more hours after birth".[10] Although the data is limited, early rescue treatment appears to be superior to late rescue treatment.[14] For the most part, neonatologists have abandoned the practice of administering the surfactant within the first few breaths to early administration of surfactant in the delivery room or the NICU.

Table 10.2. Surfactant replacement therapy: prophylaxis versus rescue[10]

Outcome	RR(95% CI)	NNT
Mortality	0.61 (0.48–0.77)	22
Pneumothorax	0.62 (0.42–0.89)	47
Pulmonary interstitial emphysema	0.54 (0.36–0.82)	40
Bronchopulmonary dysplasia or death	0.85 (0.76–0.95)	24

To date, surfactant remains the best studied drug in human neonates. Several surfactant preparations are currently approved for use in the treatment of RDS in premature infants. Exosurf®, a synthetic surfactant was the first to obtain FDA approval. However, it has been replaced with natural surfactants. Three natural surfactants are currently being used across the US. These are beractant (Survanta®), calfactant (Infasurf®) and poractant alfa (Curosurf®). Survanta® was approved by the FDA in 1991 and is derived from minced bovine lungs, whereas Infasurf® is a sterile extract of calf lungs. Curosurf®, on the other hand, is derived from porcine lung extract. All three contain surfactant proteins but their concentrations vary significantly. Surfactant protein B, which is considered the most important surfactant protein, is present only in trace amount in Survanta®. Concentration of this protein varies considerably between lots. Infasurf® contains approximately 2% protein, of which 40% is SP-B. Curosurf® contains approximately 1.3% protein and SP-B accounts for 30%. There are differences among these surfactant preparations on the amount administered, the dosing interval and the number of doses required for the treatment of RDS (Table 10.3). For the most part, these differences can be attributed to the concentration of the phospholipids and surfactant proteins. More rapid onset and sustained action are seen with preparations containing more phospholipids and SP-B.

Clinical trials comparing various surfactants followed. These trials showed the superiority of natural surfactants to first generation synthetic surfactant. The main biochemical difference between the two is the presence of surfactant proteins in the natural surfactants. However, as mentioned above, the concentration of surfactant protein B varies. There are several comparison studies involving animal derived surfactants.

Table 10.3. Commonly used surfactants and their dosing

Surfactant Preparation	Initial Dose	Phospholipid	Dosing Interval	Maximum Doses	Surfactant Protein B
Survanta	4 ml/kg	25 mg/ml	6 hours	4	trace
Infasurf	3 ml/kg	35 mg/ml	12 hours	3	0.26 mg/ml
Curosurf	2.5 ml/kg	80 mg/ml	12 hours	3	0.3 mg/ml

These studies show that all commercially available animal-derived surfactants are effective for prevention and treatment of respiratory distress syndrome. Early transient improvements in pulmonary status have been noted in some of these studies consistent with the level of SP-B. As the Committee on Fetus and Newborn concludes,[10] "it is unclear whether significant differences in clinical outcomes exist among the available products." Even though there were concerns about immunogenicity of animal derived proteins and its potential for transmitting animal borne diseases, there is no evidence to date to support this concern after nearly 25 years of use.

A second generation synthetic surfactant preparation, lucinactant (Surfaxin®), is awaiting FDA approval. The novel aspect of this preparation is that it contains the peptide KL_4 (also known as sinapultide) which mimics the essential properties of human SP-B. Pulmonary surfactant containing KL_4 is highly effective in lowering surface tension and shows resistance to degradation in *in vitro* models. KL_4-based surfactants contain the key peptide, the lipids DPPC and palmitoyl-oleyl phosphatidylglycerol, plus the fatty acid, palmitic acid. Published data from clinical trials of surfaxin® indicate that this is superior to the first generation synthetic surfactant and is similarly effective as currently available animal-derived surfactants in prophylactic treatment of RDS.[15,16]

All currently approved surfactants are to be used as liquid instillate formulations and require these neonates to be intubated first. Compatibility of KL4 with a variety of formulations (i.e. liquid instillate, aerosol, lyophilized form) has opened potential new avenues of treatment, especially for infants with less severe RDS. The availability of a less invasive method to deliver exogenous surfactant would be an attractive alternative for this population. Aerosurf® (lucinactant for inhalation) represents the first potential opportunity to effectively deliver a clinically relevant dose of surfactant without the need for intubation. Results of a phase two trials suggest that Aerosurf® is generally safe and well tolerated.[17] It retained pharmacological activity throughout the aerosolization process. If proved effective, approximately 45,000 neonates with diagnosis of RDS could benefit from this therapy.

10.3 Antenatal Steroid

Pulmonary maturation accelerates with advancing gestation. Several hormones influence lung maturation. Among these, glucocorticoids are the most important. The seminal observation regarding enhancement of pulmonary maturation by antenatal steroid was made by Liggins in 1969, while studying the role of glucocorticoids in the induction of labor.[18] He observed that fetal lambs were viable at an earlier age after the injection of the lambs with cortisol. The stage for this observation was set by a provoking suggestion by Buckingham that the lung may be an analog of developing intestine on the basis of the finding by Moog that the timing of the appearance of phosphatase in the duodenum is accelerated by cortisol. Later work by Liggins and Howie confirmed this important observation in human neonates. Results of this classic trial were published in 1972.[19] Many prospective, randomized, controlled studies followed which confirmed the findings of Liggins and Howie that maternal administration of betamethasone or dexamethasone results in accelerated maturation of the surfactant system.[20] The maturational effects of corticosteroids on other fetal organ systems such as the cardiovascular, nervous, and gastrointestinal systems have been confirmed in these randomized controlled trials. Although the optimal results are seen 24 hours following a complete course of steroid and last up to seven days, even an incomplete course is associated with some beneficial effects when compared to control infants. The magnitude of the reduction of RDS is less with premature rupture of membranes compared to intact membranes. Chorioamnionitis was considered a contraindication for administering antenatal steroid. In addition to the effect on surfactant maturation, antenatal steroid has an effect on lung architecture as well. Crawley *et al.*[20] summarized the available evidence in a meta-analysis in 1990. Data from 12 controlled trials, involving over 3000 participants, show that antenatal steroids reduce the occurrence of respiratory distress syndrome overall and in all the subgroups of trial participants. Furthermore, such therapy was also associated with reductions in intraventricular hemorrhage, necrotizing enterocolitis and neonatal death. However, clinical adaptation of this practice was slow. Only less than 20% women delivering infants weighing 501–1500 g received antenatal steroid at the time of National

Institute of Health (NIH) consensus conference in 1994,[21] which was the tipping point in the use of antenatal steroid. These experts recommended that all fetuses between 24 and 34 weeks' gestation at risk for preterm delivery should be considered candidates for antenatal treatment with corticosteroids. They also recommended antenatal corticosteroid use in pregnancies with preterm premature rupture of membranes at less than 30 to 32 weeks' gestation in the absence of clinical chorioamnionitis and in complicated pregnancies where delivery prior to 34 weeks' gestation is likely. Furthermore, they suggested that the short- and long-term benefits and risks of repeating administration of antenatal corticosteroids seven days after the initial course be evaluated in future studies. Widespread implementation of antenatal steroid use followed this consensus conference.

Although the number and timing of repeat courses remained an unanswered question, weekly course of steroid became commonplace. This practice was based on the premise that repeat courses reduced the incidence and severity of RDS supported by retrospective and preliminary prospective data. A second consensus conference was convened in 2000 to address this issue of repeat courses. The conclusion of this expert panel was that there is inadequate data from randomized, controlled studies to recommend routine use of repeat courses.[22] Results of a prospective study[23] were published in 2001. Unfortunately, this study was stopped prematurely because of lack of efficacy and concern for potential adverse neurologic effects. A recently published prospective multi-center trial also addressed several of these issues.[24] Again, the composite primary neonatal outcome was not significantly improved by repeat courses. Nevertheless, several acute morbidities were decreased with repeat courses. This study did demonstrate an adverse effect on weight and length but not on head circumference. The authors concluded that routine weekly administration of antenatal steroid is not justified, but there may be a role for less frequent dosing in a subset of women at high risk for delivering before 32 weeks. This awaits further clarification.

There is convincing evidence that prolonged postnatal steroid use is associated with significant side effects and is associated with increased incidence of cerebral palsy. There is also strong evidence in the animal model that steroid adversely affects brain growth. These evidences were the basis of the policy statement that "the routine use of systemic dexamethasone for the prevention or treatment of chronic lung disease in infants with very low birth weight is not recommended" by the Committee on Fetus and Newborn in 2002 which was reaffirmed[25] in 2006. Because of the effects of postnatal steroid on growth and brain development, there was concern about the neurological outcome of infants born to mothers given antenatal steroid. There is no strong evidence to date suggesting adverse effects of single course of antenatal corticosteroids. As mentioned above, neonatal morbidities such as intraventricular hemorrhage and necrotizing enterocolitis are decreased among infants born to women receiving one course of antenatal steroid.[20] However, it must be pointed out that there is evidence from retrospective studies that suggests that betamethasone may have less adverse neurological outcome when compared to dexamethasone. Following widespread use of weekly course of maternal steroid, evidence began emerging from both animal and human studies suggesting harmful effects of repetitive courses of steroid on birth weight and brain growth. Again, these were mostly retrospective studies. However, in the multi-center prospective study, the adverse effect on weight and length were seen primarily among infants exposed to four or more courses.[24] The mechanisms underlying this altered growth and its clinical significance is unclear, especially with no decrease in head growth. At present there are many unanswered questions.

The mechanism by which the glucocorticoids enhance lung maturation has been under investigation for decades. We know now that glucocorticoids act by binding to specific receptors in lung cells. It increases synthesis of messenger RNA and protein. At least 2% of the proteins in human fetal lungs are estimated to be regulated by glucocorticoids. They induce a number of proteins in the lung, especially the four surfactant associated proteins. Although an increase in transcription factors can be demonstrated within a couple of hours of exposure to corticosteroid, increase in new proteins generally occurs only after 12–24 hours. Optimal response is observed around 48 hours and the effect persists for at least seven days. Glucocorticoids regulate gene expression by transrepression as well. In this case corticosteroid-receptor complex interacts with transcription factors to block upregulation of cytokine-chemokine cascade. Anti-inflammatory effects are mediated through this mechanism.

Maternal corticosteroid-surfactant interaction is an important variable. Does postnatal surfactant replacement decrease the morbidity and mortality in preterm infants exposed to maternal antenatal steroid? These two therapies have an additive effect on postnatal lung function in the animal model. Lung compliance, lung volume and lung edema were improved when compared to either treatment alone. Furthermore, combined treatment resulted in a reduction in air leaks, BPD and death in the animal model. Although no randomized studies have been conducted in humans, a beneficial interaction between antenatal steroid and surfactant replacement therapy has been documented in human neonates as well. Subgroup analyses showed that infants who received both antenatal steroids and postnatal surfactant have significant reductions in mortality, severity of respiratory distress, and air leaks when compared infants who received antenatal steroids only, or surfactant only.[10,26,27]

Thyroid hormones accelerate morphological development of the lung and surfactant production in the animal model. Since there is little placental transfer of T3 and T4 in humans, maternal treatment with thyrotropin releasing hormone was the practical choice. The important question was whether the combination of antenatal steroid and TRH is superior to antenatal steroid treatment alone. Multiple studies have shown that addition of prenatal TRH to corticosteroids does not reduce the risk of neonatal respiratory disease and do not improve any of the fetal or neonatal outcomes.[28] Furthermore, prenatal TRH group had more adverse effects for both the mother and the infant.

10.4 Economic Impact

Clinical trials have shown unequivocally that surfactant replacement therapy reduces mortality. One cannot put a price on the value of life saved or lost. Even though it is an effective therapy, it has failed to reduce the incidence of chronic lung disease among survivors in part because of more immature survivors. Since it is an expensive therapy, it has an impact on allocation of resources. Objective of surfactant treatment may vary from preventing RDS, reducing morbidity from RDS, preventing mortality in immature babies, to improving long term outcomes for preterm babies. Several studies have evaluated the economic cost of a given surfactant or comparing different products. Cost depends on the choice of surfactant product, vial size and dosage. Efficiency of surfactant use depends on other variables such as use of antenatal steroid, gestation age at birth, stage of lung development, etc. Furthermore, economic impact of this intervention can be evaluated in many ways and utilizing different models. For example, cost benefit, cost effectiveness and cost utility analysis may produce different results.

A recent review by Mugford[29] on "cost effectiveness of prevention and treatment of neonatal respiratory distress (RDS) with exogenous surfactant, i.e. What has changed in the last three decades?" discusses several relevant issues on the economic impact of surfactant therapy. Earlier studies compared surfactant therapy with no surfactant therapy and showed that surfactant replacement reduced mortality and neonatal care costs. These results also indicated that surfactant for rescue treatment was a cost effective intervention compared to other health technologies of that time. Surfactant costs were not included in these calculations. Economic evaluations of surfactant treatment found an incremental cost per life gained in one study, whereas it was cost neutral in other trials. However, it must be pointed out that the groups of infants treated were not the same as indicated by the birth weights. Incremental cost per life gained was approximately £50,000 in earlier estimates.[30] Analysis of results of a very large international clinical trial of artificial surfactant estimated a much lower cost per life gained (£6375) than had been predicted by other studies including one by the same author.[29] Another study showed that beractant and calfactant were similar in terms of efficacy, safety, and total number of doses per patient but calfactant was more costly because of greater product waste. Studies of surfactant dosing and protocols for multiple uses of vials suggest that cost savings can be made without loss of effectiveness. In this era of neonatal care where surfactant replacement therapy is routine and innovations in technology has changed neonatal care, there may still be incremental savings by efficient surfactant use by minimizing waste and multiple use vials, but the next economic efficiency of providing neonatal care for preterm babies is likely to come from reducing chronic lung disease or prematurity itself.

References

1. National Center for Health Statistics Health, United States. (2007) With Chartbook on Trends in the Health of Americans Hyattsville, MD.

2. Avery ME, Mead J. (1959) Surface properties in relation to atelectasis and hyaline membrane disease. *AMA J Dis Child.* 97: 517–523.

3. Avery ME. (1995) Lung stability and surface-active agents. In: Proctor, DF, ed. A *History of Breathing Physiology.* New York: Marcel Dekker; 283–301.

4. Clements JA. (1957) Surface tension of lung extracts. *Proc Soc Exp Bio Med* 95: 170–172.

5. Whitsett J. (2004) Composition of pulmonary surfactant lipids and proteins. In: Polin, Fox and Abman, ed. Fetal and neonatal physiology Saunders, Philadelphia; 1005–1013.

6. Randell SH, Young SL. (2004) Structure of alveolar epithelial cells and surface layer during development. In: *Fetal and Neonatal Physiology.* Polin, Fox and Abman, ed. Saunders, Philadelphia; 1034–1040.

7. LM Nogee, DE deMello, LP Dehner, HR Colten. (1993) Pulmonary surfactant protein B deficiency in congenital pulmonary alveolar proteinosis, *N Engl J Med* 328: 406–410.

8. Fujiwara T, Maeta H, Chida S, Morita T, Watabe Y, Abe T. (1980) Artificial surfactant therapy in hyaline-membrane disease. *Lancet* 12(1): 55–59.

9. Enhorning G, Robertson B. (1972) Lung expansion in premature rabbit fetus after tracheal deposition of surfactant. *Pediatrics* 50: 58–66.

10. William A. Engle, MD, and the Committee on Fetus and Newborn. (2008) Surfactant-Replacement therapy for respiratory distress in the preterm and term neonate. *Pediatrics* 121: 419–432.

11. Soll RF, Morley CJ. (2001) Prophylactic versus selective use of surfactant in preventing morbidity and mortality in preterm infants. *Cochrane Database Syst Rev* (2): CD000510.

12. Liechty EA, Donovan E, Purohit D, Gilhooly J, Feldman B, Noguchi A, Denson SE, Sehgal SS, Gross I, Stevens D, *et al.* (1991) Reduction of neonatal mortality after multiple doses of bovine surfactant in low birth weight neonates with respiratory distress syndrome. *Pediatrics* 88: 19–28.

13. Hoekstra RE, Jackson JC, Myers TF, Frantz ID 3rd, Stern ME, Powers WF, Maurer M, Raye JR, Carrier ST, Gunkel JH, *et al.* (1991) Improved neonatal

survival following multiple doses of bovine surfactant in very premature neonates at risk for respiratory distress syndrome. *Pediatrics* 88: 10–18.

14. Stevens TP, Harrington EW, Blennow M, Soll RF. (2007) Early surfactant administration with brief ventilation vs. selective surfactant and continued mechanical ventilation for preterm infants with or at risk for respiratory distress syndrome. *Cochrane Database Syst Rev* Oct 17(4): CD003063.

15. Sinha S, Lacaze-Masmoneil T, Valis i Soler A, *et al.* (2005) A randomized, controlled trial of lucinactant versus poractant alfa in very premature infants at high risk for respiratory distress syndrome. *Pediatrics* 115: 1030–1038.

16. Moya F, Gadzinowski J, Bancalari E, *et al.* (2005) A multicenter, randomized, masked, comparison trial of lucinactant, colfosceril palmitate, and beractant for the prevention of respiratory distress syndrome in very preterm infants. *Pediatrics* 115: 1018–1029.

17. Finer NN, Merritt TA, Bernstein G, Job L, Mazela J, Liu G. (2006) A multicenter pilot study of Aerosurf™ delivered via nasal continuous positive airway pressure (nCPAP) to prevent respiratory distress syndrome in preterm neonates. *Pediatr Res* 59: PAS2006: 4840.138.

18. Liggins GC. (1969) Premature delivery of foetal lambs infused with glucocorticoids. *J Endocrinol* 45: 515–523.

19. Liggins GC, Howie RN. (1972) A controlled trial of antepartum glucocorticoid treatment for prevention of the respiratory distress syndrome in premature infants. *Pediatrics* 50: 515–525.

20. Crowley P, Chalmers I, Keirse MJ. (1990) The effects of corticosteroid administration before preterm delivery: an overview of the evidence from controlled trials. *Br J Obstet Gynaecol* 97: 11–25.

21. Effect of corticosteroids for fetal maturation on perinatal outcomes. NIH Consensus Development Panel on the Effect of Corticosteroids for Fetal Maturation on Perinatal Outcomes (1995) *JAMA* 273: 413–418.

22. Antenatal corticosteroids revisited: repeat courses. (2000) *NIH Consens Statement* 17: 1–18.

23. Guinn DA, Atkinson MW, Sullivan L, Lee M, MacGregor S, Parilla BV, Davies J, Hanlon-Lundberg K, Simpson L, Stone J, Wing D, Ogasawara K, Muraskas J. (2001) Single vs weekly courses of antenatal corticosteroids for women at risk of preterm delivery: a randomized controlled trial. *JAMA*, 286: 1581–1587.

24. Wapner RJ, Sorokin Y, Thom EA, Johnson F, Dudley DJ, Spong CY, Peaceman AM, Leveno KJ, Harper M, Caritis SN, Miodovnik M, Mercer B, Thorp JM, Moawad A, O'Sullivan MJ, Ramin S, Carpenter MW, Rouse DJ, Sibai B, Gabbe SG. (2006) National Institute of Child Health and Human Development Maternal Fetal Medicine Units Network. Single versus weekly courses of antenatal corticosteroids: evaluation of safety and efficacy. *Am J Obstet Gynecol* 195: 633–642.

25. Committee on Fetus and Newborn. (2002) Postnatal corticosteroids to treat or prevent chronic lung disease in preterm infants. *Pediatrics* 109: 330–338.

26. Jobe AH, Mitchell BR, Gunkel JH. (1993) Beneficial effects of the combined use of prenatal corticosteroids and postnatal surfactanton preterm infants. *Am J Obstet Gynecol* 168: 508–513.

27. Kari MA, Hallman M, Eronen M, *et al.* (1994) Prenatal dexamethasone treatment in conjunction with rescue therapy of humansurfactant: a randomized placebo-controlled multicenter study. *Pediatrics* 93: 730–736.

28. Crowther CA, Alfirevic Z, Haslam RR. (2004) Thyrotropin-releasing hormone added to corticosteroids for women at risk of preterm birth for preventing neonatal respiratory disease. *Cochrane Database Syst Rev* (2): CD000019.

29. Mugford M. (2006) Cost effectiveness of prevention and treatment of neonatal respiratory distress (RDS) with exogenous surfactant: what has changed in the last three decades? *Early Hum Dev* 82: 105–115.

30. Mugford M. (1995) Cost-effectiveness of policies for surfactant use based on the results of the OSIRIS trial: a preliminary analysis. *Neonatal Monit* 12: 10–12.

Chapter 11

Antibiotics and Other Miracle Drugs

Oommen P. Mathew*

Drugs used in neonates, infants and children today, for the most part, were tested and approved for use in adults. Gradually they found their way for use in children with similar conditions or diseases. Until recently, pregnant women and children have been purposefully excluded from clinical trials of drugs. Antibiotic usage is an example of such practices which sometimes results in terrible misadventures. This is exemplified in the development of gray baby syndrome in neonates following chloramphenicol use. This chapter will focus on drugs that have positively impacted the practice of neonatal-perinatal medicine. Some of these drugs were developed for specific conditions affecting neonates and have undergone clinical trials in this population, while others have found unique applications in this population. Surfactant therapy for the treatment of respiratory distress syndrome in preterm infants is on the top of this list (it is covered in a separate chapter) in the former category, whereas antibiotic prophylaxis during labor to prevent group B streptococcal infection in the newborn is an excellent example of the latter.

*Professor of Pediatrics, Medical College of Georgia.

11.1 Neonatal Infections

Antibiotics had an impact in the care of neonates similar to most other areas of medicine. Neonatal infection continues to be a major problem on a global basis. World Health Organization (WHO) estimates that more than four million neonatal deaths occur each year and 98% of these deaths occur in developing countries. Over a million of these neonatal deaths are estimated to be caused by infection. Antibiotic use has reduced the mortality from infection substantially in developed countries. Similarly, vaccinations for common childhood diseases such as tetanus, polio, diphtheria, and whooping cough have also significantly reduced both morbidity and infant mortality. These vaccinations are *not* initiated in the neonatal period because optimal response to vaccines is not observed during the neonatal period.

11.1.1 *Viral infections*

11.1.1.1 *Hepatitis B infection*

Hepatitis B vaccination is given during the immediate neonatal period. This exception to the general practice stems from the fact that most affected infants acquire the infection through vertical transmission occurring primarily during delivery. The risk of infants acquiring hepatitis B from asymptomatic carrier mothers is high in Taiwan, Japan and China compared to the US.[1,2] Hepatitis B infection and carrier state can be reduced significantly by administration of this vaccine, the first dose of which is given soon after birth. If maternal hepatitis status is unknown or positive, the vaccine should be given within 12 hours of birth. Hepatitis B immune globulin is used routinely in conjuction with the vaccine in the US for all infants born to hepatitis B surface antigen positive mothers. Since WHO recommended global hepatitis B vaccination, the number of countries that have included the hepatitis B vaccine into their national infant immunization programs has increased to 171 at the end of 2007 compared with 31 countries in 1992.[3] Vaccination has reduced the rate of chronic hepatitis B infection to less than 1% among immunized children in many countries where the infection rate was 8% to 15%.[3]

11.1.1.2 *Human Immunodeficiency Virus (HIV) infection*

Since the beginning of the HIV epidemic, 25 million people have died of HIV-related causes. Thirty three million people are estimated to be living with HIV worldwide in 2007, including two million children.[4] In 2007 alone, 2.7 million people became infected with the virus, and two million people died of HIV-related causes. Nearly half a million children are infected each year and most of these infants (90%) are infected through vertical transmission from the mother during pregnancy, labor or in the neonatal period through breastfeeding. Breastfeeding by HIV positive mothers is discouraged in North America and Europe. Since safe and affordable alternatives are not available in many developing countries, it is still an acceptable practice in many of these countries.

In a landmark clinical trial published in 1994, investigators were able to demonstrate that perinatal transmission can be reduced by two-thirds by treating HIV infected mothers with Zidovudine during pregnancy, labor and treatment of neonate in the first few weeks of life.[5] This quickly became the standard of care in the US but it was cost prohibitive in most developing countries where HIV was a major clinical problem. Many modified trials soon followed. A Thai trial, for example, demonstrated that Zidovudine during the last one month of pregnancy and labor alone can reduce the transmission rate by one half in non-breastfeeding mothers.[6] Similar regimen in breastfeeding mothers showed a reduction in transmission by almost 40%.[7] Cesarean section before the onset of labor and rupture of membranes reduces transmission to the infant by 50% if the mother is not receiving retroviral therapy and by 87% if she is receiving therapy.[8,9] In the US, anti-retroviral drugs are given to HIV infected women during pregnancy, labor and delivery and neonates are treated with Zidovudine soon after birth.

11.1.2 *Bacterial infection*

Epidemiology of bacterial infection in the neonatal period has changed over the years. Organisms colonizing the maternal genitourinary tract account for the vast majority of early onset neonatal infections. In the pre-antimicrobial era, Group A *Streptococcus* was the predominant organism.

After the introduction of penicillin and sulphonamides, gram negative organisms, especially *E. coli*, became the primary offending agent. *Staphylococcus aureus* was a major pathogen in the 1950s and early 1960s. We saw the emergence of Group B *Streptococcus* (GBS) in the 1970s. Today both *E. coli* and GBS remain the main source of early onset sepsis in the neonate in the US. In recent years, survival of very low birth weight infants has been associated with an increased risk of nosocomial infection during their hospital stay. These infants develop infections, typically between two and three weeks and have double the mortality of comparable very low birth weight infants without infection. Two bacterial diseases that are rather unique to neonates and how we have been able to impact them are highlighted below.

11.1.2.1 *Ophthalmia neonatorum*

Purulent conjunctivitis during the first 28 days is defined as ophthalmia neonatorum. It was a major cause of blindness in the 19th century and is still a significant problem in developing countries. It is caused, for the most part, by gonococcal and chlamydia infection. Ophthalmia neonatorum was observed in 8% of infants in the US before the introduction of ophthalmic prophylaxis. It occurs at birth, or more commonly 2–5 days after birth. There is an increased risk with prolonged rupture of membranes and in premature infants. Ophthalmia neonatorum has become a rare disease today among newborn infants, especially in the US. Two important factors account for this observation. One, antenatal screening of pregnant mothers has become routine, leading to treatment in infected women. This practice combined with the use of antibiotic prophylaxis soon after birth accounts for this reduction.

Credé introduced silver nitrate prophylaxis in 1881. Uncontrolled studies showed a dramatic decrease in the incidence with the use of silver nitrate. Many investigators touted antibiotics because it is less irritating to the eye compared to silver nitrate. It is of interest to note that New York City reported an increase in the incidence of ophthalmia neonatorum when bacitracin was substituted for silver nitrate. Comparison of erythromycin to silver nitrate followed. These trials showed that there was no significant difference between silver nitrate and erythromycin prophylaxis.[10] Today erythromycin or tetracycline ophthalmic ointment is used for prophylaxis in developed countries, whereas silver nitrate is still being used in many developing countries. Silver nitrate may have an advantage in areas where penicillinase producing gonococcal infection is a problem.

11.1.2.2 *Group B streptococcus infection*

GBS is a very common pathogen that colonizes the genital or lower gastrointestinal tract of up to one third of all pregnant women. Some of the differences in the colonization rate globally may relate to the number of cultures obtained from a single site, the frequency of testing and the techniques used. Several other factors affecting colonization also have been identified. These include age, parity, and ethnicity. In the 1970s, GBS invasive disease occurred in 2–3 per 1000 live births in the US accounting for over 10,000 cases. Mortality ranged from 23–55%. By the late 1990s, the attack rate has been reduced to less than 0.5 per 1000 births along with a reduction in mortality to approximately 10%. The reduction in 1998, for example, was estimated to be nearly 4000 early onset cases and over 200 deaths. Its incidence has been reduced even further (0.33/1000) in recent reports.[11] This substantial reduction in neonatal death is not the result of any new antibiotics but is due to the innovative use of existing antibiotics. GBS is very sensitive to penicillin, which has been available for decades. This remarkable achievement can be attributed to the antibiotic prophylaxis regimen used during labor today. We will review the evolution of this strategy.

GBS reaches the fetus *in utero* through ascending infection of the placental membrane and/or the amniotic fluid. The newborn may also acquire the organism during passage through the birth canal. GBS may promote rupture of membranes and preterm delivery. Although most of the affected neonates are term, preterm infants have much higher incidence of GBS disease. Vertical transmission occurs in nearly one half of infants born to colonized mothers. Early diagnosis and treatment of culture positive women for 1–2 weeks in late pregnancy was attempted in the early 1970s with only limited success. Intravenous antibiotics during labor were attempted next. These studies clearly showed that ampicillin prevented vertical transmission successfully. Steigman and colleagues in 1978 reported that there had been no cases of GBS for 22 years in their institution and attributed their finding to penicillin G prophylaxis for ophthalmia neonatorum.[12] Their institutional practice was to administer one dose of penicillin within half an hour of birth to all newborn infants. Subsequent prospective studies confirmed a reduction in the incidence of GBS among infants receiving penicillin prophylaxis. It also became clear that timing of prophylaxis is important and that infection that has begun *in utero* cannot be prevented by postnatal prophylaxis.

Results of antepartum and intrapartum treatment studies were initially confusing and contradictory. This was related to several factors including colonization rate which varies in different groups and changes during pregnancy. The relationship of neonatal disease to maternal colonization is less than 1% which makes it very difficult to prove a reduction in neonatal disease with any treatment regimen from a single institution in a reasonable time. However, infants born to women with GBS colonization, with preterm labor or prolonged rupture of membranes constituted a very high risk group. These infants represented approximately two thirds of all neonatal GBS diseases and 94% of all neonatal deaths due to this disease. Early evidence supporting the effectiveness of intrapartum prophylaxis in reducing invasive disease in neonates was provided by Boyer and Gotoff in 1986.[13] In this study, GBS colonized women with premature labor, prolonged rupture of membranes or maternal fever were randomly assigned to routine care or intrapartum intravenous ampicillin. None of the infants born to mothers receiving antibiotics developed invasive disease, whereas 5/79 infants in the routine care group developed invasive disease and one died. Several other studies have subsequently confirmed these results and the cost effectiveness of this strategy. For intrapartum prophylaxis to be effective in preventing the disease, the antibiotics must be administered at least four hours prior to delivery.

The American Academy of Pediatrics (AAP) and the American College of Obstetricians and Gynecologists (ACOG) published their recommendations regarding intrapartum chemoprophylaxis in 1992.[14,15] Although there were several areas of concurrence, significant differences existed between these recommendations. Both agreed that preterm labor, premature and prolonged rupture of membranes and maternal fever constituted risk factors for developing early onset neonatal disease. The primary difference was on the utilization of maternal culture results by AAP, whereas ACOG based their recommendation on risk factors alone. Neither recommendation was fully implemented by the practicing physicians. New consensus guidelines were published in 1996 by the CDC,[16] endorsed by both AAP and ACOG. These guidelines suggested that hospitals and obstetricians adopt either a risk based or culture based strategy to identify women requiring intrapartum GBS prophylaxis. Approximately 25% of pregnant women qualify for intrapartum prophylaxis by either strategy. However, it became clear in subsequent years that the culture based approach was more effective. The revised guidelines by the CDC were published in 2002,[17] which remain the gold standard today. It must be mentioned that public interest groups such as Group B Strep association, a nonprofit organization founded by parents who lost their children to GBS disease, also played an important role in the education and research on GBS disease. The current regimen has reduced neonatal colonization and infection rates significantly as well as neonatal mortality, although regional and racial differences persist. Rapid identification of GBS colonized women has been a major impediment in the implementation of the current strategy. The potential for polymerase chain reaction (PCR) based screening is that it is not only rapid but also has high sensitivity and specificity. Results can be available in less than an hour. The clinical performance characteristics of a real-time PCR assay using vaginal/rectal swabs from antepartum (35–37 weeks of gestation) and intrapartum women was evaluated in a multi-center trial.[18] These authors concluded that performance characteristics of the PCR assay exceed the threshold recommended by the CDC when compared with culture. FDA has already approved a PCR based screening test. It awaits wider implementation.

11.2 Neural Tube Defects and Folate Supplementation

Neural tube defects (NTD) are congenital malformations which arise during the development of the brain and spinal cord, and include anencephaly, myelomeningocele and encephalocele. Anencephaly is incompatible with survival, whereas the other two have a high perinatal and infant mortality. Impairments in surviving children vary in severity depending on the location of the defect, its size, extent of neural tissue damage and the degree of accompanying hydrocephalus. They often have reduced mobility and sensation, incontinence, and learning difficulties. Epidemiological and genetic studies indicate that neural tube defects are multifactorial in origin with genetic and environmental causes.[19] Geographical variations in the prevalence of NTD, both between and within countries, can be considerable. For example, the prevalence in China was six per 1000 in the Northern Province compared to one per 1000 in the Southern Province.[20] NTD may occur as isolated defects or with other birth defects. It has increased risk of recurrence in subsequent pregnancies. The epidemiological investigation of NTD identified the protective effect of maternal periconceptional supplementation with folic acid. Research efforts also indicate that gene-gene, gene-environment, as well as maternal genetics influence NTD risk, highlighting the complexity of this disease process.[19]

In 1981, Laurence showed a 60% reduction in the risk of recurrent NTD among women who took folic acid.[21] The importance of periconceptual folate supplementation in reducing NTD emerged over a long period of time. This included data from observational studies, nonrandomized intervention trials and randomized controlled trials. One of the pivotal trials was a randomized controlled trial sponsored by the British Medical Research Council which showed that folic acid supplements (4.0 mg per day) reduced the risk of having a subsequent NTD-affected pregnancy by 70% among women with a history of prior NTD-affected pregnancy.[22] Wider acceptance of folic acid supplementation slowly followed. There are numerous studies that have documented the impact of folic acid supplementation.[23–26] Periconceptual folate supplementation in China, for example, reduced NTD in the highly prevalent area from 4.8 per 1000 pregnancies to 1.0 and in the low-NTD region from 1.0 to 0.6 per 1000.[20]

CDC issued a guideline in 1991 advocating the daily consumption of 4.0 mg of folic acid, from at least one month before conception through the first three months of pregnancy for women with a prior history of NTD-affected pregnancy who are planning to start a new pregnancy.[27] In 1992, they recommended that all women of childbearing age should consume 0.4 mg of folic acid per day to reduce the risk of a NTD-affected pregnancy.[28] Women at higher recurrent risk who are planning to become pregnant can follow the 1991 guideline and consult their physicians. Folic acid fortification of all enriched cereal-grain products went into effect in January 1998 as required by the FDA.[29] According to CDC report, NTD rate has decreased 26% in the US since folic acid fortification began. The prevalence of neural tube defects in Canada has decreased by nearly half from 1.58 per 1000 births before fortification to 0.86 per 1000 births during the full-fortification period.[30] Uniform compliance is estimated to decrease the incidence of NTD by up to 70% resulting in an overall incidence of 0.6 per 1000 pregnancies and prevent this disease in approximately 2000 babies per year in the US. By reducing NTD, folic acid fortification of grain may yield a substantial economic benefit as well. The best estimate of this benefit ranges from approximately $100 million to $250 million depending on the level of fortification.

Consumption of adequate folic acid will reduce some, but not all, NTD. Further research will be needed to identify the causes of NTD that are not reduced by folic acid intake. Folic acid enters cells of certain tissues via a receptor-mediated process. The folate receptor alpha gene codes for the protein responsible for binding folate, which is the first, and only, folate-dependent step in folate transport. It appears unlikely that the beneficial effects of maternal folate supplementation acts through this mechanism. Despite extensive genetic analysis of folate cycle enzymes, and quantification of metabolites in maternal blood, neither the protective mechanism nor the relationship between maternal folate status and susceptibility for NTD are understood completely. Genotyping of samples for known polymorphisms in genes encoding folate-associated enzymes have not revealed any correlation between specific genotypes and the observed abnormalities in folate metabolism, suggesting that as yet unrecognized genetic variants result in embryonic abnormalities of folate cycling may be causally related to NTD.

11.3 Rh Hemolytic Disease and Anti-D Globulin

Approximately 85% of the US population is Rh-positive. If an Rh-negative woman conceives a child with an Rh-positive partner, there is a potential for Rh incompatibility between the mother and the fetus. Rh hemolytic disease is caused by transplacental passage of Rh-positive fetal red cells to the maternal circulation. This results in sensitization in Rh-negative women and induces the development of antibodies typically occurring late in pregnancy or soon after delivery. Therefore, the first pregnancy where it occurs is usually not seriously affected by hemolysis. In subsequent pregnancies, the antibodies cross the placenta and cause hemolysis in the Rh-positive fetus and newborn. In general, the fetus of each subsequent pregnancy exhibits more severe effects than in the previous pregnancy. Severely affected infants may die *in utero* or are born prematurely. They are often very anemic, have severe edema, ascites and pleural and pericardial effusions. Neonatal management of these severely affected infants, infants with hydrops fetalis, includes maximal cardiorespiratory support in addition to the management of severe anemia and hyperbilirubinemia. Early exchange transfusion is the cornerstone of Rh hemolytic disease management. It removes bilirubin, sensitized red cells, antibodies, and increases hemoglobin concentration and oxygen carrying capacity. Before exchange transfusion became available, mortality was extremely high for hydrops fetalis.

The greatest innovation in the care of infants with Rh hemolytic disease occurred with maternal administration of anti-D immune globulin to Rh-negative mother at the time of delivery. Alloimmunization rate after two pregnancies in Rh-negative women fell from approximately 16% to 2% with routine postpartum administration of a single dose of anti-D immune globulin and was further reduced to as low as 0.1% with the addition of routine antenatal administration in the third trimester.[31] Anti-D immune globulin is a sterile solution containing IgG anti-D manufactured from human plasma. Administration of this drug results in the lysis of fetal cells in maternal circulation thereby preventing sensitization. A single 300 microgram dose contains sufficient anti-D to suppress the immune response to 15 mL of Rh-positive red blood cells. Administration of anti-D immune globulin is now the standard of care. It should be administered to Rh-negative women any time when there is an increased risk for fetal cells to enter the pregnant woman's circulation such as miscarriage, ectopic pregnancy, chorionic villus sampling and amniocentesis. Further refinement of this therapy has resulted in the administration of anti-D immune globulin at 28 weeks to maximize benefits.[32] If given correctly, this medication is more than 99% effective in the prevention of Rh hemolytic disease. Rh hemolytic disease has become a rarity in the NICU today.

11.4 Patent Ductus Arteriosus (PDA) and Indomethacin

Lungs are fluid filled *in utero* and the vast majority of the right ventricular output bypasses the lung through the ductus arteriosus. Ductus arteriosus typically closes within the first day in most term infants. Incidence of PDA (failure to close within 72 hours) is approximately 1 in 2–5000 births. However, it is much more prevalent in preterm infants and is inversely related to birth weight. PDA is present in nearly 50% of preterm infants weighing less than 1000 g.[33] Increased frequency of PDA is seen in infants with RDS, whereas antenatal steroid administration decreases its incidence. Clinically significant PDA is associated with increased blood flow to the lungs and decreased blood flow to other organs. Clinical symptoms include heart murmur, increased precordial activity, bounding pulses, wide pulse pressure, and hypotension. Increased pulmonary blood flow results in pulmonary edema and may contribute to respiratory failure, metabolic acidosis and apnea and bradycardia. Systemic hypoperfusion may result in metabolic acidosis and predisposes these infants to necrotizing enterocolitis and renal dysfunction. If left untreated, cardiac hypertrophy with failure may develop.

Approximately 25,000 infants are treated yearly for PDA in the US. Treatment of PDA has evolved over the years. Initially, medical management was the norm in these infants. Surgical ligation became part of the management in the early 1970s. Indomethacin which inhibits cyclooxygenase (COX) systems was introduced as a treatment for PDA in the mid-1970s. It decreases prostaglandins by blocking the conversion of arachidonic acid to prostaglandins. We now know that prostaglandins, especially PGE2, are involved in the closure of ductus arteriosus. Following birth circulating PGE2 decreases due to the removal of the placental source and increased pulmonary metabolism. In full term infants, ductal constriction induces significant local hypoxia resulting in upregulation of a number of inflammatory mediators initiating a cascade of events that result in permanent closure. Only oral formulation of indomethacin was initially available. Absorption following oral administration was poor and incomplete and blood levels were unpredictable. Mortality of infants treated with indomethacin was similar to surgically treated infants. Early studies showed that it was an effective treatment for PDA.[34,35] No selective long term morbidity attributable to indomethacin treatment has been observed on follow up.[36] Ductus arteriosus is less responsive to PGE2 as gestation advances and therefore, indomethacin is less effective in closing PDA with increasing postnatal age.

Advent of echocardiography was an important milestone in the diagnosis of PDA. Today, this noninvasive imaging technique is the gold standard in evaluating the status of the PDA and its response to therapy. Management of preterm infants with PDA can be categorized into three, i.e. conservative medical management with fluid restriction and judicious use of diuretics, pharmacological closure, and surgical ligation. Indomethacin became the mainstay in medical management for at least two decades. It has been used either for prophylaxis or as treatment of symptomatic PDAs. Although no effects on mortality or reduction in CLD or NEC have been established, prophylactic use is associated with a significant reduction in symptomatic PDA.[33] A decrease in severe IVH has been documented as well.[33] Treatment of symptomatic infants with indomethacin is associated with an approximately 75% closure rate. It must be pointed out that spontaneous closure of the ductus can occur in approximately one-third of these infants and up to 35% of infants reopen their ductus after initial successful closure.[37] Surgical treatment is generally reserved for infants who have failed medical treatment or have contraindications to medical treatment. Surgical treatment, either primary or following failure of medical management, is associated with an increased incidence of chronic lung disease.[36] Early use of both indomethacin and postnatal corticosteroid is associated with an increased risk of gastrointestinal perforation.[38]

Indomethacin treatment for PDA has remained as the mainstay for a long time. Recently, ibuprofen was approved for use in neonates. Multiple trials comparing these two drugs have shown no significant differences in therapeutic effectiveness between these two drugs.[39,40] Both inhibit COX-1 and COX-2 isoforms but to a diiferent degree. Ibuprofen has less COX-1 inhibition than indomethacin. Indomethacin prophylaxis has a protective effect on intraventricular hemorrhage. Ibuprofen is associated with less renal toxicity and has less impact on mesenteric and cerebral blood flow. Thus, the safety profile is superior with ibuprofen and consequently, there is a shift in the usage of these drugs, from indomethacin to ibuprofen.

11.5 Persistent Pulmonary Hypertension and Inhaled Nitric Oxide

Respiratory failure in term and near-term infants is typically treated with supportive care such as oxygen and mechanical ventilation with excellent outcome. Although the vast majority of infants developing respiratory failure are preterm infants with immature lungs, a small fraction of term and near-term infants may develop respiratory failure due to other causes such as meconium aspiration syndrome and sepsis. In a subgroup of these infants, hypoxic respiratory failure develops due to decreased pulmonary blood flow, and they may not respond well to mechanical ventilation alone. Pulmonary vascular resistance is high *in utero* and only 7% of combined ventricular output passes through the lung. Most of the right ventricular output is diverted into the systemic circulation through the ductus arteriosus. In most term and near-term infants systemic blood pressure increases and pulmonary vascular resistance decreases following birth, resulting in increased pulmonary blood flow and improved gas exchange. In some infants, pulmonary vascular resistance may remain elevated leading to persistent pulmonary hypertension (PPHN) and hypoxic respiratory failure. The phrase PPHN was first coined by Levin *et al.* to describe a group of newborns with severe pulmonary hypertension, clear chest radiographs, and right-to-left shunting across the ductus arteriosus,[41] although the association of respiratory distress syndrome with pulmonary hypertension and right-to-left ductal shunting was shown in the early 1960s by Rudolph and co-workers. We know now that PPHN could complicate the course of other diseases of the newborn, such as meconium aspiration and pulmonary hypoplasia as well. Echocardiographic evaluation is essential in the initial evaluation and ongoing management of severe hypoxic respiratory failure due to PPHN.

Over the years, a variety of approaches to the management of PPHN were tried with limited success. The underlying premise was to decrease pulmonary vascular pressures and increase pulmonary blood flow. These measures included hyperventilation, alkalinization and vasodilator therapy. Tolazoline was one of the few vasodilator agents available at that time but its usage resulted in limited success. The main problem with this drug was that it was not a selective pulmonary vasodilator and often resulted in systemic hypotension and other side effects such as gastrointestinal hemorrhage. Extracorporeal membrane oxygenation (ECMO), a form of heart-lung bypass, remained as the only available rescue option for these infants. In this scenario, one carotid artery, a major source of blood supply to the brain, had to be tied off permanently and the infant maintained on anticoagulants for several days while waiting for PPHN to resolve. This invasive procedure is associated with significant risks such as stroke and brain hemorrhage.

Another potential treatment option developed with the discovery of endothelium-derived relaxing factor in 1980. Early studies on this compound were done without any knowledge of its chemical structure. No one in their wildest imagination could forsee its development as a treatment for PPHN at that time. Identification of endothelium-derived relaxing factor as nitric oxide (NO) soon followed. Intense research in this area led to the award of Nobel Prizes to three US scientists in 1998. NO is a free radical with very short half life (3–5 s). It is a clear, odorless gas that diffuses easily across cell membranes. Most importantly, it is a potent vasodilator. Nitroglycerin, nitroprusside and related nitro compounds relax smooth muscle by liberating NO which stimulates cyclic AMP.

Frostell *et al.* showed that inhaled NO is a selective pulmonary vasodilator in the animal model of pulmonary hypertension.[42] Improvement in oxygenation in human neonates with PPHN with inhaled NO was demonstrated subsequently. Results of multi-center trials with inhaled NO showed that it is an effective treatment for neonatal PPHN and reduces the number of neonates requiring ECMO.[43,44] Since it is a selective pulmonary vasodilator, its effect on systemic blood pressure was essentially nonexistent. No other serious side effects were noted in these studies. FDA approved the use of inhaled NO for neonatal pulmonary hypertension in 1999. It was approved in Europe in 2001. Since the FDA approval, inhaled NO has become the standard of care among term or near-term infants with hypoxic respiratory failure. Only infants who fail to respond to this therapy are considered for ECMO. Inhaled NO treatment improved short-term pulmonary outcomes and decreased ECMO utilization. Inhaled NO treatment may also play a role in stabilizing patients before ECMO is initiated.

Based on the available evidence, an initial dose at 20 ppm of inhaled NO is recommended in term newborns with PPHN. The lowest effective starting dose for inhaled NO in term newborns with PPHN has not been determined. Numerous strategies for weaning the inhaled NO have been utilized but little differences have been observed. The typical duration of inhaled NO treatment in PPHN is less than five days. One should observe for evidence of rebound pulmonary hypertension when inhaled NO therapy is discontinued. Other causes of pulmonary hypertension should be considered when inhaled NO is required for longer than five days. NO reacts with oxygen to form nitrogen dioxide, a potential toxic agent. Therefore, it is stored in inert gas such as nitrogen. Since its effects are transient, NO is administered continuously while carefully monitoring the concentration of both NO and nitrogen dioxide. In the presence of oxyhemoglobin, NO is rapidly converted to nitrate with the formation of methemoglobin. Although brief exposures to higher doses appear to be safe, sustained treatment with higher doses of NO increases the risk of methemoglobinemia.

Inhaled NO has potential clinical benefits in a number of other disease states as well. Effects of inhaled NO may be less when lung volume is suboptimal in various parenchymal diseases. Pulmonary hypertension may be exacerbated because of the adverse mechanical effects of under inflation and over inflation on pulmonary vascular resistance. Atelectasis, pneumonia and pulmonary edema may decrease the effective delivery of inhaled NO to its site of action. Inhaled NO treatment trials in patients with congenital diaphragmatic hernia found no difference in the combined endpoint of death and/or ECMO utilization between NO treated and control infants. However, it clearly plays a role in the treatment of late pulmonary hypertension in patients with CDH.

Several key observations suggest that inhaled NO is potentially beneficial in preterm infants at high risk for developing chronic lung disease. NO has been shown to improve oxygenation in preterm infants with respiratory failure. Furthermore, it improves surfactant function, reduces lung inflammation in an animal model and reduces hyperoxic lung injury. However, results of the majority of NO trials in critically ill preterm infants have not shown any longer term beneficial effects, including a large multi-center trial by Van Meurs *et al.*[45] No decrease in the rates of death or bronchopulmonary dysplasia was found with the use of inhaled nitric oxide in critically ill premature infants weighing less than 1500 g. Moreover, worse outcomes were seen in a subgroup of neonates with birth weights of 1000 g or less.[41] On the other hand, Schreiber *et al.* showed that the incidence of chronic lung disease and death among premature infants with the respiratory distress syndrome is reduced by treatment with low-dose inhaled nitric oxide.[46] This treatment also decreased severe intraventricular hemorrhage and periventricular leukomalacia.[46] A two-year follow-up study showed improved cognitive neurodevelopmental outcome in infants treated with inhaled nitric oxide as neonates.[47] Potential reasons for the disparities between the two studies include differences in gestational ages, ethnicity and severity of illness as pointed out in an accompanying editorial.[48]

Two large recent clinical trials investigated the potential benefit of NO in reducing chronic lung disease.[49,50] In both trials very small premature infants requiring mechanical ventilation were exposed to small doses of inhaled NO for relatively long periods. In one trial, NO was started within the first two days of life and maintained up to three weeks. In the other trial, similar infants were started at a later time period (7–21 days of age) on somewhat higher doses initially and reduced at weekly intervals and continued for up to 24 days. Kinsella *et al.*[49] observed no overall difference between groups in the combined primary outcome of death or bronchopulmonary dysplasia, although a reduction in the combined primary outcome and bronchopulmonary dysplasia alone was observed in a subgroup of infants (birth weight: 1000–1250 g). A secondary outcome of brain injury, defined as grade three or four intraventricular hemorrhage, periventricular leukomalacia or ventriculomegaly, was also reduced in the treated group. In contrast, Ballard *et al.*[50] reported that nitric oxide treatment improved survival without bronchopulmonary dysplasia and reduced the duration of oxygen therapy and hospitalization without increasing the complications of prematurity. It must be pointed out that the improvement in primary outcome was limited to infants in whom the treatment was initiated between seven and 14 days. Given the expense ($3000 per day and up to $12,000 for a 30-day period) and the lack of benefits in critically ill neonates, this treatment regimen cannot be considered cost effective. Questions still remain on the most effective dose, duration, and time of initiation of inhaled NO in less critically ill infants.

11.6 Summary

Several drugs such as surfactant, inhaled NO and anti-D immunoglobulin were developed for unique problems in the neonate, whereas other drugs such as indomethacin and penicillin, although available for decades, found unique applications in neonates. Still others such as Zidovudine and hepatitis B vaccine have reduced the transmission of HIV and HBV from mother to infant and prevent life long illness and even death. It is impossible to imagine the practice of neonatology today without these miracle drugs.

References

1. Stevens CE, Beasley RP, Tsui J, Lee WC. (1975) Vertical transmission of hepatitis B antigen in Taiwan. *N Engl J Med* 292: 771–774.
2. Bradley JS. (2006) Hepatitis. In: Remington JS, Klein OJ, Wilson CB, Baker CJ. eds. *Infectious Diseases of the Fetus and Newborn Infant*. Elsevier Saunders Philadelphia; 823–843.
3. Hepatitis B. http://www.who.int/immunization/topics/hepatitis_b/en/index.html
4. UNAIDS. 2008 Report on the global AIDS epidemic.
5. Connor EM, Sperling RS, Gelber R, *et al.* (1994) Reduction of maternal-infant transmission of human immunodeficiency virus type 1 with zidovudine treatment. *N Engl J Med* 311: 1173–1180.
6. Shaffer N, Bulterys M, Simonds RJ. (1999) Short courses of zidovudine and perinatal transmission of HIV. *N Engl J Med* 340: 1042–1043.
7. Dabis F, Msellati P, Meda N, Welffens-Ekra C, You B, Manigart O, Leroy V, Simonon A, Cartoux M, Combe P, Ouangré A, Ramon R, Ky-Zerbo O, Montcho C, Salamon R, Rouzioux C, Van de Perre P, Mandelbrot L. (1999) 6-month efficacy, tolerance, and acceptability of a short regimen of oral zidovudine to reduce vertical transmission of HIV in breastfed children in

Côte d'Ivoire and Burkina Faso: a double-blind placebo-controlled multi-centre trial. DITRAME Study Group. DIminution de la Transmission Mère-Enfant. *Lancet* 353: 786–792.

8. Riley LE, Green MF. (1999) Elective caesarean delivery to reduce the transmission of HIV. *N Engl J Med* 340: 13, 1032.

9. The International Perinatal HIV Group. (1999) The mode of delivery and the risk of vertical transmission of human immunodeficiency virus type 1—a meta-analysis of 15 prospective cohort studies. *N Engl J Med* 340: 977–987.

10. Hammerschlag MR, Cummings C, Roblin PM, Williams TH, Delke I. (1989) Efficacy of neonatal ocular prophylaxis for the prevention of chlamydial and gonococcal conjunctivitis. *N Engl J Med* 320: 769–772.

11. Centers for Disease Control and Prevention. (2007) Perinatal Group B Streptococcal Disease After Universal Screening Recommendations — United States, 2003–2005. *Morb Mortal Wkly Rep* 56(28): 701–705.

12. Steigman AJ, Bottone EJ, Hanna BA. (1978) Intramuscular penicillin administration at birth: prevention of early-onset group B streptococcal disease. *Pediatrics* 62: 842–844.

13. Boyer KM and Gotoff SP. (1986) Prevention of early onset of neonatal group B streptococcal disease with selective intrapartum chemoprophylaxis. *N Eng J Med* 314: 1665–1669.

14. Group B streptococcal infections in pregnancy. (1992) *ACOG Tech Bull* 170: 1–4.

15. Committee on infectious diseases and committee on fetus and newborn. (1992) Guidelines for prevention of group B streptococcal infection by chemoprophylaxis. *Pediatrics* 90: 775–778.

16. Centers for Disease Control and Prevention. (1996) Prevention of perionatal group B streptococcal disease: a public health perspective. *MMWR Morb Mortal Wkly Rep* 45: 1–24.

17. Centers for Disease Control and Prevention. (2002) Prevention of perionatal group B streptococcal disease: revised guidelines from CDC. *MMWR Morb Mortal Wkly Rep* 51: 1–22.

18. Edwards RK, Novak-Weekley SM, Koty PP, Davis T, Leeds LJ, Jordan JA. (2008) Rapid group B streptococci screening using a real-time polymerase chain reaction assay. *Obstet Gynecol* 111: 1335–1341.

19. Mitchell LE. (2005) Epidemiology of neural tube defects. *Am J Med Genet C Semin Med Genet* 135C(1): 88–94.

20. Berry RJ, Li Z, Erickson JD, Li S, Moore CA, Wang H, Mulinare J, Zhao P, Wong LY, Gindler J, Hong SX, Correa A. (1999) Prevention of neural-tube defects with folic acid in China. China-U.S. Collaborative Project for Neural Tube Defect Prevention. *N Engl J Med* 341: 1485–1490.

21. Laurence KM, James N, Miller M, *et al.* (1981) Double blind randomized controlled trial of folate treatment before conception to prevent recurrence of neural-tube defects. *Br Med J* 282: 1509–1511.

22. MRC Vitamin Study Research Group. (1991) Prevention of neural tube defects: results of the Medical Research Council Vitamin Study. *Lancet* 338: 131–137.

23. Werler, Shapiro S, Mitchell AA. (1993) Periconceptional folic acid exposure and risk of occurrence neural tube defects. *JAMA* 269: 1257–1261.

24. Shaw GM, Schaffer D, Velie EM, *et al.* (1995) Periconceptional vitamin use, dietary folate, and the occurrence of neural tube defects in California. *Epidemiology* 6: 219–226.

25. Czeizel AE, Dudas I. (1992) Prevention of the first occurrence of neural tube defects by periconceptional vitamin supplementation. *N Eng J Med* 327: 1832–1835.

26. Smithells RW, Nevin NC, Seller MJ, *et al.* (1983) Further experience of vitamin supplementation for the prevention of neural tube defect recurrences. *Lancet* 1: 1027–1031.

27. Centers for Disease Control and Prevention. (1991) Use of folic acid for prevention of spina bifida and other neural tube defects — 1983–1991. *MMWR* 40: 513–516.

28. Centers for Disease Control. (1992) Recommendations for the use of folic acid to reduce the number of cases of spina bifida and other neural tube defects. *MMWR* 41 (No. RR-14).

29. Food and Drug Administration. (1996) Food standards: amendment of standards of identity for enriched grain products to require addition of folic acid. *Federal Register* 61: 8781–8797.

30. De Wals P, Tairou F, Van Allen MI, Uh SH, Lowry RB, Sibbald B, Evans JA, Van den Hof MC, Zimmer P, Crowley M, Fernandez B, Lee NS, Niyonsenga T. (2007) Reduction in neural-tube defects after folic acid fortification in Canada. *N Engl J Med* 357: 135–142.

31. Bowman, JM. (1988) The prevention of Rh immunization. *Transfus Med Rev* 2: 129.

32. American College of Obstetricians and Gynecologists. (1999) Prevention of Rho(D) alloimmunization. American College of Obstetricians and Gynecologists Practice Bulletin No. 4. Washington, DC.

33. Schmidt B, Davis P, Moddemann D, Ohlsson A, Roberts RS, Saigal S, Solimano A, Vincer M, Wright LL. (2001) Trial of Indomethacin Prophylaxis in Preterms Investigators. Long-term effects of indomethacin prophylaxis in extremely-low-birth-weight infants. *N Engl J Med* 344: 1966–1972.

34. Yanagi RM, Wilson A, Newfeld EA, Aziz KU, Hunt CE. (1981) Indomethacin treatment for symptomatic patent ductus arteriosus: a double-blind control study. *Pediatrics* 67: 647–652.

35. Gersony WM, Peckham GJ, Ellison RC, Miettinen OS, Nadas AS. (1983) Effects of indomethacin in premature infants with patent ductus arteriosus: results of a national collaborative study. *J Pediatr* 102: 895–906.

36. Madan JC, Kendrick D, Hagadorn JI, Frantz ID 3rd. (2009) National Institute of Child Health and Human Development Neonatal Research Network. Patent ductus arteriosus therapy: impact on neonatal and 18-month outcome. *Pediatrics* 123: 674–681.

37. Herrera C, Holberton J, Davis P. (2007) Prolonged versus short course of indomethacin for the treatment of patent ductus arteriosus in preterm infants. *Cochrane Database Syst Rev.* April 18: (2): CD003480.

38. Stark AR, Carlo WA, Tyson JE, Papile LA, Wright LL, Shankaran S, Donovan EF, Oh W, Bauer CR, Saha S, Poole WK, Stoll BJ. (2001) National Institute of Child Health and Human Development Neonatal Research Network. Adverse effects of early dexamethasone in extremely-low-birth-weight infants. National Institute of Child Health and Human Development Neonatal Research Network. *N Engl J Med* 344: 95–101.

39. Van Overmeire B, Smets K, Lecoutere D, Van de Broek H, Weyler J, Degroote K, Langhendries JP. (2000) A comparison of ibuprofen and indomethacin for closure of patent ductus arteriosus. *N Engl J Med* 343: 674–481.

40. Patel J, Roberts I, Azzopardi D, Hamilton P, Edwards AD. (2000) Randomized double-blind controlled trial comparing the effects of ibuprofen with indomethacin on cerebral hemodynamics in preterm infants with patent ductus arteriosus. *Pediatr Res* 47: 36–42.

41. Levin DL, Heymann MA, Kitterman JA, Gregory GA, Phibbs RH, Rudolph AM. (1976) Persistent pulmonary hypertension of the newborn infant. *J Pediatr* 89: 626–630.

42. Frostell C, Fratacci MD, Wain JC, Jones R, Zapol WM. (1991) Inhaled nitric oxide. A selective pulmonary vasodilator reversing hypoxic pulmonary vaso-constriction. *Circulation* 83: 2038–2047.

43. Kinsella JP, Truog WE, Walsh WF, Goldberg RN, Bancalari E, Mayock DE, Redding GJ, deLemos RA, Sardesai S, McCurnin DC, Moreland SG, Cutter GR, Abman SH. (1997) Randomized, multicenter trial of inhaled nitric oxide and high-frequency oscillatory ventilation in severe, persistent pulmonary hyper-tension of the newborn. *J Pediatr* 131: 55–62.

44. Davidson D, Barefield ES, Kattwinkel J, Dudell G, Damask M, Straube R, Rhines J, Chang CT. (1998) Inhaled nitric oxide for the early treatment of persistent pulmonary hypertension of the term newborn: a randomized, double-masked, placebo-controlled, dose-response, multicenter study. The I-NO/PPHN Study Group. *Pediatrics* 101:325–334.

45. Van Meurs KP, Wright LL, Ehrenkranz RA, Lemons JA, Ball MB, Poole WK, Perritt R, Higgins RD, Oh W, Hudak ML, Laptook AR, Shankaran S, Finer NN, Carlo WA, Kennedy KA, Fridriksson JH, Steinhorn RH, Sokol GM, Konduri GG, Aschner JL, Stoll BJ, D'Angio CT, Stevenson DK. (2005) Preemie Inhaled Nitric Oxide Study. Inhaled nitric oxide for premature infants with severe respiratory failure. *N Engl J Med* 353: 13–22.

46. Schreiber MD, Gin-Mestan K, Marks JD, Huo D, Lee G, Srisuparp P. (2003) Inhaled nitric oxide in premature infants with the respiratory distress syndrome. *N Engl J Med* 349: 2099–2107.

47. Mestan KK, Marks JD, Hecox K, Huo D, Schreiber MD. (2005) Neurodevelopmental outcomes of premature infants treated with inhaled nitric oxide. *N Engl J Med* 353: 23–32.

48. Richard JM, Michele CW. (2005) Inhaled nitric oxide for preterm infants — who benefits? *NEJM* 353: 82–83.

49. Kinsella JP, Cutter GR, Walsh WF, *et al.* (2006) Early inhaled nitric oxide therapy in premature newborns with respiratory failure. *N Engl J Med* 355: 354–364.

50. Ballard RA, Truog WE, Cnaan A, *et al.* (2006) Inhaled nitric oxide in preterm infants undergoing mechanical ventilation. *N Engl J Med* 355: 343–353.

Chapter 12

Impact of Surgical Innovations

Oommen P. Mathew*

Like many other areas of medicine, surgical treatment options over the years have evolved and expanded for neonatal diseases. The intent of this chapter is not to catalog these innovations but to highlight the impact of few important ones. I have chosen the treatments of retinopathy of prematurity, hypoplastic left heart syndrome and transposition of great arteries, as well as minimally invasive and fetal surgeries for this purpose.

12.1 Retinopathy of Prematurity (ROP)

ROP is a common blinding disease in children in developed countries and is becoming increasingly prevalent in the developing countries, accounting for approximately 50,000 blind children globally. It has emerged in three waves. The first wave occurred in the late 1940s and 1950s. ROP, known as retrolental fibroplasia (RLF) then, was the leading cause of blindness in children in the US. During this first epidemic 7000 infants are estimated to have lost their vision from RLF. Formation of scar tissue behind the lens leading to detachment of the retina is the cause of blindness in these infants. In addition, vision of thousands of other infants was affected by this disease. Several publications in the 1950s suggested a strong association between oxygen use and RLF. These included prospective controlled studies on the use of oxygen. The first such controlled study by Patz and

---

*Professor of Pediatrics, Medical College of Georgia.

colleagues showed that use of high concentration of oxygen in low birth weight infants was associated with a higher incidence of RLF.[1] This led to the recommendation in 1954 by the Pediatric Advisory Committee that infants receive oxygen only as needed and then in concentrations not to exceed 40%. However, it must be noted that RLF was not exclusively a disease of low birth weight infants exposed to oxygen therapy. RLF has been reported in preterm infants not exposed to oxygen, as well as in term infants. A clear decrease in RLF followed the restrictive use of oxygen in preterm infants. This era, unfortunately, was also marked by an increase in mortality as well as neurological morbidity in neonates.

A re-emergence of ROP was noted in the late 1970s. One of the important changes during this period is the increased survival of low birth weight infants. The two major risk factors of ROP are prematurity and the use of oxygen. Oxygen toxicity was not the primary factor in this re-emergence of ROP. The clinical practice of oxygen therapy had changed during his period; close monitoring of blood oxygen levels has become the norm and hyperoxemia was being minimized. Phelps estimated the number of ROP blinded infants in the US in 1981 to be 883 compared to 397 in 1971.[2] A third epidemic is now emerging primarily in Eastern Europe, Latin America, India and China. Babies in these countries are being exposed to risk factors which are now largely controlled in industrialized countries.

12.1.1 *Pathogenesis*

The severity of the disease increases with decreasing gestational age. Premature birth interrupts normal retinal vascular development. Postnatal tissue oxygen levels are significantly higher than those present *in utero*, oxygen therapy can further increase tissue oxygen levels. ROP has two phases. The first phase begins with delayed retinal vascular growth after birth and partial regression of existing vessels, and the second phase consists of hypoxia-induced pathological vessel growth.[3] Hypoxia induces the release of factors stimulating new and abnormal blood vessel growth. Both oxygen-regulated and non-oxygen-regulated factors contribute to the development of ROP (Fig. 12.1). Vascular endothelial growth factor (VEGF) is an important oxygen-regulated factor, whereas insulin-like growth factor (IGF-1) is a non-oxygen-regulated growth factor. Suppression of VEGF by

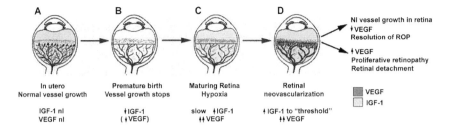

Fig. 12.1. Schematic representation of IGF-1/VEGF control of blood vessel development in ROP. (Reproduced with permission from Ref. 4.)

oxygen in phase I of ROP inhibits normal vessel growth. Elevated levels of VEGF in phase II of ROP induce pathological vessel proliferation. IGF-1 levels are low after preterm birth. Low IGF-1 levels may prevent normal vessel growth in phase I. As levels of IGF-1 rise in phase II of ROP, it indirectly regulates VEGF stimulated pathological neovascularization. Serum levels of IGF-1 in premature babies directly correlate with the severity of clinical ROP.[4] There is hope that restoration of IGF-1 to normal levels might prevent ROP.

12.1.2 *Classification*

ROP is classified using an international classification system which was developed during the cryotherapy trials. This International Classification of Retinopathy of Prematurity (ICROP) was published in two parts, the first in 1984 and later expanded in 1987, and it was modified recently.[5] This classification brings uniformity to the findings for screening and treatment of premature infants. Examinations identify the scope of vascularization, the degree of abnormal vessel growth, and the amount of the eye that is affected. In this classification, the retina is divided into three zones (Fig. 12.2), i.e. a central zone at the posterior pole of the eye with a radius of twice the distance from the optic disc to the macula (zone 1), a circle outside zone 1 with a radius from the optic nerve to the nasal ora serrata (zone 2), the remaining temporal crescent of retina (zone 3). The extent of the disease is indicated by the number of clock hours and the severity of the disease is subdivided into five stages. In stage 1, a flat white line demarcates the vascular and avascular retina, whereas in stage

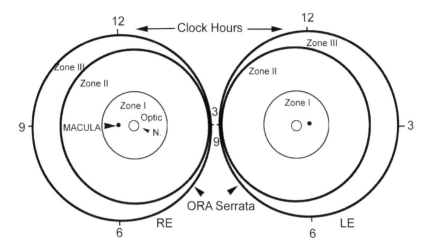

Fig. 12.2.   International classification of ROP.

2 a ridge of fibrous tissue protrudes into the vitreous. In stage 3, new blood vessels and fibrous tissue grow along the ridge. Partial retinal detachment constitutes stage 4, while total retinal detachment is stage 5. Primary treatment modalities include cryosurgery and laser photocoagulation. Although these treatments have reduced the incidence of blindness, visual outcomes after treatment are still not optimal.

12.1.3 *Treatment*

Our understanding of the pathogenesis and treatment has improved dramatically over the years. Cryotherapy and laser photocoagulation have given hope to neonates with ROP who would otherwise be blind. Initial treatment with cryotherapy produced conflicting results. This was in part related to the stage of the disease treated and whether or not the avascular zone was included in the treatment. Success rate improved dramatically only when the avascular zone was treated. A tissue temperature of –5°C is required for ablation. For cryotherapy in preterm infants probe temperature of –55°C is optimal compared to –65°C to –85°C in adults. Lower temperature can result in over treatment with increased complications such as hemorrhage, retinal tears and freezing of sclera, choroid and retina. Other complications of cryotherapy are lid edema, laceration and conjunctival and vitreous hemorrhage. Cryotherapy reduces the incidence of retinal detachment by causing regression of preretinal neovascularization.

A randomized clinical trial of cryotherapy was begun in 1986. Transscleral cryotherapy to the avascular retina was applied in one eye when there was threshold retinopathy in both eyes. Threshold ROP was defined as five consecutive or eight cumulative clock hours of extraretinal fibrovascular proliferation, in zone I or II, in the presence of plus disease. Nearly 10,000 low birth weight infants (≤ 1250 g) at 23 centers in the USA were enrolled in the CRYO-ROP trial. Among these infants, 291 progressed to threshold disease and were randomly assigned to either cryotherapy or control groups. Cryotherapy was performed within 72 hours. At three months, unfavorable outcome, defined as posterior retinal detachment, posterior retinal fold, or retrolental tissue that obscured the view of the posterior pole, was reduced from 43% in the control eyes to 21.8% in the cryotherapy treated eyes.[6] One year unfavorable outcome was similar (47% versus 26%).[7] Masked Teller Acuity Card assessment of grating acuity indicated an unfavorable functional outcome in 56% of the control eyes compared to 35% of the treated eyes indicating that cryotherapy reduces the risk of unfavorable retinal findings and functional outcome from threshold retinopathy of prematurity.[7] These results remained valid at 10 years at which time eyes that had received cryotherapy were much less likely than control eyes to be blind showing long-term safety and efficacy of cryotherapy in preserving visual acuity in eyes with threshold ROP.[8]

With the advent of laser, there was a shift from cryotherapy to laser photocoagulation even before adequate randomized controlled trials showed its superiority. This was in part related to the lower complications rate of laser therapy. Furthermore, it is more precise, technically easier to administer, and has less ocular and systemic side effects. Subsequent controlled studies have indeed confirmed that laser therapy is overall more superior to cryotherapy.[9,10] Although diode laser photocoagulation produces better long-term structural outcome and visual acuity compared with cryotherapy for the treatment of threshold ROP, refractive errors are not significantly different between the two groups.[11] Recent studies have shown that laser-treated eyes were significantly less myopic than cyrotherapy-treated eyes.[12] Early treatment of high-risk prethreshold ROP

Prethreshold ROP treatment

Zone	Stages				
	1	2	3	4	5
I			New		
I w/plus	New	New			
II					
II w/plus		New	No min hours		
III					
III w/plus			No min hours		

☐ Observation   ▥ Treatment

Fig. 12.3. Criteria for intervention in early treatment (prethreshold) ROP trial.[13]

reduces unfavorable outcomes even further (Fig. 12.3). Grating acuity results showed a reduction in unfavorable visual acuity outcomes with earlier treatment from 20% to 14%.[13] Unfavorable structural outcomes were reduced from 16% to 9% at nine months.

Retinal detachment and blindness occur despite timely and complete peripheral retinal laser therapy in a subset of infants. As mentioned earlier, the growth of abnormal blood vessels in ROP is stimulated by VEGF. The availability of FDA-approved drugs for anti-VEGF treatment in adults has triggered off-label and compassionate use of these drugs in neonates with promising results. Available drugs include pegaptanib sodium (Macugen) for partial blockage of VEGF-A, or drugs such as ranibizumab (Lucentis) and bevacizumab (Avastin), which cause complete blockage of VEGF-A. As VEGF is required in the developing retina for normal angiogenesis, the goal is to block the excessive levels of VEGF trapped within the overlying vitreous. At the 2008 Joint Meeting of the American Academy of Ophthalmology and European Society of Ophthalmology, Banker and his colleagues presented the results of anti-VEGF therapy in 21 babies. Fourteen eyes received laser and then anti-VEGF injections, 12 eyes received anti-VEGF injection only, and six eyes received anti-VEGF, then laser treatment. In all cases the abnormal blood vessels resolved without further treatment, and no adverse results were seen on follow-up exams.

Anti-VEGF treatment appears to provide rapid, effective treatment for ROP and was simpler and safer to provide to medically fragile babies. As abnormal vessels receded, normal retinal vessels slowly grew in their place. Larger, randomized clinical trials will be necessary to establish the safety and efficacy of anti-VEGF therapy. Such studies are currently underway.

12.1.4 *Screening*

Screening guidelines of preterm infants for ROP was originally published in 2001 and revised in 2006.[14] These guidelines are endorsed by the American Academy of Pediatrics Section on Ophthalmology, the American Academy of Ophthalmology, and the American Association for Pediatric Ophthalmology and Strabismus. As per these screening guidelines all preterm infants with birth weight less than 1500 g, or less than 28 weeks gestational age and infants with birth weight between 1500–2000 g or greater than 30 weeks gestational age with unstable clinical course should be screened for ROP. First exam should be performed at 31 weeks postmenstrual age for infants < 28 weeks at birth and at four weeks chronological age for 28–32 weeks gestational age infants. Follow-up examinations are performed at intervals of one to three weeks until the growth of retinal vessels are completed to the ora serrata. Follow-up examination within one week or less is recommended for infants with stage 1 or 2 ROP in zone 1 or stage 3 ROP in zone 2. Recent reports show the incidence of any ROP around 20% among infants with birth weight <1500 g and 27% among infants with birth weight <1200 g.[15] Among patients with any ROP, the proportion who underwent laser photocoagulation was approximately 10% during the initial hospital stay. At present, the disease causes approximately 500 new cases of blindness per year in the USA. It is anticipated that with continued screening, new guidelines for intervention and promising new forms of therapy, this number will decrease further.

12.2 Hypoplastic Left Heart Syndromes (HLHS)

HLHS consists of hypoplasia of the left ventricle with mitral atresia or stenosis, aortic atresia or stenosis and hypoplasia of the ascending aorta. Extracardiac anomalies are reported in up to 25% of cases, sometimes associated with chromosomal anomalies such as Turner's syndrome. It accounts for 1% to 3.8% of all congenital cardiac malformations. Generally these infants are full term and initially appear healthy. With closure of the ductus arteriosus, the systemic perfusion decreases, resulting in hypoxemia, acidosis, and shock. The second heart sound is loud and single and often the liver is enlarged secondary to congestive heart failure. A small subset of patients presents with cardiogenic shock and profound cyanosis at birth, because of an inadequate or absent atrial communication and are likely to die in the absence of an intervention. HLHS was a uniformly fatal disease, accounting for the majority of neonatal deaths due to congenital heart disease. Significant advances in the surgical and medical management of this disease have resulted in dramatic improvements in survival during the last three decades. HLHS should be managed on the basis of cardiac morphology, donor availability, and family wishes. Today parents have distinctly different management options, e.g. staged reconstruction, heart transplantation and occasionally compassionate care. Early prenatal detection of HLHS offers another option, i.e. termination of pregnancy.

Prenatal detection rate of HLHS has increased substantially. Hypoplasia of the left ventricle leads to dilation of the right ventricle. The systemic blood flow is provided through the ductus arteriosus. Management of HLHS diagnosed *in utero* varies considerably. In one study, 16 of 32 parents opted for termination of pregnancy and four fetuses died *in utero*. Five parents elected compassionate care, and seven patients received a palliative reconstructive procedure.[16] In another study, pregnancy was terminated in 11 of 33 fetuses. Fourteen of 22 live-born infants underwent surgery, and eight parents elected compassionate care.[17] In a very recent study from Australia, marked difference in parental decision was documented between prenatal and postnatal diagnosis of HLHS. When the diagnosis of HLHS was made prenatally, 96% infants underwent surgery, whereas only 47% infants underwent surgery when the diagnosis was made postnatally.[18]

Treatment for HLHS continues to evolve. This has resulted in improved short- and long-term survival. Staged reconstruction and heart transplantation constitute the available surgical options. For infants undergoing staged reconstruction, the Norwood procedure is performed in the newborn period, followed by a hemi-Fontan operation at 4–6 months of age, and a modified

Fontan operation at one to two years of age. The US hospital discharge data for HLHS from 1988–1997 was reviewed in a recent article.[19] Among 1986 cases of HLHS patients, the in-hospital mortality rate was 41%, which decreased from 54% in 1988 to 38% in 1997. Patients treated with the Norwood procedure increased from 8% in 1988 to 34% in 1997. The percentage of infants discharged from the hospital without surgery or transferred to another hospital remained relatively unchanged during this period. No difference in gender, race, type of insurance, or income was noted between patients treated with the Norwood procedure compared with those who received comfort care.

In a recent study, survival rate over a 14 year period for "low-risk" patients managed with Norwood staged palliation was 80% at hospital discharge after stage 1, and 69% at one year.[20] At present several centers worldwide report less than 10% surgical mortality for stage 1. Patients without significant non-cardiac abnormality or prematurity less than 35 weeks or mechanical and circulatory support prior to stage 1 was classified as "low-risk" patients in this study.[20] Other recognized risk factors are chromosomal anomalies, abnormal tricuspid valve with severe regurgitation and intact atrial septa. In another recent publication, the five-year actuarial survival for patients who underwent operations was 61%.[21]

Several factors have contributed to the increased survival rate. A recent modification of the Norwood procedure is the placement of a right ventricle to pulmonary artery conduit instead of a systemic artery to pulmonary shunt (modified BT shunt) as the source of pulmonary blood flow. This modification has improved postoperative stability, and decreased inter-stage mortality.[18,22] Others have reported that routine postoperative use of ventricular assist device has been useful in meeting increased cardiac output demands following Norwood operation with resultant stable postoperative period, less aggressive ventilator or inotrope support.[23] Several modifications of Fontan's operation have been utilized. One is a fenestrated Fontan operation. A new approach for Fontan completion is the catheter-facilitated (i.e. non-surgical) placement of a stent covered with a thin layer of Goretex from the inferior vena cava to the hemi-Fontan baffle.

With increasing survival of infants with HLHS, the focus has shifted to health status and neurodevelopmental outcome. Although these children enjoy a number of sports activities, they tire easily and do not perform at a very high intensity level. Their limited ability to increase cardiac output during exercise as well as the blunted heart rate response due to sinus node dysfunction often contributes to this problem. Increased risks for thrombo-embolism, as well as protein loosing enteropathy have been recognized in a minority of survivors.

Neurological outcome of the survivors are of immense interest as well. By school-age many of these children exhibit neurodevelopmental problems.[24] Increased incidence of cerebral palsy and attention deficit/hyperactivity disorders have been documented in these infants. Rogers and colleagues found that majority of children with HLHS had major developmental disabilities.[25] More recent reports have been more encouraging. For example, Goldberg and colleagues[26,27] reported that mean IQ scores were within the normal range for subjects with HLHS at three to seven years of age. Nevertheless, overall data seem to suggest that median scores are lower than that reported in the general population. It must also be noted that median Mental Developmental Index and Psychomotor Developmental Index were significantly lower among HLHS children treated with heart transplantation than expected in the general population.[28] Additionally, structural abnormalities of brain are being recognized even before the surgical intervention among infants with HLHS. These include holoprosencephaly, agenesis of corpus callosum, subtle signs of brain dysgenesis and even periventricular leukomalacia. Such emerging data seem to point towards a neurological vulnerability among these infants and it may even begin *in utero*.

Some cardiac centers perform transplantation for management of HLHS. Overall, 25% of infants with HLHS died while waiting. The primary cause of death was cardiac failure.[29] Few patients underwent Norwood/Fontan-type surgeries as interim palliation. Nearly two-third of patients underwent cardiac transplantation with the majority receiving the organ within two months. Post-transplant actuarial survival was 72% at five years. Survival following transplantation has improved because of advances in the pre- and post-operative management, as well as new options for immunosuppression. The future for children with HLHS is encouraging as evidenced by the remarkable achievements made to date and the continued interest.

12.3 Transposition of the Great Arteries (TGA)

TGA is the most common congenital cyanotic heart disease presenting in the early neonatal period. This congenital cardiac malformation is characterized by atrioventricular concordance and ventriculoarterial discordance. Aorta originates from the morphological right ventricle and the pulmonary artery originates from the morphological left ventricle. In simple transposition, which accounts for 50% of the cases, the ventriculoarterial discordance is an isolated finding. Complex transposition includes all the cases with other coexisting malformations. When we say D-TGA or L-TGA, we are referring to the ventricular looping. The spatial relationship is described as A, D, or L. In cyanotic TGA the ventricular looping is normal (D), therefore commonly called D-TGA. In the so called "congenitally corrected" TGA the ventricular loop is L, therefore L-TGA. This is, of course, non-cyanotic, since this preserves the normal serial relationships of the pulmonary and systemic circulations. In D-TGA aortic valve is to the right relative to pulmonary valve and in L-TGA aortic valve is to left of the pulmonary valve.

Today the definitive diagnosis relies on echocardiography, which is one of the greatest advances in noninvasive cardiac imaging during the last few decades. Before this, cardiac catheterization was necessary for most infants with clinically significant cardiac defects. Two-dimensional echocardiography displays anatomy and Doppler allows the estimation of pressure and flow. Echocardiography in experienced hands is a reliable diagnostic tool, providing high sensitivity and specificity. In addition, it has become very useful for intraoperative and fetal cardiac imaging, as well as in routine care of critically ill neonates. Echocardiography has reduced the need for catheterization to cases that require clarification of certain anatomic and hemodynamic aspects or when the patient is a candidate for catheter intervention. CT or MR imaging can also offer additional details. Three-dimensional magnetic resonance imaging especially has added another dimension to noninvasive imaging. Volumes of irregular shaped heart chambers and blood flow from leaking valves can now be quantitated using this technique. 2D Doppler echocardiography is preferable for intracardiac anatomy, whereas MRI appears to be superior for defining extracardiac anatomy.

Infants with TGA usually do not survive the neonatal period without surgical intervention. The initial aim in the management of the affected newborns is to assure acceptable intracardiac mixing. The presence of an atrial or a ventricular septal defect may provide satisfactory mixing. Intravenous prostaglandin E1 infusion is often used to maintain ductal patency leading to an increase in pulmonary blood flow, which in turn increases left atrial pressure promoting left to right atrial flow. However, prostaglandin action is often modest and insufficient to assure a satisfactory oxygenation of the systemic blood. Rashkind balloon septostomy has become an important tool in the pre-operative management of these babies. This technique consists of placing a balloon-tipped catheter in the left atrium through the oval foramen and pulling back into the right atrium after inflation, tearing the atrial septum. This procedure is often echocardiographically guided to avoid radiation. It is considered successful when an atrial septal defect is at least 5 mm in diameter and there is an increase in the oxygen saturation. Rashkind balloon septostomy is often an effective and safe procedure ensuring adequate interatrial mixing.

Definitive treatment involves surgery. The early history of the surgical approach utilized atrial switch operations. These operations (Mustard or Senning) resulted in normal systemic oxygen saturation and carried low operative risk. However, significant long term complications such as right ventricular dysfunction and symptomatic arrhythmias were not uncommon among survivors. Not infrequently, these infants required pacemakers for their cardiac arrhythmias. These complications were not unexpected, since it involved extensive atrial surgery and continued functioning of right ventricle as the systemic ventricle or pump. The arterial switch procedure, on the other hand, restores the aorta and pulmonary artery to their normal anatomic positions and normalizes the physiology in infants with transposition of great vessels. Establishment of the left ventricle as the systemic ventricle and maintenance of sinus node function were important factors that contributed to the development of this procedure. Since the original description of the arterial switch operation in 1975,[30] it has become the procedure of choice and is performed typically in the first two weeks of life.

Surgical repair of TGA is performed via a median sternotomy incision during cardiopulmonary bypass, Operative mortality was initially higher than the atrial switch operations. Arterial switch has been performed in infants with intact ventricular septum, with ventricular septal defects and double outlet right ventricle. It was performed initially as a single stage operation or in two stages. Two-stage correction had several disadvantages. For the most part, it is done today as a single stage procedure. Mobilization and translocation of coronary arteries remain the most challenging part of this operation. At present, arterial switch operation is performed with extremely low early mortality rates, negligible late mortality rates, and infrequent need for reoperation. Reported 10-year survival exceeds 90%.[31] Longer term complications include supravalvar pulmonary stenosis, aortic root dilation and valvar regurgitation, bronchopulmonary collateral arteries, coronary insufficiency, and myocardial perfusion abnormalities.[32] Late mortality occurs in 1–2% of hospital survivors and is mostly secondary to acute myocardial infarction.[32]

Outcome measures up to 15 years are now available. Long-term survival exceeds 90%. The vast majority of the patients was unlimited in their physical activity and received no medication.[31] Neurocognitive outcome in children with TGA has been below expectation in several areas. These include IQ, language, visual-motor integration, and oromotor control. However, quality of life and health status as perceived by children eight to 15 years after TGA repair is excellent when compared with published normative data.[33,34] Long-term follow-up studies will be necessary to determine whether the theorized benefits of the anatomic repair are realized.

12.4 Minimal Access Surgery

Endoscopic surgeries are beginning to transform surgical treatments for infants who would otherwise have faced much more complex surgical interventions. Advances in miniaturization of instruments and hands on experience have enabled the surgeons to perform a vast array of operations in the neonate and small children utilizing these techniques. There are several reports documenting the experience with video assisted surgery in neonates. However, most of these reports involve relatively small numbers. Although operative mortality is rare, anesthetic incidents during insufflation such as oxygen desaturation, transient hypotension, hypercapnia, hypothermia, and metabolic acidosis are well recognized adverse events.[35] Ponsky and Rothenberg[36] recently reported the largest number of infants undergoing such procedures in one institution — 649 children weighing 5 kg or less underwent minimally invasive surgery during the period from 1993 to 2007. Among the 43 different procedures performed, Nissen fundoplication accounted for nearly one half. Pyloromyotomy (104 cases), PDA ligation (26 cases), tracheoesophageal fistula repair (22 cases), duodenoduodenostomy (20 cases), Hirschsprung's disease (18 cases), colonic pull-through for imperforate anus (10 cases), and congenital diaphragmatic hernia repair (10 cases) accounted for the vast majority of remaining cases. There were no surgery-related deaths. Intraoperative complication rate was less than 1% and the overall complication rate was 3%. Advances to full feeds following laparoscopic surgery were significantly sooner than with conventional surgeries. These data suggest that minimal invasive surgery in neonates is both feasible and safe.

12.5 Fetal Surgery

Open hysterotomy was the procedure of choice for fetal surgery initially. Onset of preterm labor and premature rupture of membranes pose the greatest risks for both the mother and the fetus following this procedure. Minimal access surgical techniques are being increasingly employed, utilizing modifications of existing endoscopic techniques and development of novel fetoscopic instruments. This has given rise to innovative surgical options for life-threatening fetal diseases such as severe congenital diaphragmatic hernia, twin-to-twin transfusion syndrome and obstructive uropathy. Developments in some of these conditions are highlighted in this section.

12.5.1 *Lower urinary tract obstruction*

Posterior urethral valves and urethral obstruction account for the majority of fetal lower urinary tract obstructions.[37] It is a disease of high mortality and morbidity and is associated with cystic renal dysplasia leading to progressive renal dysfunction. Severe oligohydramnios, predisposing the fetus to pulmonary hypoplasia and positional limb abnormalities are not uncommon. Male fetus is typically affected. Mortality rate with oligohydramnios may be as high as 80%, and 25–30% survivors develop end-stage renal disease requiring dialysis or transplantation.

The initial surgical approach to reversing the obstruction and optimization of renal function involved open hysterotomy. The first successful *in utero* decompression for hydronephrosis was performed in 1981. However, it was associated with maternal morbidity as well as preterm labor and its sequelae. No new cases of open fetal surgery have been reported during the last two decades. Today percutaneous vesico-amniotic shunting is the most commonly used technique. It involves the placement of a double pig-tailed catheter in the fetal bladder under ultrasound guidance to allow drainage of fetal urine to the amniotic cavity. Review of 169 cases of successful percutaneous shunt placements over 14 years found a survival rate of 47%, with nearly half of survivors developing end-stage renal disease.[38] Shunt-related complications were common. Mechanical or laser endoscopic ablation of posterior urethral valves offers another therapeutic option.[39] Even though fetal decompression therapy for lower urinary tract obstruction has been practiced for more than 25 years, there is still a lack of high-quality evidence to support this clinical practice. A randomized controlled trial of vesicoamniotic shunting in moderate to severe lower urinary tract obstruction is now in progress.

12.5.2 *Congenital diaphragmatic hernia (CDH)*

CDH is a developmental defect resulting in the failure of the posterolateral, anterior or crural diaphragm to fuse with the chest wall. Eighty five percent of lesions are left-sided, 13% right-sided and 2% bilateral. The majority of cases of CDH have an isolated defect. Survival is dependent on the degree of lung hypoplasia and pulmonary hypertension. Survival rates are between 50% and 70% for isolated CDH (see Ref. 40 for a review). Variable degrees of respiratory insufficiency and pulmonary arterial hypertension are common. Aggressive hyperventilation and hyperoxygenation and emergency repair were the cornerstones of neonatal management before the 1990s, whereas today we practice gentle ventilation, ECMO and delayed surgery with improvement in outcome.

Initial attempts of *in utero* anatomical repair were abandoned because of poor results. The observation that fetuses with congenital high airway obstruction syndrome display greater lung growth was the impetus for the concept of lung growth triggered by tracheal occlusion, which was initially performed by laparotomy and fetal neck dissection. Subsequently, an endotracheal balloon occlusion utilizing fetoscopy was developed. Its effects depend on the timing and duration. A balloon is typically inserted at 26–28 weeks and then removed at 34 weeks. This procedure has proven safe and reproducible. In the randomized controlled trial cases, tracheal occlusion did not improve survival compared to optimal neonatal care.[41] It must be noted, however, that nearly all cases had moderate hypoplasia. Fetuses with moderate hypoplasia are expected to have reasonable outcomes even without fetal intervention. In a subsequent trial, only fetuses with severe hypoplasia were selected for fetal intervention.[42] Survival till discharge in this group is between 50% and 60%. There were no maternal complications but iatrogenic preterm rupture of the membrane occurred in 25% of patients. More than 75% of patients delivered beyond 34 weeks. Major predictors of survival were gestational age at delivery and lung size prior to fetal tracheal occlusion.[43] Short-term morbidity in survivors is better than expected from the severity of lung hypoplasia. Severe developmental delay following tracheal occlusion appears to be small.

12.5.3 *Twin–twin transfusion syndrome*

Twin–twin transfusion syndrome occurs in approximately 10% of monochorionic twin pregnancies and is associated with high morbidity and mortality.[44] Transfusion of blood from the donor twin to the recipient twin via placental vascular anastomoses is the underlying phenomenon. As a consequence, the donor twin develops hypovolemia, oliguria, oligohydramnios, and growth restriction. The recipient twin develops polyhydramnios and hydrops. Discordance of amniotic fluid between the two sacs (vertical pocket 8 cm or greater in the recipient and 2 cm or less in the donor) is the widely accepted diagnostic criterion for twin–twin transfusion syndrome.[45] Serial amniocentesis or selective fetoscopic laser coagulation of the communicating vessels are the two available treatment options. The aim of amnioreduction is to minimize the amniotic fluid discordance between the two sacs and to prevent preterm delivery. However, it requires repeated invasive procedures to remove large volumes of amniotic fluid and increases the risk of adverse perinatal outcomes. The goal of laser therapy, on the other hand, is to interrupt blood flow through placental vascular anastomoses. This procedure can only be done at highly specialized centers. Recently a meta-analysis comparing the two treatments was published and included approximately 400 cases of twin–twin transfusion syndrome.[46] The results of this meta-analysis show that endoscopic laser coagulation is associated with a higher survival rate and a lower neurologic morbidity when compared to serial amnioreduction.

In summary, significant advancements have been made in the field of fetal and neonatal surgery during the last few decades. These innovations in surgical techniques have saved thousands of lives and improved patient outcome in countless others.

References

1. Patz A, Hoech LE, DeLaCruz E. (1953) Studies on the effect of high oxygen administration in retrolental fibroplasias. I: Nursery pbseervations. *Am J Ophthalmol* 35: 1245–1253.
2. Phelps DL. (1979) Retinopathy of prematurity: an estimate of vision loss in the United States. *Pediatrics* 67: 924–926.
3. Flynn JT, Chan-Ling T. (2006) Retinopathy of prematurity: two distinct mechanisms that underlie zone 1 and zone 2 disease. *Am J Ophthalmol* 142: 46–59.
4. Hellström A, Perruzzi C, Ju M, Engström E, Hård AL, Liu JL, Albertsson-Wikland K, Carlsson B, Niklasson A. (2001) Low IGF-1 suppresses VEGF-survival signaling in retinal endothelial cells: direct correlation with clinical retinopathy of prematurity. *Pro Natl Acad Sci USA* 98: 5804–5808.
5. International Committee for the Classification of Retinopathy of Prematurity. (2005) The International Classification of Retinopathy of Prematurity revisited. *Arch Ophthalmol* 123: 991–999.
6. Cryotherapy for Retinopathy of Prematurity Cooperative Group. (1988) Multicenter trial of cryotherapy for retinopathy of prematurity: preliminary results. *Pediatrics* 81: 697–706.
7. Cryotherapy for Retinopathy of Prematurity Cooperative Group. (1990) Multicenter trial of cryotherapy for retinopathy of prematurity. One-year outcome — structure and function. *Arch Ophthalmol* 108: 1408–1416.

8. Cryotherapy for Retinopathy of Prematurity Cooperative Group. (2001) Multicenter Trial of Cryotherapy for Retinopathy of Prematurity: ophthalmological outcomes at 10 years. *Arch Ophthalmol* 119: 1110–1118.

9. Connolly BP, McNamara JA, Sharma S, Regillo CD, Tasman W. (1998) A comparison of laser photocoagulation with trans-scleral cryotherapy in the treatment of threshold retinopathy of prematurity. *Ophthalmology* 105: 1628–1631.

10. Ng EY, Connolly BP, McNamara JA, Regillo CD, Vander JF, Tasman W. (2002) A comparison of laser photocoagulation with cryotherapy for threshold retinopathy of prematurity at 10 years: part 1. Visual function and structural outcome. *Ophthalmology* 109: 928–934.

11. Paysse EA, Lindsey JL, Coats DK, Contant CF Jr, Steinkuller PG. (1999) Therapeutic outcomes of cryotherapy versus transpupillary diode laser photocoagulation for threshold retinopathy of prematurity. *JAAPOS* 3: 234–240.

12. Connolly BP, Ng EY, McNamara JA, Regillo CD, Vander JF, Tasman W. (2002) A comparison of laser photocoagulation with cryotherapy for threshold retinopathy of prematurity at 10 years: part 2. Refractive outcome. *Ophthalmology* 109: 936–941.

13. Good WV. (2004) Early Treatment for Retinopathy of Prematurity Cooperative Group. Final results of the Early Treatment for Retinopathy of Prematurity (ETROP) randomized trial. *Trans Am Ophthalmol Soc* 102: 233–248.

14. Section on Ophthalmology American Academy of Pediatrics; American Academy of Ophthalmology; American Association for Pediatric Ophthalmology and Strabismus. (2006) Screening examination of premature infants for retinopathy of prematurity. *Pediatrics* 117: 572–576. Erratum in: *Pediatrics* 118: 1324.

15. Chiang MF, Arons RR, Flynn JT, Starren JB. (2004) Incidence of retinopathy of prematurity from 1996 to 2000: analysis of a comprehensive New York state patient database. *Ophthalmology* 111: 1317–1325.

16. Verheijen PM, Lisowski LA, Plantinga RF, Hitchcock JF, Bennink GB, Stoutenbeek P, Meijboom EJ. (2003) Prenatal diagnosis of the fetus with hypoplastic left heart syndrome management and outcome. *Herz* 28: 250–256.

17. Tworetzky W, McElhinney DB, Reddy VM, Brook MM, Hanley FL, Silverman NH. (2001) Improved surgical outcome after fetal diagnosis of hypoplastic left heart syndrome. *Circulation* 103: 1269–1273.

18. Tibballs J, Cantwell-Bartl A. (2008) Outcomes of management decisions by parents for their infants with hypoplastic left heart syndrome born with and without a prenatal diagnosis. *Paediatr Child Health* 44: 321–324.

19. Chang RK, Chen AY, Klitzner TS. (2002) Clinical management of infants with hypoplastic left heart syndrome in the United States, 1988–1997. *Pediatrics* 110: 292–298.

20. Jacobs JP, O'Brien SM, Chai PJ, Morell VO, Lindberg HL, Quintessenza JA. (2008) Management of 239 patients with hypoplastic left heart syndrome and related malformations from 1993 to 2007. *Ann Thorac Surg* 85: 1691–1696.

21. Kern JH, Hayes CJ, Michler RE, Gersony WM, Quaegebeur JM. (1997) Survival and risk factor analysis for the Norwood procedure for hypoplastic left heart syndrome. *Am J Cardiol* 80: 170–174.

22. Maher KO, Gidding SS, Baffa JM, Pizarro C, Norwood WI Jr. (2004) New developments in the treatment of hypoplastic left heart syndrome. *Minerva Pediatr* 56: 41–49.

23. Ungerleider RM, Shen I, Yeh T, Schultz J, Butler R, Silberbach M, Giacomuzzi C, Heller E, Studenberg L, Mejak B, You J, Farrel D, McClure S, Austin EH. (2004) Routine mechanical ventricular assist following the Norwood procedure — improved neurologic outcome and excellent hospital survival. *Ann Thorac Surg* 77: 18–22.

24. Sarajuuri A, Jokinen E, Puosi R, Eronen M, Mildh L, Mattila I, Valanne L, Lönnqvist T. (2007) Neurodevelopmental and neuroradiologic outcomes in patients with univentricular heart aged 5 to 7 years: related risk factor analysis. *J Thorac Cardiovasc Surg* 133: 1524–1532.

25. Rogers BT, Msall ME, Buck GM, Lyon NR, Norris MK, Roland JM, Gingell RL, Cleveland DC, Pieroni DR. (1995) Neurodevelopmental outcome of infants with hypoplastic left heart syndrome. *J Pediatr* 126: 496–498.

26. Goldberg CS, Schwartz EM, Brunberg JA, Mosca RS, Bove EL, Schork MA, Stetz SP, Cheatham JP, Kulik TJ. (2000) Neurodevelopmental outcome of patients after the fontan operation: a comparison between children with hypoplastic left heart syndrome and other functional single ventricle lesions. *J Pediatr* 137: 646–652.

27. Ikle L, Hale K, Fashaw L, Boucek M, Rosenberg AA. (2003) Developmental outcome of patients with hypoplastic left heart syndrome treated with heart transplantation. *J Pediatr* 142: 20–25.

28. Bordacova L, Docolomanska D, Masura J.(2007) Neuropsychological outcome in children with hypoplastic left heart syndrome. *Bratisl Lek Listy* 108(4–5): 203–206.

29. Chrisant MR, Naftel DC, Drummond-Webb J, Chinnock R, Canter CE, Boucek MM, Boucek RJ, Hallowell SC, Kirklin JK, Morrow WR, Pediatric Heart Transplant Study Group. (2005) Fate of infants with hypoplastic left heart syndrome listed for cardiac transplantation: a multicenter study. *Heart Lung Transplant* 24: 576–582.

30. Jatene AD, Fontes VF, Paulista PP, *et al.* (1975) Successful anatomic correction of transposition of the great vessels: a preliminary report. *Arq Bras Cardiol* 28: 461–464.

31. von Bernuth G. (2000) 25 years after the first arterial switch procedure: midterm results. *Thorac Cardiovasc Surg* 48: 228–232.

32. Massin MM. (1999) Midterm results of the neonatal arterial switch operation. A review. *J Cardiovasc Surg (Torino)* 40: 517–522.

33. Dunbar-Masterson C, Wypij D, Bellinger DC, Rappaport LA, Baker AL, Jonas RA, Newburger JW. (2001) General health status of children with D-transposition of the great arteries after the arterial switch operation. *Circulation* 104: 1138–1142.

34. Culbert EL, Ashburn DA, Cullen-Dean G, Joseph JA, Williams WG, Blackstone EH, McCrindle BW, Congenital Heart Surgeons Society. (2003) Quality of life of children after repair of transposition of the great arteries. *Circulation* 108: 857–862.

35. Kalfa N, Allal H, Raux O, Lardy H, Varlet F, Reinberg O, Podevin G, Héloury Y, Becmeur F, Talon I, Harper L, Vergnes P, Forgues D, Lopez M, Guibal MP, Galifer RB. (2007) Multicentric assessment of the safety of neonatal videosurgery. *Surg Endosc* 21: 303–308.

36. Ponsky TA, Rothenberg SS. (2008) Minimally invasive surgery in infants less than 5 kg: experience of 649 cases. *Surg Endosc* 22: 2214–2219.

37. Quintero RA, Johnson MP, Romero R, *et al.* (1995) *In utero* percutaneous cystoscopy in the management of fetal lower obstructive uropathy. *Lancet* 346(8974): 537–540.

38. Coplen DE. (1997) Prenatal intervention for hydronephrosis, *J Urol* 157: 2270–2277.

39. Welsh A, Agarwal S, Kumar S, Smith RP, Fisk NM. (2003) Fetal cystoscopy in the management of fetal obstructive uropathy: experience in a single European center. *Prenat Diagn* 23: 1033–1041.

40. Elisa D, Leonardo G, Tim VM, Jacques J, Mieke C, Dominique VS, Roland D, Luc DC, Philipp K, Steffi M, Veronika B, Anne D, Eduardo G, Kypros N, Jan D. (2008) Prenatal diagnosis, prediction of outcome and *in utero* therapy of isolated congenital diaphragmatic hernia. *Prenat Diagn* 28: 581–591.

41. Harrison MR, Keller RL, Hawgood SB, *et al.* (2003) A randomized trial of fetal endoscopic tracheal occlusion for severe fetal congential diaphragmatic hernia. *N Engl J Med* 349: 1916–1924.

42. Jani J, Gratacos E, Greenough A, *et al.*, The FETO Task Group. (2005) Percutaneous Fetal Endoscopic Tracheal Occlusion (FETO) for severe left sided congenital diaphragmatic hernia. *Clin Obstet Gynecol N Am* 48: 910–922.

43. Jani J, Nicolaides KH, Gratacos E, Vandecruys H, Deprest J, The FETO Task Group. (2006). Fetal lung-to-head ratio in the prediction of survival in severe left-sided diaphragmatic hernia treated by fetal endoscopic tracheal occlusion (FETO). *Am J Obstet Gynecol* 195: 1646–1650.

44. Ville Y, Hecher K, Gagnon A, Sebire N, Hyett J, Nicolaides K. (1998) Endoscopic laser coagulation in the management of severe twin-to-twin transfusion syndrome. *Br J Obstet Gynaecol* 105: 446–453.

45. Quintero RA, Morales WJ, Allen MH, Bornick PW, Johnson PK, Kruger M. (1999) Staging of twin-twin transfusion syndrome. *J Perinatol* 19: 550–555.

46. Rossi AC, D'Addario V. (2008) Laser therapy and serial amnioreduction as treatment for twin-twin transfusion syndrome: a metaanalysis and review of literature. *Am J Obstet Gynecol* 198: 147–152.

.

Index